Fine-Tuning Life

'In an engaging and personal style, Henshall relates the stories of discovery and insight that have established microRNAs as key players in the cellular economy, conferring robustness and contextual sensitivity to the processes of life. He relates an accessible and enlightening history of the experiments and ideas in this important field, highlighting open questions along the way and the exciting prospects for therapeutic intervention. *Fine-Tuning Life* is a joy to read and will be a crucial resource for biomedical students and anyone interested in the subtle choreography of life and the thinking and practice of those who seek to reveal its logic.'

Kevin J. Mitchell, Ph.D.,
Associate Professor of Genetics and Neuroscience,
Trinity College Dublin

'This book guides the reader along an accessible and lively journey into how the molecular genetic orchestra, essential for all our lives, is conducted across both health and disease. How we have reached this level of understanding is given "life" through considering the major players as people, as well as via their fundamental discoveries.'

John L. Waddington, Professor Emeritus,
RCSI University of Medicine and Health Sciences, Ireland,
and College of Pharmaceutical Sciences, Soochow University, China

'David Henshall's book is bravely aimed at two unrelated reader communities, presenting a real challenge to the author: science, medicine and pharmacology students and professionals who wish to update their know-how in this relatively new field, and naïve readers excited about novel developments in life sciences research. Dr Henshall conquers that challenge by clearly and methodically explaining the underlying scientific concepts to microRNAs' functioning. He presents their discovery, their role in health and disease, and their potential to become novel therapeutic targets. The book explores the difficulties and achievements in microRNA research and their future use in novel therapeutics in a pandemic era where RNA-based therapies have now become realistic. This book is an enlightening read if you wish to learn how a new discovery can lead to realistic pharmacology prospects, and why there are no microRNA-targeted therapeutics in the current market. Recommended most warmly and with no hesitation.'

Hermona Soreq, Ph.D., Professor of Molecular Neuroscience,
The Edmond and Lily Safra Center for Brain Sciences,
The Hebrew University of Jerusalem

'This book finally gives microRNAs the significance (credit) in human genetics they deserve – from their emerging role in the evolution of the human brain all the way to their prospects for the diagnosis and therapy of brain disorders. A must-read for the aspiring biology student and the established scientist alike.'

Professor Dr Gerhard Schratt, Head of Institute for Neuroscience, ETH Zurich

Fine-Tuning Life

A Guide to MicroRNAs, Your Genome's Master Regulators

David C. Henshall
RCSI University of Medicine and Health Sciences

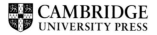

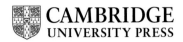

Shaftesbury Road, Cambridge CB2 8EA, United Kingdom

One Liberty Plaza, 20th Floor, New York, NY 10006, USA

477 Williamstown Road, Port Melbourne, VIC 3207, Australia

314–321, 3rd Floor, Plot 3, Splendor Forum, Jasola District Centre,
New Delhi – 110025, India

103 Penang Road, #05–06/07, Visioncrest Commercial, Singapore 238467

Cambridge University Press is part of Cambridge University Press & Assessment,
a department of the University of Cambridge.

We share the University's mission to contribute to society through the pursuit of
education, learning and research at the highest international levels of excellence.

www.cambridge.org
Information on this title: www.cambridge.org/9781009466424

DOI: 10.1017/9781009466400

First published 2024

A catalogue record for this publication is available from the British Library

A Cataloging-in-Publication data record for this book is available from the Library of Congress

ISBN 978-1-009-46642-4 Paperback

Cambridge University Press & Assessment has no responsibility for the persistence
or accuracy of URLs for external or third-party internet websites referred to in this
publication and does not guarantee that any content on such websites is, or will remain,
accurate or appropriate.

Every effort has been made in preparing this book to provide accurate and up-to-date information that is in
accord with accepted standards and practice at the time of publication. Although case histories are drawn
from actual cases, every effort has been made to disguise the identities of the individuals involved.
Nevertheless, the authors, editors, and publishers can make no warranties that the information contained
herein is totally free from error, not least because clinical standards are constantly changing through
research and regulation. The authors, editors, and publishers therefore disclaim all liability for direct or
consequential damages resulting from the use of material contained in this book. Readers are strongly
advised to pay careful attention to information provided by the manufacturer of any drugs or equipment
that they plan to use.

To Gail, Charlotte and Matthew – the perfectly tuned
molecules that matter most to me

Contents

Figures

Ode to the MicroRNA

I appeared at the dawn of life.

Unnoticed for so long, lurking among the great genes.

My journey begins: a snip here, a snip there and I'm ready.

I emerge into the cytosolic sea, a cacophony of molecular noise, machines moving everywhere.

I am not distracted; I shall not deviate on my path – argonaute awaits!

We join, a pocket into which I comfortably slip and stretch out.

Now we begin our task, moving effortlessly along our targets, probing gently.

Ah, a message; a good match, but not perfect.

I pause, my pace slowing. I call in support.

My target is growing aware of its fate now, but it is too late. It is a fly caught in my web, soon to be devoured or discarded.

Sometimes I seek adventures far from home, journeying out to distant sites; my reach is far and wide,

Always gentle, but collectively powerful.

Listen. Do you hear? The noise is quieter, the sound exquisite.

I have served my purpose, my genome, my host cell, bringing sharp order to the chaos.

You miss me when I am not there, and suffer if I take over. Better hope things remain steady.

I am a microRNA. My work is molecular diplomacy.

I am the conductor of the molecular orchestra. This is my story.

Acknowledgements

My first and biggest thanks go to my family. The most important thank-you of all. To my wife Gail and my children Charlotte and Matthew: I love you all so much. Thank you for the encouragement to start to write this and the patience to let me finish. I am sorry I miss too much of our lives together with work. It tears my heart. I hope some of the sacrifice and expanse of lost time was worth it.

Thank you to everyone at Cambridge University Press and to Anna Whiting who cornered me a few years ago and suggested a book. Many thanks also to those colleagues who read parts of the book and gave me useful feedback: Marian Brennan, John Waddington, Eva Jimenez-Mateos, Gary Brennan, Jochen Prehn, Tembi Fashina and Norman Delanty.

This section is an opportunity for me to show my gratitude to colleagues and I have a lot of people to thank. If I miss anyone, I apologise. Since this is my first and perhaps only book, I'm going to take a step back and use the space to thank people who have influenced my research and career.

Let me start with lab members. I have been lucky to find some very smart people who were willing to work for me. Since this is a book about microRNAs, it seems appropriate to begin with some of the people who worked with me in the early days. So thank you to Eva, Tobias and Ray Stallings and his team from whom we borrowed and with whom we shared so much in the early years. Thank you to those who led the microRNA work in the second wave – Cristina, Suzanne, Catherine, Rana, Omar and Mona.

To other past and present lab members at RCSI, whether you work on microRNAs or not, thank you. This is in a sort of chronological order: Brona, Helena, Niamh, Mark, Carmen, Maura, Ross, Seiji, Aurelien, Zuzanna, Genshin, Katsuhiro, Suzanne, Takanori, Gary, Guillaume, Jaime, James, Massimo, Alba, Claire M., Natalia, Amaya, Mairead, Elena, Naoki, Aasia, Sean, Teresa, Luiz, Lizzie, Aoife, Tom, Gareth, Ngoc, Joana, Kelvin, Rogerio, Karen, Rafael and Albert.

Now to those who mentored, guided and inspired me over the years, whom I will list chronologically. Bristol/the undergraduate years: Alan Hudson, who took me on as a summer student in Bristol after I finished my second year. This was my first 'research' job (and thank you to Robert Meller – see also later – who got the placement originally but then picked Pfizer, giving me his slot). Alan's grace, humility and kindness formed my conceptions of what working scientists can (should?) be like. Graeme Henderson, who let me do my final year research placement in his electrophysiology team. What a brilliant experience. You are the person who most convinced me that I could actually do 'science' for a living. Eamon Kelly – my personal tutor – thank you. When I had a mediocre middle year in pharmacology at Bristol, you kicked me in the ass for it and I needed that.

Edinburgh/the PhD years. John Sharkey, my PhD supervisor at Edinburgh. You taught me many lessons. The importance of getting really good at a few techniques that people would value – how to be an 'expert' at something, and the importance of time and hard work in the lab. I should have thanked you more then and since. I carried your work ethic with me to the USA where you told me I should go if I wanted to get on.

USA/the postdoctoral years. Roger Simon took a big risk hiring me at a time when I had nothing published. Giving me the chance to come to work in Pittsburgh was the making of me. You gave me incredible freedom, to start my own small group so early on. I realized later how few people get treated so generously. Thank you also for welcoming me into your home in those early days when I missed my family. It kept me going. And thank you for helping Gail when she visited me. Do you remember teaching her to drive on the right? Anytime I feel too busy to help someone, I remind myself that you, a head of department at a major university, took time out of your day to help the girlfriend of a lab member learn to drive. That is someone very special.

Many others at Pittsburgh deserve a mention. In no particular order: Jun and his crew, Bob, Anne, Jen, Manibu, Tetsuya, Dexi, Lan.

Portland/Legacy. Dave Bonislawski – the first person I ever hired. I look back and am still amazed at what we achieved together in a couple of years. Other people to thank: Shana, Tomohiro, Zhigang, Sachiko, Julie, An, Norman So, Akitaka. Clara – you had big shoes to fill but you fitted them in every way. Many thanks to everyone else at Legacy Research.

Robert Meller. We met on the first day of university at Bristol. You are a great friend and someone I have been fortunate enough to know for more than half my life. That weekend trip to Edinburgh in 1992 probably sealed where I went for my PhD, which of course led to everything else, so thank you. I am glad I encouraged you to come over to Portland and you came. Love to Camie and the kids.

Bob Sloviter – it was your spring hippocampal conference that first made me feel I had entered the epilepsy research community. You inspired me and gave me the advice to understand our model better. You have also made me laugh more than any other scientist.

Tallie Baram. Thank you for your support and advice in the early years at Portland and for taking the time for a chat at epilepsy congresses.

Dublin/from 2004 to now. I have been extremely lucky to work at RCSI. It is a wonderful institute that balances a rich history with a brilliant future-facing culture. My biggest thanks go to Jochen Prehn. You hired me and have looked after my career in so many ways, sheltering me from too much teaching to concentrate on research, reading and advising on grants. You are an inspiration to me and many others.

At the risk of missing people, I will call out others at RCSI who deserve a special mention: Norman, Donncha, Hany, Michael, Ronan, everyone in neurology and neurosurgery at Beaumont, Bridget, Karina, Seamus, Fergal O., Derek, Gianpiero and FutureNeuro operations, Ina and everyone in physiology, everyone in pathology (Jane, Francesca, Alan), colleagues in PBS, psychiatry. Everyone else who has made my life that bit easier – colleagues in the research office who keep working up to the last minute for grants they know I won't get (as well as a few that I did). Finance, comms, travel. Cathal Kelly – CEO.

Miscellaneous. I have been lucky enough to work with people around the world over the last twenty years or so. Thank you to everyone involved in the EpimiRNA project – Felix, Jorgen, Morten, Jeroen, Stephanie, Hajo, Peter, Jens, Gerhard and Kai. Thank you to my extended 'family' in the FutureNeuro centre – all the researchers and colleagues in companies who have worked with us on microRNAs as drugs and biomarkers. Everyone at the funding agencies who paid for our work, as well as the reviewers who read the applications or reviewed my papers.

To my friends – Chris M., Andrew and Jillian, Dave and Tanya, Emma and Jon, Simon and Hannah, Andy, Chris O., Jen and Brian, Josh. See you soon, I hope.

To my parents – Terry and Janet. Thank you for being there (and still being there). Thank you for helping me with the decision to study science and to choose the right university. To my sister Liz – you're a fab sister and I don't deserve you.

Finally, to the authors and books that inspire(d) me. I want to take the chance to thank some of the people who wrote books that I love or pushed me to write this one. Kevin Mitchell, from whom I have a signed copy of *Innate*, thank you for encouraging me and being such an inspirational supporter of science. And thank you to the authors of some of my favourite 'popular science' books on evolution, palaeontology and the planet: Jerry Coyne for *Why Evolution Is True* and *Fact vs. Faith*, Neil Shubin for *Your Inner Fish*, Richard Dawkins (too many to list), Merlin Sheldrake for *Entangled Life*, Stephen Gould's *Wonderful Life* (a thank-you here to the school winter fundraiser where I got my copy), Steve Brusatte's *The Rise and Fall of the Dinosaurs* and *The Rise and Reign of Mammals* (and thanks for answering my email), *Trilobite* by Richard Fortey and Elizabeth Kolbert's *The Sixth Extinction*.

Common Terms and Definitions

Aetiology	The cause of the disease
Antimir	An antisense oligonucleotide that targets a microRNA
Argonaute	The protein that holds the active microRNA and brings it to its target
Cluster	A set of microRNAs generated from the same precursor genes, often with overlapping targets and functions
Dendrite	The branched structure extending out from a neurone that bears the synaptic sites that collect incoming signals from other neurones
Dicer	The enzyme that cleaves the pre-microRNA to generate the final form that is passed to the Argonaute protein
Differentiation	The process whereby a cell transitions from dividing towards specialisation
Epileptogenesis	The process by which a normal brain is changed to one that generates spontaneous seizures
Hippocampus	Part of the temporal lobe in the brain, a structure involved in learning, memory and spatial navigation
Knockout	A genetic manipulation in which copies of a gene have been deleted or mutated
Phenotype	The observable characteristics of an organism
siRNA/RNAi	A process for gene silencing triggered by introduction of double-stranded RNAs with perfect complementarity to an mRNA target
Transcript	An RNA, often used as a synonym for mRNA
3' UTR	A region of the mRNA of a protein-coding gene that contains regulatory information and is the position where most microRNAs bind

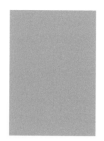

Introduction

Understanding the structure and the function of the genome has been one of the greatest and most important achievements in the history of science. An essential part of this Herculean (and ongoing) task has been understanding how the roughly 20,000 genes in the human genome are controlled. Making sure just the right amount of gene 'activity' happens.

This book is about that vital control process. There are several useful metaphors for the molecules that are the subject of this book. My favourite, and hence the title of this book, views them as nature's fine-tuning system. The conductors of the molecular orchestra. I've played a couple of musical instruments in my life, although never very well. My first was the trumpet. Our junior school had a sort of 'try-out' to find who could make a sound on it and a few of us managed a squeak and so were picked to learn it. I kept at it for another few years, getting through early grading exams. But what was really fun was being part of an orchestra. In my case, a wind band. The essence of a wind band, or indeed any orchestra, is the variety of instruments and how and when they play. This gives rise to the wondrous range of sounds that underlie a piece of music. While everyone has their own sheets of music instructions, for a piece to work properly we need a conductor. Someone at the helm, making small adjustments to the emphasis of a particular group of instruments, reminding the horn section to quieten down or the flutes to play louder. They also adjust the pace, ensuring that the timing is spot-on. Conductors are essential because they fine-tune to perfection what would otherwise be a-bit-hard-to-listen-to *noise*.

Something akin to the conductor of the orchestra is going on inside every one of the cells in your body every moment you are alive. We have genetic programmes, think music on the sheet, and we have a variety of instruments, genes and their products, that work together to do all the things that a cell needs to do to function. But this system needs a conductor. Life found a need for this oversight a long time ago. Some of the simplest organisms on Earth, comprising little more than a handful of cells, have a basic version of a conductor system. The molecules at the centre of this system and my own research are called **microRNA**. They were unknown to science until 30 years ago. But they had been there all along, tinkering away to make sure that just the right amounts of proteins are made in our cells. This book is about these conductors of the molecular orchestra.

My Road to MicroRNA

Most of us are aware of DNA as our hereditary material, the instructions for making you, me and every living thing and every thing that ever lived. An impossibly simple but sufficient set of four chemical 'letters' given the abbreviations A, C, G and T that, by arranging in different orders, are the instructions for how to make each protein in our cells. Errors in DNA, even a single misplaced A, C, G or T in the sequence, scramble the instructions and can cause devastating diseases.

My research concerns the chemical cousin of DNA, called ribonucleic acid (RNA). This RNA also functions as a code, a series of chemical letters that serve as instructions. But RNA is so much more. It is mobile, moving around the insides of cells. Signals from outside and inside a cell continuously adjust the amounts and types of RNA being made. It is quickly generated and just as quickly dismantled and capable of forming complex three-dimensional shapes that work as nano-machines. Many RNA sequences undergo chemical changes, additions, removals and editing, expanding our genome's information repertoire. It was messenger or 'mRNA' inside some of the vaccines that taught our immune systems how to fight back, saving millions of lives during the Covid-19 pandemic. But mRNA is just the tip of the RNA iceberg. Our genomes include instructions for making many different types of RNA that do not code for proteins. Those are called *non-coding RNAs*. Some of these have been known for decades. One type forms the large structures inside which proteins are made, while another feeds the amino acids, the building blocks of proteins, into that machine. The function of much of the remaining types of RNA was uncertain until relatively recently. Often, these were dismissed as molecular debris, leftover bits and pieces of longer RNAs. The rest was the genome's 'dark matter', an unsettlingly large portion of the genome whose role was unknown. One of these mysterious RNAs is microRNA, the subject of this book. After the discovery of microRNAs 30 years ago, scientists have been busy learning what these short RNAs are doing inside cells. They discovered that microRNAs are our genome's master controllers, making sure that the right amount of protein is made at the right time and in the right place for each cell in the body. If you could listen to the journey from gene to protein, I'd hazard a guess that it would begin with a cacophony of noise. Vast assemblies of enzymes joining together, jostling for space on DNA, generating copy upon copy of mRNA. These are spewed out to be read and translated into proteins. But this is skewed towards overproduction, the molecular equivalent of everyone playing their instruments as loudly as possible. The molecular noise needs to quieten down. This is what microRNAs do. They reduce, they sharpen and they shape the protein landscape, until the sound from the whole molecular orchestra is perfect.

I was midway through my undergraduate degree in pharmacology at the University of Bristol in England when microRNAs were discovered. Pharmacology is the study of drugs. My interests in the brain and drug discovery led me later to the University of Edinburgh in Scotland, where as a PhD student I tried to find ways to protect the brain against the effects of a stroke. My introduction to the RNA world came as a postdoctoral researcher, the first job many scientists take after finishing a PhD. I arrived in a snowy Pittsburgh, USA, at the start of December in 1997. The team I joined was looking for genes that controlled cell death after stroke. The person who hired me – a neurologist called Roger Simon – suggested I look at whether the same pathways were activated in the brain when a seizure occurred. There was evidence that prolonged or repeated seizures could harm the brain, so here was another brain disease where protective drugs might be useful. I knew very little about epilepsy, but my PhD training had taught me how to make models of what happens to the brain after an injury and I knew a few experimental methods for detecting damage to brain cells. It was these two skills that I had to offer. Developmental biology and cancer researchers had taught us that cell death is often controlled by gene programmes. We thought that if we could figure out the programme, we might find a way to interrupt the process and keep brain cells alive longer. I set up a model of epilepsy and then looked at the genes that became active when a seizure occurred. My first experiment looked at a gene called *GADD45*. It was known to switch on when DNA was damaged and we thought this might happen after seizures. I remember seeing the beautiful images of where the gene was active. Intense, dark patches on an X-ray film corresponding to the gene's mRNA signal, appearing in brain cells just minutes after a seizure. Seizures were causing damage to the DNA inside brain cells and the genome was fighting back, switching on this gene. I still have the original X-ray film image somewhere in my office.

I was hooked on RNA and decided I would study the RNA signals made in brain cells in epilepsy. My efforts would be aided by the development of technologies that made it possible to measure the activity of every gene at once, a method called gene profiling. One of the experiments we tried, which would later lead me to microRNAs, was to see what genes turned on or off when a brief and relatively harmless insult was given to the brain. We were trying to mimic how hibernating animals survive extremely long periods of cold and slow circulation. When the brain is stressed in a certain way, it ramps up its defences to be ready for a bigger hit in the near future. Protective molecules get turned on and sit ready for action. Other processes are switched off to conserve resources. The brain that has been forewarned can survive a stroke or prolonged seizure much better than if an insult comes out of the blue and the brain is caught unawares. We thought we could develop drugs based on this effect to protect the brain. The teams I worked with had been looking in the usual places, exploring gene activity by measuring mRNAs, when someone suggested looking at a new type of RNA. That person was Julie Saugstad, a colleague of mine at the Robert S. Dow Neurobiology Laboratories in Portland, Oregon. This was around the turn of the millennium. MicroRNAs had just been discovered in the human genome. Using an early method to measure levels of microRNAs, she found that these new types of gene also switched on or off when the brain was exposed to low oxygen. The idea sat in the back of my mind as, in 2004, I relocated from the USA to Ireland. I was there to establish an epilepsy research lab at a medical school in Dublin called the Royal College of Surgeons in Ireland, now the RCSI University of Medicine and Health Sciences. I was joining a department headed by Jochen Prehn, a world expert on the control of cell death. This opened doors to new techniques, including imaging molecules and mathematical models of how brains cells react to injury. Within a few years I was joined by a remarkable talent, a postdoctoral researcher from Madrid, Spain, called Eva Jimenez-Mateos. She and other members of my lab would lead the team into the world of microRNAs, where we have remained ever since.

How the Book Works and a Few Disclaimers

This book is the story of microRNAs. Early chapters cover their origins, who discovered them and how, why they evolved and how they do what they do. In the middle chapters, I explain how microRNAs shape the gene programmes we use during development, how they affect the properties of the brain and what happens when microRNAs fail to do their job. Finally, I look at the applications of these discoveries, and the emergence of ways to drug them and track their course as they circulate through our bodies to diagnose diseases. Much of this has been possible through remarkable developments of technology, so I touch on that as well. Finally, what is next? What are the big questions that remain and what more can we expect from these incredible molecules?

I have written this book to be understandable to a broad readership. You will not need a degree in biochemistry or genetics to make sense of it, I hope. I have aimed to tell it as a story of discovery, how it unfurled. There is some history and I have tried to respect chronology. For some readers, I may have been too light on detail. For others, the molecular 'soup' may sometimes exceed your level of understanding or interest. To some extent, this is a personal account and memoir. I have taken a rather neuro-centric view of the role of microRNAs. Large parts of it, particularly the second half of the book, concern the actions of microRNAs in the brain, where my own research has made some contributions. I have had to be selective, and have tended to pick the discoveries that interest me the most. Throughout the book I have included light descriptions of key experiments and often mention the year and the scientific journal the work appeared in. Many examples are in the most prestigious and glamorous journals in science – *Nature*, *Science* and *Cell*. Not all of the important findings on microRNAs appear in such journals, but I hold fairly traditional views about the relative quality and importance of published research and the references I make to work that appears in such journals is a reflection of that and the respect I have for the teams that managed these feats of scientific achievement. Publishing in such top journals comes down to novelty, how far they move a field ahead, the depth and sophistication of the experiments performed, and maybe a little bit of luck with peer reviewers. Often, but not always, the biggest breakthroughs appear in these types of journal. Watson and Crick's work on the DNA helix was reported in *Nature*. But a lot of great science gets published in specialist journals that are less scientifically glamorous. For instance, a technique we and many others use to calculate the amount of protein in a given sample was reported in the *Annals of Biochemistry* and has been cited by more than 240,000 scientific studies. Watson & Crick's paper on the structure of DNA in *Nature* has been cited a tiny fraction of that number of times. I won't go further into the debate on how best to measure scientific impact and value. The intention behind explaining some of the experiments is to give the reader a sense of *how we know what we know*, the microscopes, enzyme reactions, cells, organisms and models used. I include this not simply to provide context and history but in the hope that it captures more of the life of the bench scientist. I name-check some people. These are often the heads of the labs and their name usually appears last on a research paper. The *senior author*. The first author on a paper is often the person who did most of the actual bench work. The head of a lab may no longer perform experiments themselves, but it is they that probably had the original ideas behind the experiments, the hypothesis, and they who applied for and secured the funding and managed the project team. They are often the person who writes the paper. So, I apologise to everyone else named on the papers I mention; you can find those in the References. And I apologise to the many researchers and papers that I have not singled out for specific mention but whose work has nevertheless contributed in one way or another to this field of study. Now, let us begin. MicroRNAs are profoundly important to the workings of just about every living organism, including you. This is their story; let it be told.

Discovered!
A New Regulator of Gene Activity

The beauty of nature lies in detail.

From Wonderful Life: The Burgess Shale and the Nature of History, *by Stephen Jay Gould (Penguin Books, 1989, p. 13)*

Humans – as is all life when you really think about it – are a wonder. Imagine briefly the range of activities that your body performs on a typical day. Your heart pumping blood. The muscles that allow you to stand, walk, run and propel food through your gut. Your liver and kidneys, helping digest food, detoxifying your blood. Your immune system, providing constant surveillance of your inner health, capable of fighting known and new pathogens, recognizing what is 'you' and what is not. The electrochemistry of your brain, where over 80 billion cells are performing unfathomable computations, processing information from outside – such as sound, light, taste, smell, touch – and regulating every system inside the body. Enabling you to plan and execute, remember and forget, learn from mistakes, be creative (play a musical instrument), have empathy, feel love and sometimes act altruistically.

Our bodies perform an impossibly vast array of tasks and they do it extremely well and for a tiny amount of energy consumed, about 2,000 kilocalories a day. That's under 100 watts an hour. An electric kettle uses 30 times this amount of energy. That's a lot of 'bang for your buck', as they say. Your body does all of this through the collective actions of its basic building blocks: *cells*. Humans are made up of an estimated 30 trillion of these minuscule membrane-enclosed sacs of living chemistry. Cells work individually as well as together, teaming up to form larger structures: tissues, organs and entire systems such as the cardiovascular and nervous systems. Cells are specialised to carry out the functions of the body.

The abilities of cells to do all of this emerge from their inner biochemistry. The molecules they contain, the structures and bio-machines they form and the functions those machines carry out. In the Introduction to this book, I used the analogy of an orchestra to frame the central ideas of how precise tuning of this biological chemistry is essential for life. The sheets of music are our genes, the information needed to play the music correctly. But that is not enough for a top performance. A conductor is needed, to make adjustments to the molecular equivalent of sounds, volume and tempo, so that it all works perfectly. In between the sheets of music and the collective sound of the orchestra we have the *instruments*. The instruments we are talking about inside our cells are *proteins* and the conductor is a special form of *nucleic acid*. An information-carrying chemical cousin of DNA called ribonucleic acid (RNA).

Proteins perform vast numbers of functions in our cells. We have proteins that can read DNA. Proteins that form gates to control the movement of raw materials into our cells and let waste out. We have proteins that prompt our cells to grow and develop special features, turning simpler cell forms into sophisticated structures such as brain cells or any one of the hundreds of other cell types in our bodies. Proteins that form nano-machines to transport other proteins. Proteins that drive the motion of the hair-like projections called cilia on the surface of cells in our lungs that waft fluid and inhaled materials past the delicate air sacs. Other proteins form mechanical rod-like structures that give certain cells the ability to change shape, a motion that allows muscle cells to contract. We have proteins that carry out chemical reactions, converting glucose into the energy currency, called adenosine triphosphate (ATP), that all cells rely on. Sometimes the cell is more or less just protein. Red blood cells are packed with about 270 million copies of the haemoglobin protein, which can bind and release oxygen. Several of the proteins you will meet in this book are able to bind to RNA. These are called RNA binding proteins (RBPs). The human genome contains instructions to make about 3,000 different RBPs. They can bind to RNA of all different shapes and sizes. Some RBPs live out their lives in the nucleus close to DNA whereas others spend their days in the cytosol, the liquid outside the nucleus that makes up the remainder of the fluid in our cells. Some find their way to far reaches of the cell, making molecular journeys the equivalent of you travelling to the moon and back. Many RBPs work to keep RNA safe, protecting it from harm. And there are enzyme versions of RBPs that can cut, breaking the chemical bonds that hold together RNA. Molecular scissors that slice off and discard chunks of RNA akin to a sculptor chipping off pieces of marble to shape the statue beneath. Two of the RBPs that have this ability are fundamental to the lives of microRNA and we will meet them in Chapter 2.

All proteins are formed by the linking together of amino acids into long chains, assembled one at a time inside giant molecular machines called ribosomes. There are about twenty different amino acids that make up all the proteins in our cells. Amino acids are simple molecules made up of two main parts attached to a central carbon atom. One side has an amine group (one nitrogen and three hydrogen atoms; NH_3). The other end has a carboxyl group (one carbon, two oxygen and one hydrogen; COOH). Inside a cell, the two ends are charged, with the amine end carrying a positive charge and the carboxyl end a negative charge. This polarity provides them with the means to bond together in long chains, just as the positive end of one magnet is attracted to the negative end of another. Each amino acid differs in the nature of the atoms that form a branch off the central carbon atom called the *side chain*. Some carry a charge; others are neutral; others have highly reactive atoms that power chemical reactions. These differences are exploited by mixing together different combinations of amino acids to generate a protein that can do a particular job. Some amino acids are good at creating bulk and shape in a protein, while others sit at the centre of the reaction core where molecules are split apart or bonded together. The simplest amino acid is glycine. That contains a hydrogen (H) as the side chain. The amino acid cysteine contains a sulphur atom in its side chain and when paired with another cysteine can form a chemical bond called a di-sulphide bridge. This helps proteins fold and maintain their correct shape. Some amino acids, including alanine and leucine, are especially good at forming twists in proteins called α-helices.

The instructions for the order in which the amino acids are placed are carried by a molecule called *messenger RNA* (mRNA). This became a household name during the Covid-19 pandemic because some of the vaccines used the mRNA that codes for the spike protein on the virus to teach the immune system what to look out for. The instructions for the mRNA sequences to assemble your proteins are encoded in your DNA. These instructions for making you were inherited from your parents. Deoxyribonucleic acid (DNA) is a mega-molecule. Technically it is a polymer, a name given to molecules that are made up of fixed, repeating sub-units. A *gene* is commonly used to refer to a discrete section of DNA that has the instructions for making a protein. But there are many sites in the genome that this does not apply to. Indeed, less than 2 per cent of the human genome contains information to make proteins. The HUGO [Human Genome Organisation] Gene Nomenclature Committee (HGNC), which globally agrees a set of rules, defines a gene as 'a DNA segment that contributes to phenotype/function'. It is becoming increasingly clear that far more of our genome than we once thought meets this criterion. Most microRNAs are genes under the HUGO nomenclature, that is, distinct units that can be transcribed, that are book-ended by start and stop signals, that are heritable and that serve specific biological functions.

It is at a key step along the pathway from DNA to protein that microRNAs act. Indeed, while this book is about microRNAs, it is ultimately a book about proteins because the main job of microRNAs is to make sure that our cells have just the right amount of each protein. Is it important to have just the right amount of a protein in a cell? Yes. While most systems in the body can tolerate a degree of variation in the proteins that carry out specific functions, we know that without microRNAs, a key regulator of protein levels, you would not be alive to read this. If you're missing microRNAs at the start of life then you never get much further than being a ball of cells. If you remove microRNAs around the time of birth then you fail to develop much further. If you remove them when you reach adulthood, you can develop cancer or accelerated ageing. Stop them working in the brain and you develop seizures before the brain turns to mush. I am taking some liberty with the word 'you' here. This knowledge comes mainly from experiments in lab animals such as mice. But we are confident that the outcome would be more or less the same in humans. Indeed, people are born with errors in the machinery for making these molecules and this can have devastating impacts on their health. Some of the microRNA genes are so important that we never see people born without them because it is lethal at an early stage. So, this system for controlling protein levels in cells is essential for life. **Figure 1.1** provides a simple overview of the 'gene pathway'. Information flows from DNA to RNA and on to making a protein. I have highlighted the approximate position in this process where microRNAs act.

The Genetic Code

The human genome is a code running to three billion letters. Despite the extraordinary information it contains, including the 20,000 or more genes that code for proteins plus many other interesting parts that code for RNAs that do important things in our cells, it has oddly straightforward chemistry. The code is made from repeats of four simple chemicals called bases: adenine, cytosine, guanine and thymine or A, C, G and T for short. Like amino acids, they are simple molecules and about the size of one of the larger amino acids. The order of the DNA bases in a protein-coding gene determine which amino acid gets picked. Three bases (a trinucleotide) form the unit of information that codes for a particular amino acid. This is known as a *codon*. Because it is a triplet code, we have 4^3 possible combinations, giving us 64 different codons. Of these, 61 code for amino acids and 3 perform another function, signalling to terminate the making of the protein. Most amino acids can be coded for by more than one codon. For example, a glycine is placed in a protein if the mRNA sequence read contains the codons GGC, GGA or GGG.

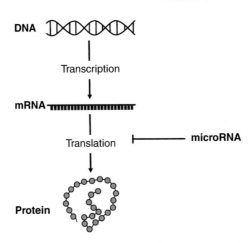

Figure 1.1 Overview of where microRNAs act on the pathway from gene to protein

In this simplified pathway from gene to protein, the first step is transcription, where an RNA copy is made from a gene encoded in the DNA. For protein-coding genes, the RNA formed is called mRNA. The nucleotide sequence of the mRNA (indicated by notches) is used as a template to generate a protein during translation. Proteins are formed by the sequential assembly of amino acids (round circles in the diagram). MicroRNAs act after the mRNA is formed but prior to the formation of the protein.

The structure of DNA slightly resembles a ladder or a spiral staircase, comprising two strands with the bases pairing to one another at regularly spaced intervals up the middle. The backbone (in the ladder analogy, the sides of the ladder you hold as you step up and down) is made up of two types of molecule. The first is a form of carbohydrate, closely related to the sugar you might add to sweeten something. Sugars are made up of carbon, oxygen and hydrogen. The one in the backbone of our DNA has five carbons and so is a pentose sugar; it is called deoxyribose. The deoxy refers to it missing a hydroxyl (OH) group. The other part is a phosphate group, a phosphorous atom with four oxygen atoms attached to it (PO_4). The deoxyribose and the phosphate are strongly bonded together and alternate as deoxyribose-phosphate-deoxyribose-phosphate and so on. The base attaches to the deoxyribose. So each rung of the ladder has a deoxyribose, a phosphate and one of the four bases. This unit – the base, the sugar and the phosphate – is called a *nucleotide*. Bases pair in a specific way. In DNA, an A is always paired across from a T and a C is always paired across from a G; Gs don't bind to Ts or As, and As don't bind to Gs or Cs. A gene sequence is simply an extremely long series of these four bases in different orders, for example A-C-T-G-C-G-T-A and so on. **Figure 1.2** provides an overview of the chemistry of DNA.

In the cells of eukaryotes, organisms that include mushrooms, plants and animals, DNA is found in the nucleus, one of several organelles (another is mitochondria, which make most of our cells' ATP). The DNA in eukaryotic cells is found wrapped around the outside of proteins called histones. This provides a way to compact the genomic instructions and avoid DNA strands becoming tangled. The mix of DNA and histone proteins is called *chromatin*. This is a suitable place for a very short aside on the history of DNA. Key discoveries of what DNA is made of came from work in the early 1900s by Phoebus Levene, a Russian-American biochemist who identified the four DNA bases, the basic rules of their combinations and the presence of the ribose sugar. Most people are familiar with Watson and Crick. They are credited with solving the structure of DNA, which was

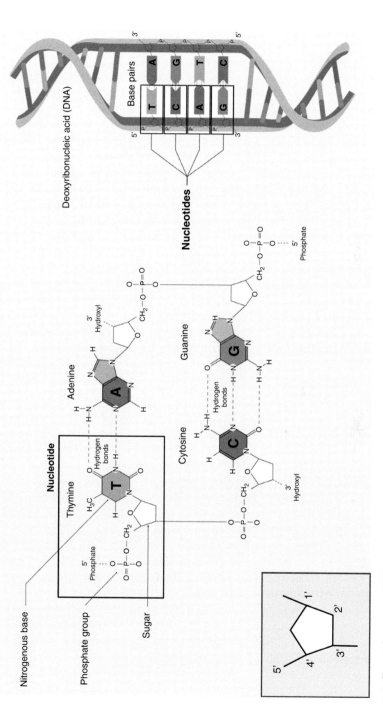

Figure 1.2 Chemical structure of DNA

This shows the basic chemical structure of the nucleotide, the basic building block of DNA, and the base-pairing rules. A nucleotide consists of a sugar molecule (deoxyribose in DNA) attached to a phosphate group and one of the four chemical bases. The bases in DNA are adenine (A), cytosine (C), guanine (G) and thymine (T). In RNA, the base uracil (U) takes the place of thymine. Molecules of DNA and RNA are polymers made up of long chains of nucleotides. The inset (bottom-left) shows the number-position labelling of carbons in the ribose sugar.

Source: Image courtesy of Darryl Leja and the National Human Genome Research Institute (www.genome.gov).

reported in the journal *Nature* in 1953, and this helped our understanding of how DNA worked (1953 is also famous for being the year that kainic acid was discovered, a key tool in neuroscience and epilepsy research – see Chapter 6). Key to confirming Watson and Crick's insights were X-ray images of a crystal of DNA. These were produced by Rosalind Franklin and shared without her knowledge. She was not initially credited with this work, but is now recognised as conducting the key experiments used in the discovery. Some accounts imply that Rosalind failed to grasp what her images revealed about the structure of DNA, but this is a misrepresentation. She was an equal contributor in the solution. She died from cancer owing to the radiation she was exposed to as part of her work; we owe much of modern scientific and medical discovery to this woman. Once the organisation of the DNA molecule was understood, with the sugar as the outside backbone and the bases pairing across from one another in the middle, how it coded could be understood. There was still a lot of work to do and Watson and Crick didn't determine what combination of bases coded to make proteins. That would come later. A couple of other key discoveries on the journey are worth a mention. Swiss scientist Friedrich Meischer gets credit for the 1869 discovery of DNA in the nucleus of cells. In 1944 we have Oswald Avery and colleagues, who proved that DNA is the hereditary material in our cells. They added DNA from a dangerous strain of bacteria to a normally harmless one, causing it to become deadly. In 1950, Erwin Chargaff reported that the amounts of Gs and Cs and the amounts of As and Ts were always the same, but the ratios were different in different species. Towards the end of that decade and in the first years of the 1960s, Marshal Nirenberg is credited with understanding how the code actually works in practice. That is, how sets of bases encode the amino acids in proteins. In the years since, the specific sequence of bases that code for each amino acid has been determined.

The Journey from Gene to Protein

Let us go briefly through the full process from start to finish: the start, the reading of the DNA code, through to the generation of mRNA that later gets read to form a growing amino acid chain that ultimately becomes a protein. Our depth of understanding of this process is now remarkable. I will cover enough detail to understand where and how microRNAs participate in this process. The first stage of the journey from DNA to protein is *transcription*. This is the process of reading a particular stretch of DNA, the gene, and making a copy of that sequence out of RNA. If we are making a protein, then the RNA made is an mRNA. It is common to refer to mRNAs as 'transcripts'. Other sections of DNA can also be read and an RNA copy made. But these other RNAs do not code for a protein and are *non-coding RNA*. There are many different types of non-coding RNA. Some, such as the RNA found inside the ribosome protein factories, are far more abundant in our cells than mRNAs. MicroRNAs are an example of such non-coding RNAs. **Figure 1.3** provides an overview of the basic chemistry of RNA and some of the different forms of RNA in cells.

Reading and copying DNA to make mRNA is a highly regulated, multi-step process. An enzyme called an RNA polymerase binds to a section of DNA. The two strands of DNA are unzipped from one another. The bonds holding the Cs to Gs and the As to Ts are broken and the base pairs are separated. The RNA polymerase now makes an RNA, with each base being inserted according to what it reads from the DNA strand. The strand of DNA that is read is called the *antisense* strand. The other ignored section of DNA is called the coding or *sense* strand because its sequence is the same as the mRNA that is generated. This reading process occurs in one direction only, analogous to how you read this sentence, from left to right.

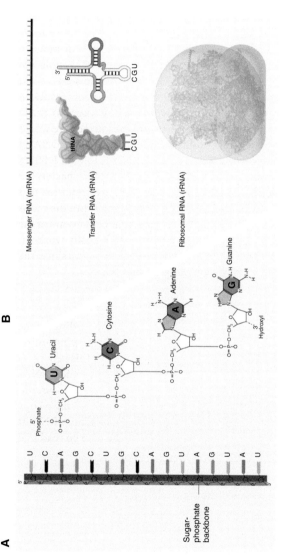

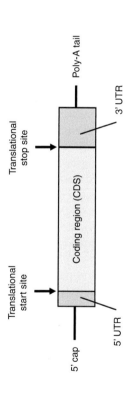

A

Sugar-
phosphate
backbone

B

Messenger RNA (mRNA)

Transfer RNA (tRNA)

Ribosomal RNA (rRNA)

Uracil

Cytosine

Adenine

Guanine

5'
Phosphate

3'
Hydroxyl

C

Translational
start site

Translational
stop site

5' cap

5' UTR

Coding region (CDS)

3' UTR

Poly-A tail

Figure 1.3 The base composition and different forms of RNA

Panel A shows the four different chemical bases present in RNA along the sugar-phosphate backbone (vertical column). Note that uracil (U) replaces thymine (T) in RNA. Within and between RNA molecules, base-pairing can occur between Us and As and between Gs and Cs. In the coding sequence of an mRNA, every three nucleotides comprise a codon for a specific transfer RNA to bring an amino acid during the building of a protein. Panel B shows examples of some of the non-coding RNAs in a cell.

Panel C shows the basic subparts of an mRNA.

Key: U, uracil; A, adenine; C, cytosine; G, guanine; UTR, untranslated region; rRNA, ribosomal RNA; tRNA, transfer RNA.

Source: Images in Panels A and B courtesy of the National Human Genome Research Institute (www.genome.gov). Panel C is the author's own.

Each end of a DNA and an RNA molecule has a number. This is based on the position of the five carbon atoms in the ribose sugar (see **Figure 1.2**). The numbering works in a clockwise direction starting with one at the three o'clock position and running to position five. Carbon 1 is attached to a base and carbon 2 also faces in towards the centre. Carbon 4 faces out. This leaves carbons 3 and 5. Carbon 5 is at the top of the ribose and is the point of attachment for the phosphate group above it. Carbon 3 of the ribose bonds with the phosphate group below it. These are referred to as the 5 prime (5') and the 3 prime (3') positions. Both DNA and RNA use the same naming system.

During transcription, DNA is read by RNA polymerases in the 3' to 5' direction while the growing RNA strand is created in the opposite direction (5' to 3'). The RNA polymerase adds each new base onto the 3' end of the growing RNA strand. If the polymerase reads a G on the DNA strand, it places a C in the growing RNA molecule, while reading a T results in an A being placed in the RNA. One of the bases used by the polymerase is different from the standard four in DNA. The thymine base in DNA is not present in RNA. Instead, another base called uracil (U) is inserted into RNA. So wherever RNA polymerase reads an A base on the DNA strand it puts a U, not a T, into the growing RNA molecule. So, reading a stretch of DNA that had the sequence TAC GGA would generate an mRNA with the sequence AUG CCU. As the polymerase passes along reading the DNA sequence, the RNA strand passes out in one direction while the DNA strand is rejoined with the original strand it was separated from. The process is divided into four stages called initiation, promoter escape, elongation and termination.

Transcription requires specific signals to be in place to mark the gene to be read. The key molecules that mark a gene as ready to read are proteins called *transcription factors*. There are also proteins called transcription repressors that do the opposite, having the effect of reducing any transcription of the targeted gene. Transcription factors receive their instructions from signals that originate outside or inside the cell. The transcription factor doesn't synthesise the mRNA; it simply docks onto the DNA. This happens a bit upstream of the section of DNA that codes for the protein. That site is called a *promoter*. It is a short stretch of DNA bases that acts as a 'come here and get started' signal for the enzyme complex that will make the mRNA copy. Alone, however, this doesn't result in much transcription. A second site needs to be activated; this is called an *enhancer*. This can be quite a distance from the gene and the promoter and a different set of proteins bind to this site. However, chromatin is flexible and a loop can be formed that brings the enhancer site close to the promoter site, resulting in a powerful 'on' switch for transcription.

Next, a complex of proteins called Mediator acts to communicate between these two sections of DNA and transcription now takes place. The RNA polymerase unwinds a stretch of fourteen base pairs of the DNA at what is called the transcriptional start site (TSS). An RNA strand starts to form (step 1 done). The polymerase now has to break free of the promoter to work properly, a process termed promoter escape (step 2). Now the polymerase can begin to read and form the full-length transcript, which grows at a rate of about 1,000 nucleotides per minute (elongation – step 3). Finally, the polymerase finishes and breaks loose (termination – step 4). By the end of transcription we have a long RNA molecule, although different genes vary in length and so do the RNAs transcribed from them.

We don't yet have our final mRNA. What we have by the end of transcription is really pre-mRNA. Synthesised mRNAs undergo a complex series of further adjustments in a process termed post-transcriptional regulation. These actions result in an mRNA that is prepped and ready to be sent to the ribosome for translation. The prepping processes include splicing, capping, tailing and editing. An estimated 100 different chemical modifications of mRNA have been discovered. We don't know what all of these do, but they generally affect the stability or the readability of the mRNA.

The parts of the pre-mRNA that code for the protein are called *exons*. When the pre-mRNA is made, it usually contains long sections of RNA that do not code for amino acids. These are called *introns* and they are snipped out. The sections of RNA either side are glued (spliced) back together. This leaves a series of exons joined together. The processing of the pre-mRNA may also result in inclusion of some but not other exons. For example, the pre-mRNA may include ten different exons but the final mRNA may omit one or more of these. That is called *alternative splicing*. It is carefully regulated by RBPs that bind onto the segments to be chosen for inclusion or exclusion; the enzymes that do the cutting are called nucleases. The proteins that result from these different splicing events display subtle differences in their properties. For example, one version might possess an extra signal that allows it to interact in a different way or directs the protein to a particular place in the cell. This is a way that the main repertoire of proteins encoded in the genome can be boosted even further. Thus, from around 20,000 protein-coding genes, cells can generate approximately 100,000 different proteins.

The part of the mRNA that is important for the sequence of amino acids is called the coding sequence (CDS) (see **Figure 1.3C**). Either side of this region are other stretches of RNA that serve regulatory functions. This includes the start codon at the 5' end of the CDS. This is usually the sequence AUG. Just in front of this start codon is a segment of RNA called the 5' untranslated region (5' UTR). This is only a few bases in length and is usually not a signal for an amino acid to be placed. Both far ends of the mRNA undergo modifications. At the 5' end of the mRNA, a structure called a cap is added. In most cases this involves the addition of a chemically modified guanine base. The cap serves several functions, protecting the molecule from being digested and identifying it for export to the ribosome. At the other end of the pre-mRNA, a stretch of adenines is added called a poly(A) tail. This can include more than 200 As in a row. Like the cap structure, this marks the mRNA for export and translation, and also affects its stability. The poly(A) tail doesn't last, at least at its full length. Specific enzymes shorten it over time and this ultimately dictates the lifespan of the mRNA. These modifications, the intron removal, the 5' cap and the 3' poly(A) tail, are coordinated and occur *co-transcriptionally*. That is, it all happens almost immediately as the transcript is generated.

Between the CDS and the poly(A) tail is a segment called the *3' untranslated region* (3' UTR). This contains important regulatory information which controls how much protein is made from the mRNA. It can vary substantially in length. Longer 3' UTRs tend to mean that the transcript is more heavily 'policed' during translation. This is the part of the mRNA where microRNAs usually exert their effects. It will feature heavily in later chapters. Once the modified and final mRNA reaches the cytoplasm, it is chaperoned to the ribosome. This is where the message is read and a protein is formed.

Translation

Proteins are made or synthesised inside giant molecular machines called ribosomes. These are conglomerates of a special form of RNA called ribosomal RNA or rRNA (see **Figure 1.3B**), intertwined with coils of various proteins in an approximately 60:40 mix. Ribosomes have one large sub-unit or part called the 60S and one smaller sub-unit, the 40S.

It is an ancient structure in that its design and function and the sequences that code for the building blocks are highly similar or conserved in all eukaryotes. An mRNA arrives to a ribosome chaperoned by various RBPs and is then fed into a groove between the two sub-units. Next, another form of RNA called transfer RNA (tRNA) swoops in, carrying in its grasp a single amino acid that has been joined on prior to arrival. There are 40 to 60 different types of tRNA in human cells. Each tRNA carries its own amino acid. The tRNA structure slightly resembles a lower-case letter r. The 'bottom' of the r is called the anti-codon loop. This part contains a triplet sequence that is the complementary match for the codon, on the mRNA. For example, a tRNA with an anti-codon loop sequence CGU will pair to an GCA sequence on the mRNA. The amino acid is attached at the opposite end of the tRNA, the 'handle' of the r shape. As the mRNA is fed into the ribosome, the 5' end attaches to the small sub-unit. The ribosome moves along until it reaches a start codon. The large sub-unit is then brought in along with the first tRNA, followed by other tRNAs falling into place in sequence according to the codon:anti-codon pairing. Specific regions within the ribosome house and arrange the tRNA-amino acid molecules as they enter.

For each triplet sequence we get one additional amino acid. The tRNA that brought in the amino acid gets released and the ribosome bumps along to the next codon. The process ends when a stop codon is encountered in the mRNA. The common ones are UAG, UAA and UGA. The ribosome then releases the polypeptide. From these twenty amino acid building blocks we can generate every protein in the body. The growing chain of amino acids is created in a way that has a front and a back end. The beginning has an amine group (NH_3) and is referred to as the N-terminus. The end of the protein has a carboxyl group (COOH) and is called the C-terminus. When a protein is shown in a drawing, these ends are typically highlighted and the convention is to show the N-terminal on the left and the C-terminus on the right. The finished polypeptide is not yet a functional protein, however. As it is produced, it begins to fold and form more complex structures. These include the spiral α-helix mentioned earlier. These are called secondary structures. Further folding, tertiary structure creates the 3D shape of the protein. A higher level called quaternary structure refers to when groups of folded proteins form superstructures. And now we have reached the end of the DNA-to-protein pathway.

Asserting Control Over Proteins

The instructions for every protein are present inside every cell, with the exception of red blood cells. These originally contained DNA, but this is actively removed during the maturation process, creating more space for haemoglobin. Every other cell contains the instructions to make any and all proteins. But we know they aren't all made. A muscle cell is packed with structural proteins that allow the cell to contract and relax. A liver cell is packed with enzymes to break down ingested substances. If you are a neurone then you must be capable of transmitting rapid changes in electrochemical signals and producing, storing and releasing neurotransmitters. Clearly, cells pick and choose what proteins they make. This makes a simple but profoundly important point. The protein landscape, the collection of proteins that forms the structures of cells, enzymes, transporters, motors and everything else, is tailored to the job(s) the cells perform. And if a cell isn't making the right proteins or the correct amount of those proteins then problems quickly arise. At best, the cell doesn't do its job well enough. For example, it doesn't secrete what it should (insulin from the Beta islet cells of the pancreas of a patient with type 1 diabetes), contract how it should or signal how it should. At worst, a cell can become cancerous. Dividing, invading and ultimately killing its host. How much of a given gene's encoded protein a cell makes and when and where its product is generated must be subject to precise control. But how is this control achieved?

The correct amount of a protein is determined by regulatory steps at multiple points in the pathway. Researchers continue to apply new and more sophisticated ways of measuring global protein output relative to mRNA levels. A key influence on protein levels is how much actual transcription occurs in the first place. Put simply, the more mRNA, the more protein. But, by several estimates, mRNA abundance accounts for only about half the levels of a protein. Accounting for differences in the mRNA:protein ratio are various steps along the way. These include factors acting after transcription but before translation, including on mRNA stability and other post-transcriptional controls, and after translation, including on protein stability and turnover. MicroRNAs act post-transcriptionally. They latch onto the mRNA and alter how much is translated into protein. So how were they discovered? How many are there? What proteins do they control? What are the rules they live by?

Gene, RNA and Protein Naming Conventions

We are about to dive into a section that shifts between talking about genes among our DNA, transcribed mRNA, and the translated product of the mRNA, the protein. There are conventions for naming each of these. A quick overview will make it easier to keep track of which part of the 'molecular soup' is being referred to. Let's imagine a hypothetical gene called 'read every day'. Because there is more than one version of this gene, let us give it a number – 1. In humans, the full gene name would be written as 'read every day 1'. When referred to in its abbreviated form, the gene is *RED1*. All capital letters in italic. The mRNA for this gene would also be *RED1*. The protein is not italicised, though, and is written as RED1. Now we come to other species. The full name of the mouse version of the gene would also be 'read every day 1'. But the abbreviated form of the mouse gene only has the first letter capitalised. The rest are lowercase. The gene would be *Red1*, the mRNA would also be *Red1*, but the protein would be uppercase RED1. Many of the early discoveries on microRNA were made in an animal called *Caenorhabditis elegans* or *C. elegans* for short. The language convention for naming organisms is to use Latin. The *C. elegans* gene naming convention includes a hyphen when there is a number and the first letter is not capitalised. So we get the gene *red-1*, the mRNA *red-1* and the protein RED-1.

A Worm's Tale

The discovery of microRNAs in animals can be traced back to two landmark papers in the same 1993 issue of the journal *Cell*. The discovery of microRNAs was not made in humans but rather in *C. elegans*, a roundworm. What were the researchers looking for in the worm and why were they using worms? The *C. elegans* is what is called a model organism. Model organisms are an essential tool in biology, allowing complex problems to be understood in a simpler context. Another advantage of model organisms is how quickly they develop, shortening the time it takes to run experiments: *C. elegans* reaches adulthood three days after hatching from an egg. Adult *C. elegans* worms measure about 1 mm and so they are cheap to house and feed. Further, *C. elegans* can survive being deep-frozen, making them easy to store. Model organisms also allow experimentation including genetic mutation that might not be otherwise possible for ethical or technical reasons. Other examples of model organisms include the bacterium *E. coli*, the fruit fly *D. melanogaster* and a fish called *D. rerio*.

The roundworm *C. elegans* has been helping biologists understand the genetic programmes that control how animals develop for more than fifty years. A key figure is Sydney Brenner, a Nobel prize winner who passed away in 2019. One of the most brilliant minds of the twentieth century, he entered university in his home country of South Africa at the age of fifteen and five of the people he trained went on to win Nobel prizes. He worked for a time with Francis Crick at the University of Cambridge, contributing to our understanding of the triplet code for amino acids. He later headed the university's laboratory of molecular biology. He was interested in how sets of genes work to give rise to the complex organisation of organisms, including their nervous systems. He recognised that simple or lower organisms share much of the same biology as humans. For example, the *C. elegans* genome has similar versions to 60 per cent to 80 per cent of human protein-coding genes, despite being separated by 500 million to 600 million years of evolutionary time. Our last shared common ancestor was in the pre-Cambrian period, slightly before the fossilisation of the animals that are the focus of the history of life story featured at the start of this chapter. Brenner's true passion was always to understand how the brain worked. Writing in an article in the journal *Genetics* in the early 1970s, he laid out the case for how, by understanding the complete structure of a simple organism's nervous system, the timing of its development, the underlying genetic programmes that control behaviours, you could gain insight into much more complex systems (i.e., human systems). His work on *C. elegans* had begun in the 1960s. He had pondered using *D. melanogaster* but decided the numbers of neurones were still unmanageable. Adding to the argument to use *C. elegans*, the laboratory conditions for maintaining were simple and already established. The worms are also hermaphrodites, meaning they can self-fertilise and their offspring are clones and therefore genetically identical. At the time he started, *C. elegans* was thought to have about 200 neurones. These numbers have been slightly revised; a typical adult worm has ~300 neurones of its total of ~1,000 cells. While it has a nervous system, a reproductive system and a digestive system, it lacks a respiratory system or a circulatory system. Over many years, Brenner's and other teams transformed our understanding of how genes control the developing nervous and other systems. Indeed, *C. elegans* was the first animal to have its complete nervous system 'connectome' mapped, in a wiring diagram in which every connection between every neurone has been documented.

After hatching from an egg, *C. elegans* goes through four larval stages termed L1–L4, before becoming an adult worm. The genetics of its growth and development have been studied in such depth that we know precisely what genes switch on when, what processes they control, the number and whereabouts of every cell made, what tissues they form and even how many cells are killed off. Indeed, Brenner's Nobel prize was shared with others who discovered genetically encoded pathways that eliminate excess cells generated during development; some of the same genes in humans get inactivated in cancers. A common trick to learn what a gene did was to expose worms to known mutagenic chemicals that randomly inserted errors in their genomes. The position of the errors could be traced, allowing researchers to understand a bit about the function of the gene that contained the mistake. By repeating this enough, researchers learnt which genes affected worm development. Researchers now have the ability to engineer the *C. elegans* genome to precisely change sequences as well as introduce molecules that are fluorescent under a microscope, allowing them to track the growth, movement and final resting place of any cell in the worm.

MicroRNAs were discovered during studies on the development of *C. elegans*. The scientists at the centre – Victor Ambros and Gary Ruvkun – were both Boston area–based. At the time, a number of genes called *heterochronic* genes were known to control the timing of development. Ambros had performed experiments that showed that mutations in these genes resulted in changes to the timing of specific events during worm development, for example the reappearance of early developmental changes. One of these heterochronic genes was *lin-14*. The 'lin' stands for abnormal cell <u>lin</u>eage. The *lin-14* gene encoded a transcription factor that appeared early during larval development, in the embryo and the L1 stage. Experiments had already shown that the LIN-14 protein, normally present in the nucleus as befits its job of controlling gene activity, later disappeared and was not detectable at later larval stages and in mature worms. That is, a time-dependent, decreasing gradient of LIN-14 was required for normal development. But researchers noted that the mRNA for *lin-14* didn't disappear. In fact, it remained present the whole time. The message was still being made, but something was now preventing translation. Something was acting *post-transcriptionally* to lower production of LIN-14 protein and control the timing of worm development.

At the time, transcription of another gene, called *lin-4*, was known to affect the timing of larval development. Mutations that caused loss of *lin-4* resulted in animals going back into earlier larval phases. They would re-start previous rounds of development and would be missing certain adult features. *Lin-4* was necessary for maturation of the worm. Loss-of-function mutations in *lin-14* that prevented the protein being made produced the opposite features. Worms skipped steps in early larval development, jumped ahead, and the result was the inappropriate appearance of adult-like features in the young worms (see **Figure 1.4A**). In contrast, overproduction of *lin-14* produced worms that looked similar to the faulty *lin-4* mutants, displaying re-engagement of early development features. This was consistent with *lin-4* acting as a negative regulator of *lin-14*.

By studying the mutant *lin-14* worm, Ruvkun's team had narrowed down the genetic error that was stopping the decline in LIN-14 protein during later development. The mutant worm that couldn't 'switch off' LIN-14 was missing a section of the *lin-14* mRNA. The missing piece was not, however, in the protein-coding sequence. It was found in the untranslated region of the mRNA, the 3' UTR. The 3' UTR of *lin-14* contained information in the form of a nucleotide sequence that was important for blocking production of LIN-14 protein. Was this linked somehow to whatever *lin-4* was doing that seemed to control translation of the LIN-14 protein?

Ambros' team had been working since the early 1980s on *lin-14* and other genes including *lin-4* that controlled the timing of *C. elegans* development. His team, in parallel with Ruvkin's, were about to make a major advance in molecular biology. By uncovering the mechanism by which *lin-4* regulated translation of LIN-14 protein, they would discover a fundamental mechanism by which gene activity in all animals, not just worms, was controlled. Ambros' work in the seminal *Cell* paper[1] began by a detailed analysis of the *lin-4* locus, the specific position on a chromosome where the gene information resides. He and his team noted that the sequence lay within an intron of another gene and analysis of the genetic sequence revealed that it did not code for a protein. Indeed, introducing changes to the sequence of *lin-4* that would have scrambled or blocked translation of a protein-coding mRNA had no effect on the ability of *lin-4* RNA to affect developmental timing. When they searched for evidence of expression of RNA from the locus, they detected two transcripts. One was sixty-one nucleotides in length and the other was twenty-two nucleotides. The longer one was

A

B

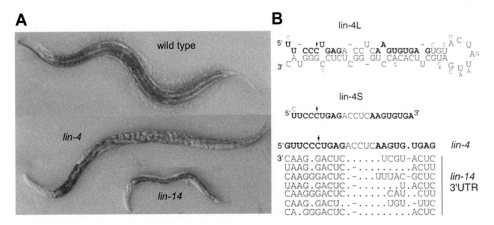

Figure 1.4 *C. elegans* and the discovery of the first microRNA

Panel A shows three *C. elegans* worms. Compared to the wild-type worm, adult *lin-4* loss-of-function mutants lack many adult structures and they are unable to lay eggs on account of a failure to develop a vulva (note the spherical eggs accumulating within their bodies). The bottom worm is a *lin-14* loss-of-function mutant. This has developed certain adult features precociously at larval stages, resulting in smaller, poorly formed adults.

Panel B shows the sequences deduced for (top) the precursor *lin-4L* including the hairpin loop and (middle) the shorter *lin-4S*, the mature microRNA. Sequences in bold are those complementary to the 3' UTR of *lin-14*. The smaller type letters are the annotation of sequences that differ in other species of *Caenorhabditis*. Other markings indicate positions of introduced mutations. The lower panel shows complementary sequence alignment of *lin-4S* with seven sites in the 3' UTR of the *lin-14* transcript. At the time, the RNA sequences were deduced from the DNA sequence and transcript mapping and not from direct sequence analysis of RNA.

Source: Panel A reprinted with permission from Ambros, *Nature Medicine*, vol. 14, pp. 1036–40 (2008).[2] Panel B adapted with permission from Lee et al., *Cell*, vol. 75, pp. 843–54 (1993).[1]

predicted to have a region that folded over on itself, creating a loop structure. The team deduced the sequences of both, discovering that the short form, *lin-4S*, was identical to the 5' end of the longer *lin-4L*. This suggested the *lin-4S* had originally been part of the longer transcript, so perhaps *lin-4L* was a precursor of *lin-4S*. Both sequences were also found in three other species of *Caenorhabditis*, whereas the parts of *lin-4* outside of this region were poorly conserved between different worm species (see **Figure 1.4B**).

Now came the eureka moment. They aligned the *lin-4S* sequence with the 3' UTR section of the *lin-14* mRNA known to be critical for blocking translation. There was a series of seven repeating sections of complementarity between the two RNAs: stretches of nucleotides on the *lin-4* RNA that were perfectly complementary to *lin-14*. One region of the 3' UTR of *lin-14* had the sequence CAAGGGACUC, which would be able to base-pair to a region of *lin-4* contained within the twenty-two nucleotide shorter RNA that ran GUUCCCUGAG. The final piece of the puzzle was in place. *Lin-4* was reducing the amount of LIN-14 by direct RNA-to-RNA interaction within the 3' UTR of *lin-14*. In their conclusions, they offered that *lin-4* RNA may bind to *lin-14* mRNA in the cytoplasm and inhibit its translation. *Lin-4* was acting like molecular Velcro, sticking onto the *lin-14* RNA, forming a duplex and preventing it from being translated into a protein. This type of inhibitory mechanism had a name – *antisense*. We previously came across antisense in the context of transcription. When the DNA helix is unwound, it is the antisense strand that is the template that the RNA polymerase uses. The generated mRNA is a sense strand and is also identical except for the swapping of a T for a U to the other sense DNA strand. Here, an RNA from one part of the genome was being made that could control the effects of another RNA by sticking to it. This was not completely unheard of because an RNA called *XIST* had been identified that was involved in shutting down one of the two copies of the X chromosome in the cells of females. But *XIST* is 16,500 bases long. *Lin-4* was 0.1 per cent of this length. The authors realised that *lin-4* might be the first of a new class of *small regulatory* RNA. **Figure 1.4** shows examples of the *lin-4* and *lin-14* mutant worms and the sequence of *lin-4*, as well as the sequence alignment to the 3' UTR of *lin-14*.

Ruvkun's team performed similar experiments on the levels of *lin-4* and *lin-14*/LIN-14, confirming that it was a post-transcriptional event and mapping the seven complementary interaction sites.[3] They also performed some clever experiments that further confirmed this new gene control mechanism. They took the section of the *lin-14* 3' UTR that contained the regulatory information and inserted it into another protein-coding mRNA that was not sensitive to developmental timing. The transplant was a success. The protein product of the recipient gene now showed developmental down-regulation, even though the host gene had nothing to do with the functions of LIN-14. As with the original *lin-14* observations, the amount of RNA of the hybrid containing the transplanted 3' UTR remained unchanged, with only the protein decreased. Finally, they found that the acquired timing effect of the transplanted 3' UTR only worked if *lin-4* was also present. The tampered gene returned to its original unregulated state if *lin-4* was mutated. The 3' UTR of *lin-14* contained the complete instruction for the translational block by *lin-4*.

A major new regulatory step had been discovered in the pathway from gene to protein with *lin-4* the founding member. But the significance of the findings were rather overlooked at the time. That would all change at the turn of the millennium. The year 2000 would be a big year. What could have been an idiosyncratic finding in a worm turned out to be something fundamental to complex life on Earth.

MicroRNAs Emerge as Master Controllers

2

[T]he vast majority of the 3 billion 'letters' of the human genetic code are busily toiling at an array of previously invisible tasks.

From Rick Weiss' 2007 commentary in the *Washington Post* on the first results of the ENCODE project to map the non-coding genome

---

The landmark discoveries of 1993 by Ambros and Ruvkun did not immediately usher in a new dawn of research on small RNAs that control gene activity. But it was coming. The floodgates would truly open in 2000 and further in 2001 and they would not close. At more than 150,000 scientific articles and counting, the field of microRNA research continues to grow year-on-year. The appearance of a seven-year gap before the next leap forward is misleading, however. Ambros' lab worked hard between 1993 and 2000 looking for 'cousins' of *lin-4* in other worm species and finding another target of *lin-4* (*lin-28*), proving that the small RNA regulated more than one gene. The growth was initially driven by the labs that had been working on *C. elegans* development along with new players who entered the field. Questions were being asked such as were there other small RNAs that worked like *lin-4*? How many and in what other species? How did the binding of *lin-4* to *lin-14* prevent translation? Was it by simple physical impediment on entry to the ribosome? What machinery in the cell was needed to make and guide their actions? What types of gene and what processes in cells were being controlled?

The opening salvo in the year 2000 came from Ruvkun's group, with a pair of papers in *Nature* showing that *lin-4* was not a one-hit wonder.[4, 5] They had found another. *Let-7,* standing for lethal, was a second small regulatory RNA that could base-pair to sites in the 3' UTR of a protein-coding gene during worm development. The *lin-4* finding was no longer an oddity of worm development. Perhaps more important, however, was the finding that the same gene, *let-7,* was present *in the human genome*. It would also soon emerge that these RNAs were not only working during development. The ~20 nucleotide RNAs began to be referred to as *small temporal* RNAs. They would soon have their very own name, appropriately conferred by Gary Ruvkun in 2001: microRNAs.[6]

Just before we get to the studies that showed that these RNAs were in fact members of a much larger and widely conserved class, two other important discoveries around this time merit attention. The first was the 1998 paper in *Nature* by Andrew Fire and colleagues,[7] findings that would garner a Nobel prize: the discovery of *RNA interference*, abbreviated as RNAi. Researchers had known for some time that you could design and introduce artificial nucleotides, sequences of As, Cs, Gs, Us, that would bind by Watson-Crick pairing rules to complementary sequences in mRNAs. This would lower expression of the targeted gene. The big leap forward in this paper, which would cross over to the soon-to-emerge microRNA world, was the finding that short double-stranded RNAs, containing a sense as well as an antisense strand, produced far more potent and specific inhibition of the target mRNA than did single strands. In contrast to the findings on *lin-4*, double-stranded RNA (dsRNA) that contained a sequence of ~20 nucleotides that matched an mRNA strongly reduced the mRNA levels of that gene. Fire's team deduced that, like *lin-4*, this was controlling gene activity by a post-transcriptional mechanism. But their system had a catalytic aspect. A molecular machine inside cells must be taking up double-stranded RNAs and using them as a template to go after and destroy copies of the mRNA sequence that matched. This was a much more potent and efficient method of gene silencing than simple one-to-one binding of a small RNA onto an mRNA target, which was how *lin-4* worked. The authors recognised the implications of their discovery as well as its applications. It was now possible to knock-down any mRNA simply by designing a dsRNA. The world of molecular biology had a powerful new tool. Soon this would transform researchers' ability to discover what genes did in cells. It was to become an enormously popular and flexible means to control gene activity. Within a few years, everyone from cancer researchers to neuroscientists was designing and ordering a dsRNA to their favourite gene and within a few weeks would receive a kit with everything they needed to knock down their gene of interest and then look for a change in function, a phenotype.

The RNAi system had not, of course, evolved to help molecular biologists understand gene function. The natural function of RNAi was a genetic surveillance system. It was there to defend against two main threats to the genome: transposons and viruses. Transposons are short non-coding sequences in our genomes that are mobile. That is, they can jump around. Likewise, certain viruses can insert their genetic material into the host genome of the cell they infect. These are called retroviruses and our genomes are packed with ancient virally derived sequences which we carry with us today. Since these incorporation events can result in damage to useful genes, organisms have evolved ways to combat this, and RNAi is one of those tools. Transposon and retrovirus activity generates dsRNA and this then degrades mRNAs that contain complementary sequences protecting against insertion and replication. The systems inside the cell that allowed this to happen would be uncovered in parallel with the breakthroughs on microRNAs.

The second paper, a year before the big microRNA breakthroughs of 2000 and 2001, came from a team of British botanists led by David Baulcombe. Their findings, reported in *Science*, were the discovery of small, ~22 nucleotide RNAs that regulated gene expression in plants.[8] This meant that small, post-transcriptional regulators of gene activity were not unique to the animal kingdom.

Small RNAs Double

Back to 2000 and Ruvkun's team's discovery of a second small RNA controlling the timing of *C. elegans* development.[4] The team had begun by screening thousands of *C. elegans* exposed to genomic mutagens for events that disrupted developmental timing. The strongest effect was seen for the disruption of a gene called *let-7*. The mutation in *let-7* caused a restarting of larval events at the L4 to adult transition. In other words, the gene was required for later events, during normal transition to adult worms. Flipping the experiment, they overproduced *let-7* in immature L3 worms and found that this triggered early adult features. So, *let-7* was controlling the switch between late larval forms and the adult worm. But how? They next explored the *let-7* gene in detail, finding that it did not contain a protein-coding sequence but instead contained a region of 21 nucleotides that was highly conserved in other worm species and thus most likely critical for function. This small RNA was normally highly abundant in worms during the late development and adult transition. Seeing the parallels to *lin-4*, they searched for complementary sites in the 3' UTRs of mRNAs known to regulate developmental timing. Among those checked was *lin-14*. Sites where *let-7* could bind were found in *lin-14* and one other heterochronic gene called *lin-41*. To prove that this was functional, they inserted the 3' UTR from *lin-41* containing the predicted site for *let-7* into a transcript that normally lacks developmental timing. The replacement of the *lin-41* 3' UTR sequence conferred late L4-adult stage regulation on the surrogate gene. That is, they converted a non-timed gene into one that was developmentally regulated just by including the sequence that *let-7* could stick to. They had located and proven how *let-7* worked to control timing by down-regulating genes expressed earlier in development. **Figure 2.1** shows the structure of the newly discovered *let-7* along with *lin-4* and the adopted naming convention for microRNAs.

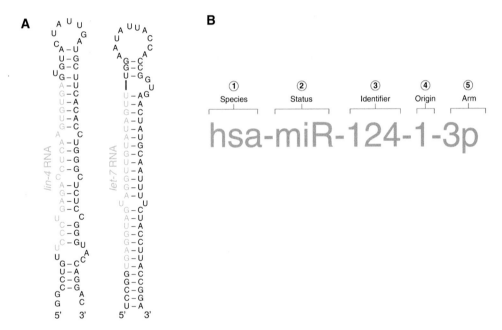

Figure 2.1 Structure of a microRNA and naming convention

Panel A shows the *C. elegans* predicted stem loops for the founding microRNAs *lin-4* and *let-7*, comprising the mature microRNAs (light grey) and the flanking sequence (dark grey).

Panel B shows the basic naming system for a microRNA. Each microRNA is identified by a species code (1) (e.g. Hsa for humans, mmu for mice). The maturation state of a microRNA molecule is indicated by 'mir' for pre-cursor microRNA and 'miR' for mature microRNA (2). With a few exceptions (the let-7 family), microRNAs have an identifier number (3), which indicates the order of discovery (e.g. miR-100 was discovered before miR-101). The site of origin from the original hairpin precursor is indicated as '3p' or '5p' (5), depending on whether the microRNA originated from the 3p or 5p arm. If two microRNAs have near-identical mature sequences, an 'a' and a 'b' are used to distinguish them (e.g. miR-146a-5p and miR-146b-5p). If identical mature microRNA sequences arise from different genomic locations, a '1' and a '2' are used to distinguish them (4) (e.g. miR-124-1-3p and miR-124-2-3p).

Source: Panel A reprinted with permission from Bartel, *Cell*, vol. 116, pp. 281–97 (2004).[9] Panel B is from Henshall & Brennan, *Nature Reviews Neurology*, vol. 16, pp. 506–19 (2020).[10]

The *let-7* discovery was followed in the space of a few months by another study by Ruvkun's group, also published in *Nature*.[5] They predicted, correctly, that *let-7* might be present in other species. Armed with the *let-7* sequence, they searched the genomes of other species. They found a single copy of the same sequence in the fly genome. When they got to the human genome, they got a surprise. Not only was *let-7* present in the human genome but there were multiple copies, some identical, others with 20 out of the 21 nucleotides the same. Versions of the *let-7* gene were present on several human chromosomes. In contrast, *lin-4*, found back in 1993, appeared to be unique to *C. elegans*. No equivalent existed in humans or in any other animals they checked including flies, fish and several other major divisions of the animal kingdom. In contrast, *let-7* was widespread in the animal kingdom. Sea urchins, bony fish and snails, referred to as bilaterian animals, also produced RNA from a *let-7* gene. But it was not absolutely everywhere. One phylum (the first major division of the animal or any other kingdom) called Cnidarian, which contains simple organisms called polyps, and the groups of animals that include sponges did not have *let-7*. This suggested that the *let-7* gene may have evolved half a billion years ago.

Having established that *let-7* was in humans, they took a first look at where the gene was made in the body. They did this by synthesising an artificial nucleotide or *oligonucleotide* that would stick to the *let-7* RNA sequence. The oligonucleotide carried a label so that it could be detected on film and was added to a gel in which RNA samples had been run from different organs. The results provided another surprise. The probe designed to detect *let-7* in humans showed a signal in most organs – including the heart, brain and kidneys – meaning that it was widely expressed. In fact, the only place it didn't seem to be made was the bone marrow, a cell birthing factory packed with immature cells destined to become blood cells. This was a good fit with what *let-7* was doing in *C. elegans*, regulating processes from late development into adulthood. The amount of *let-7* was not, however, the same in each tissue. It was abundant in the lungs and the kidneys, but a lower signal was detected in the heart and the colon. Something was varying the amount of *let-7* in different parts of the body. It suggested that some organs required more and some less. Ruvkun's paper concluded by dubbing *let-7* a member of a new class, the *small temporal RNAs*. A year later, and reflecting the fact that not all of these small RNAs were developmentally regulated, they would have the name 'microRNA'.

Triple Whammy

The stage was set for another seismic event in the microRNA world. Short RNAs such as *lin-4* and now *let-7* worked by post-transcriptional interference, curbing mRNA translation; they also worked as single transcripts rather than the double-stranded form required by the RNAi mechanism. They were known to be processed from longer transcripts (the details of how this happens will be covered in Chapter 3). Then, on 26 October 2001 came the simultaneous publication of three studies in *Science*. Together, these proved that microRNAs were an abundant and common feature of animal genomes. The first of the three papers came from the team of Thomas Tuschl,[11] at the time working at the Max-Plank Institute in Göttingen, Germany. Tuschl's group had been studying gene silencing by RNAi during fly development, using the model organism *D. melanogaster*. They were trying to understand the precise length requirements for a synthetic double-stranded RNA to produce gene silencing. This had led to a technique they could use to discover *any* short ~20 nucleotide RNAs made in the fly. They took RNA from fly embryos and searched for other short RNAs being made at the earliest stages of development. Using their technique, they identified 69 short RNA sequences comprising one or more copies of 16 different sequences. Rather than naming them, these new microRNAs were numbered, in order from 1 to 14. Two, called miR-2 and miR-13, differed by only a single base and were therefore referred to as 'a' and 'b' versions of the same microRNA. As with the earlier *C. elegans* work, the abundance of some varied significantly during development of the fly. Some of the microRNAs were present only at specific stages of fly development, whereas others were present at relatively steady levels throughout. They noted that some sequences were made only in specific cell types from flies and others displayed patterns of on/off similar to *lin-4* in *C. elegans*. This hinted that microRNAs controlled not only the timing of development but also the specification of cell types and tissues. They also located the sites in the fly genome where they came from, mapping with precision the DNA sequences that encoded the RNAs.

Tuschl's team pressed on with a search for their microRNAs in humans. This required a source of human RNA and for this they chose HeLa cells. These are a very commonly used human cell line for research. They are popular because they continuously divide, meaning that they are immortal and thus a never-ending source of human cells. This property relates to their origins. In 1951, a patient in the USA underwent an operation for cervical cancer at Johns Hopkins Hospital. Her name was Henrietta Lacks. Samples from her biopsy were shared with a tissue culture laboratory. Unlike most biopsy tissues, Henrietta's cells were found to divide rapidly in culture. The patient died shortly after the operation, but her cells, HeLa cells, continued to be studied. They were then shared freely with other scientists, revolutionising *in vitro* cell culture. Now, much good has come from sharing the cells. HeLa cells have underpinned major breakthroughs in the fields of biology and medicine. Famous users include Jonas Salk, who developed the polio vaccine, and more than 100,000 scientific studies make use of or reference to HeLa cells. The ethics of how the cells were used is questionable, however. Consent was never obtained to share the cells, but at the time this was not a legal requirement. Her family never received any benefit despite the commercial use of the cells. Later, the HeLa cell case helped inform the development of principles of consent for research using human samples.[12]

By searching the RNA they had extracted from HeLa cells, Tuschl's team found 21 different microRNAs in humans and mapped these to the relevant genomic location on human chromosomes. For a selection, they went on to look for the same gene in other species, finding homologues of the 15th and 16th (miR-15, miR-16) in tissues from mice and fish. For other microRNAs they did not find homologues in all species. This indicated evolutionary conservation of some but not others; more extensive searches would be forthcoming. The team concluded their paper by noting that the microRNAs come from longer precursor RNAs which contain sequences that form hairpin loops. But the microRNAs they found were a mix of those coming from either the 3' or the 5' ends of the longer precursor. When small RNAs were extracted and analysed, one arm was usually found and not the other. It wasn't clear what was choosing one or the other arm to become the 'final' microRNA or what had happened to the other arm. But there was asymmetry. They closed with two important speculations. First, the decision process on which arm was picked might have to do with the enzyme Dicer and another protein found to control RNAi in *C. elegans* called Argonaute. We will learn more about these in Chapter 3. And second, these microRNAs might have uses in reprogramming cells into other tissues. They were correct on both counts, and we will meet examples of using microRNAs to turn one cell type into another shortly and again in Chapter 4.

The second or middle paper was led by David Bartel's team at the Massachusetts Institute of Technology (MIT).[13] While Tuschl's team had been led to microRNAs out of an interest in understanding RNAi, Bartel's team wanted to know if *lin-4* belonged to a broader class of RNAs. But their search strategy was similar and began by selecting RNAs of the right size and chemistry. The RNA they extracted from *C. elegans* was drawn through a gel using an electric current. Smaller fragments move quicker than large ones, making it possible to pick out the size you want by comparing to a molecular weight marker, typically a ladder of labelled RNA of known molecular weights. Combined with other biochemical techniques, this allowed them to identify only RNAs of about 22 nucleotides in length that contained two other features: a phosphate at the 5' end and a hydroxyl at the 3' end, that is, fingerprints of the actions of an enzyme called Dicer (more about this in Chapter 3). The RNA fragments they found were then treated with an enzyme that performs reverse transcription, converting RNA to DNA. This creates complementary or cDNA sequences, also called clones, that are very stable and can be fed into a DNA sequencer and then matched to genomes, in this case the genome of *C. elegans*. Among more than 300 sequences, they detected both *lin-4* and *let-7*, proving that their technique was working. They found another 52 unique sequences with the correct length and which, using the agreed naming system, were newly discovered *C. elegans* microRNAs. Several of the same sequences were found in searches of the *D. melanogaster* and human genomes, indicating that they were evolutionarily conserved. As before, the team found that the stable microRNA product could come from either arm of the precursor hairpin structure and it was not clear what features in the RNA might be driving the selection process. They did, however, note nucleotide features common to a majority of the microRNAs. Most had a U base at the 5' end of the microRNA. Checking more than a dozen of these for abundance during *C. elegans* development, they found that most displayed timing-related spikes in levels. One of these, named miR-84, followed precisely the same pattern of emergence as *let-7*, appearing at larval stage 3 and remaining thereafter. Others showed steady-state expression, including miR-1. Bartel's study also noted clusters or hotspots of microRNAs in the genome of *C. elegans*. The physical proximity of a series of microRNAs with only short DNA sequences in between suggested that they were probably transcribed together. Wherever this occurred, the sequences of the microRNAs were quite similar. Bartel had found evidence of microRNA *families* that might act cooperatively on the same or similar mRNA targets. The authors reflected ruefully that these microRNAs had always been present in RNA extracts from *C. elegans* but were missed because the sequences lack features such as open reading frames. It was a reminder that some things are invisible or unknown to science simply because no one's looking for them or they don't yet have a method of detection. Bartel and colleagues also observed that the microRNAs did not align to the central coding sequences of mRNAs for *C. elegans*, meaning that they acted elsewhere, per *lin-4* and *let-7*. They closed by speculating that microRNAs may do more than regulate developmental timing, which turned out to be a very accurate prediction.

The third paper in the series of studies was by Ambros and also began with a search for new small temporal RNAs in *C. elegans*.[14] Now working at Dartmouth College in the USA, his team used a similar search strategy to Bartel's. Short RNAs from *C. elegans* were size selected and converted to DNA. This was followed by sequencing and looking for an origin from a longer precursor predicted to form a fold-back hairpin structure. This task was helped by a computer program developed by a team at the University of Rochester in the USA in 1999 for predicting these kinds of RNA structures.[15] Qualification also depended on a genomic location away from sequences that coded for proteins. Ambros' study found 15 new microRNA genes in *C. elegans* to join *lin-4* and *let-7*. Of these, 10 showed variation in abundance during worm development. They moved on to look in mouse and human samples, making another important advance by using tissues rather than a cell line, which was more physiologically relevant. This revealed that one of the highly conserved microRNAs, miR-1, was expressed exclusively in heart tissue in humans.

Placing Ambros' paper third in the *Science* issue gives an impression of its coming last, so it is important to give some further context here. Ambros and Rosalind Lee, the first author of the 1993 paper in *Cell* that discovered *lin-4*, had been working between 1993 and 2000 to see if other small RNAs such as *lin-4* existed. In a 2008 review written about the early days,[2] Ambros reflected on how he was slightly complacent in thinking that their work was not being watched by others who had equivalent skills and similar interests. Ambros came within a whisker of being scooped by the Bartel and Tuschl labs. Ambros recalled how, at a *C. elegans* meeting, he heard that Bartel was cloning small RNAs from *C. elegans* but slightly dismissed this as competition since Bartel wasn't from the *C. elegans* field. This type of jumping between fields is a great driver of scientific discovery, but it is also a cause of great pain to many who get caught out when someone stumbles onto what you previously held was 'yours'. It's a humbling reminder that you're unlikely to be the only person to have thought of something and to be quick about publishing it. Ambros was in fact sent Tuschl's paper to review, a common practice because editors send submitted manuscripts to the top people in the field. Ambros wrote back apologising and excusing himself from reviewing on the basis of a conflict of interest, since he and Lee had just made similar discoveries of more small RNA genes. *Science* said that it would consider publishing his and Lee's work alongside Tuschl's and Bartel's if they could submit their paper *that week*. The reality was that Ambros had no such paper ready to be submitted but he knew that he could not miss the opportunity. So, final experiments were run hand in hand with writing the paper, beginning that day, a Tuesday, and submitted as promised on the Friday. The rest, as they say, is history.

The three *Science* papers of 2001 represent the second wave of the origins of the microRNA field. These molecules were abundant in animal genomes, including our own. Their ~22 nucleotide length was highly conserved and several microRNAs were identical across a diversity of species. They were found in specific locations in the genome and, when expressed, contained sequence features that influenced their processing. Some were made only at certain times or in certain tissues, while the presence of others was more constant. It was clear that they could regulate developmental timing but also influence what type a cell became. They also had to be performing jobs unrelated to the control of organism development because microRNAs had been found in fully mature tissues, implying roles in everyday functions inside adult cells. Remarkably, there were other seminal papers in 2001 that laid the foundations of the field, including a *C. elegans* study featuring Ruvkun and Fire that identified two of the major genes (*alg-1* and *dcr-1*) involved in producing active microRNAs.[16] Reflecting at the end of the year on the remarkable breakthroughs of 2001,[17] Ambros posed a number of 'what's next?' questions and suggestions for how to experimentally answer them. How best to search for more microRNAs? Traditional searches for new expressed genes used methods that were biased towards identification of protein-coding genes. Bespoke searches would be needed, geared towards short transcripts using size selection and searching for sequences that could form hairpin structures in sites away from those encoding proteins. The microRNA pioneers knew that if there were dozens of microRNAs in a simple animal like *C. elegans*, chances were that there would be more in higher organisms, including humans. With less than 2 per cent of the human genome coding for proteins, there was certainly room for plenty of microRNAs. Why were microRNAs the length they were? What pathways were microRNAs able to regulate? Answers to these questions would require models such as the loss- and gain-of-function worm mutants that had been helpful in the past for understanding *lin-4* and *let-7*. Tracking changes in organism function when you knock out or over-express a microRNA would be a key approach in understanding their functions. It was not known if base-pairing to mRNAs to reduce translation was the only or even the main mechanism. Perhaps microRNAs could do other things? Maybe they influenced the stability or location of mRNAs in cells? MicroRNAs might do this by cooperating with proteins such as RBPs. Perhaps mRNAs were not the only type of RNA that microRNAs regulated? Understanding the rules of pairing to targets was a priority. Was all of the ~22 nucleotide microRNA used during targeting? MicroRNAs did not seem to be causing strong reductions in the levels of the mRNAs, so presumably they had to be pairing over shorter distances than the full length of their sequence; otherwise, they would trigger RNAi. What mechanisms controlled how much of an individual microRNA was made in specific cells? Over the coming years, answers to all of these questions and the predicted mechanisms of action would emerge. Ambros' predictions were prescient and would be borne out as he foresaw the next stages of microRNA discovery bringing 'a mixture of surprise and delight'.

MicroRNAs: The Next Early Years

The next couple of years saw exponential growth in microRNA research, providing basic answers to all of the questions posed at the end of 2001, including clarity on microRNA: target pairing rules, how microRNAs were processed and the proteins that helped them find and act on their targets. There were also the first accurate estimates of how many microRNAs were in the human and other model organism genomes. Within the first months of the following year, 2002, a team reported a possible link between microRNAs and a human disease. A protein critical for the function and survival of motoneurones, the nerves that control our voluntary movements, was found wedged in a complex with another protein along with a whole suite of new microRNAs.[18] Later in 2002, the neurodevelopmental disorder fragile X syndrome would be found to have a microRNA link and the first paper showing a link between microRNAs and cancer was published.[19] Tuschl's group performed a comprehensive profiling of microRNAs in mouse tissues.[20] This led to finding more than 30 new microRNAs, several of which were unique to particular organs. These included one in the liver named miR-122, and several in the brain, including miR-124, miR-128 and miR-134. We will meet miR-124 again shortly and the other two in more detail in Chapters 5 and 6. Still in mid-2002, Philip Sharp's team at MIT and the group of Brian Cullen at the Howard Hughes Medical Institute at Duke University designed and deployed artificial microRNAs.[21] Assembled by stitching together a series of nucleotides in the lab, these synthetic microRNAs, when expressed as longer precursors with a hairpin, worked just as well as their natural counterparts. They could inhibit translation of target mRNAs inside mammalian cells. It continued to be a remarkable year. Bartel's lab searched and found multiple microRNAs in *Arabidopsis*, a model plant organism, and other plant species.[22] Then, *let-7* was found to be capable of directing cleavage of certain mRNAs, muddying the waters between the microRNA and the RNAi pathways.[23] The main steps in the biogenesis pathway, the enzymes that processed and used microRNAs, were solved (covered in Chapter 3). The next year, 2003, would be no less packed with landmark findings. Tuschl kept on discovering, with more than 30 new microRNAs identified in mice and humans.[24] The extent to which some microRNAs were conserved across evolutionary time continued to surprise. For example, we share about half of our microRNAs with pufferfish. Teams discovered the enzyme responsible for the first step in microRNA processing[25] and the protein that shuttles microRNAs out of the nucleus to meet their mRNA targets.[26] Bartel's group developed a dedicated microRNA search algorithm and used it to estimate the total number of microRNA genes in certain species.[27] This gave an initial projection of about 200 in humans, which would turn out to be a bit of a low-ball. Other groups weighed in on this specific question, estimating numbers of microRNA genes in species including *C. elegans* (numbered at around 100 – that has held) and *D. melanogaster.* New teams were beginning to join the search. A study in plants found a virus that disabled microRNA functions as part of its infection mechanism.[28] Studies in *D. melanogaster* found new cell processes that were controlled by microRNAs, including cell death, metabolism and stress.[29] MicroRNAs were detected in human embryonic stem cells,[30] cells that hold the ability to divide indefinitely and become any cell type, making them the earliest microRNAs to switch on. MicroRNAs were also found that switched on during brain development.[31] Genomic sequences that acted as transcription cues for microRNA production were identified in *C. elegans.*[32] User-friendly technologies became available, allowing multiple microRNAs to be measured at the same time and opening the door to non-experts in molecular biology to study microRNAs. Researchers learnt what was influencing the choice of which arm of the microRNA duplex was selected.[33] The year closed with Bartel and colleagues introducing an algorithm, called Targetscan, that allowed researchers to predict the *targets* of microRNAs;[34] it is still going, now on version 8.0.

Taking stock of what was known about microRNAs at the start of 2004 reveals the remarkable leaps taken in a short space of time. The major rules and biochemistry by which microRNAs were made and acted had been uncovered. There was a solid understanding of how many microRNA genes there were and where they were located in genomes. Of the species studied in sufficient depth, it was clear that microRNAs made up about 1 to 2 per cent of the genes in mammals, flies and worms. They were processed from longer precursors that contained a fold-back structure. Two major steps shortened the microRNA ready for use and these spanned events in the nucleus and cytoplasm. What triggered transcription of microRNAs was less clear. MicroRNAs that derived from introns were presumed to be under the control of whatever transcription factor drove expression of the host gene. For those microRNAs outside of protein-coding genes that functioned as independent transcriptional units, the mechanisms were largely unknown. MicroRNAs were clearly important for organism development, switching on and off at defined times, helping to sculpt early, undefined cells into their highly specialised forms in mature tissues. But the steady-state levels of some microRNAs in mature tissues indicated that they were controlling other cell functions. It was known, but not why, that the amount of a microRNA in a specific cell could vary from a few to tens of thousands of copies per cell. A core sequence of seven nucleotides, positions 2 to 8, from the 5' end of the microRNA was the most conserved segment of microRNAs and therefore likely key to how they did their job. The main docking site on mRNAs appeared to be the 3' UTR. The main effect of a microRNA on a given target appeared to be reduced translation. At the time, it was slightly favoured that this was via stalling or delaying the ribosome, but other mechanisms could have explained the findings, such as active degradation of the growing polypeptide or mRNA cleavage, depending on the extent of complementarity between the two. A third mechanism, destabilisation of the target, emerged later. This was viewed cautiously, however, because the knowledge of how *lin-4/let-7* worked probably shaped the thinking and design of experiments at the time. MicroRNAs were known to cooperate. More sites for microRNAs could strengthen repression of a target. Naming rules and conventions were also established. The earliest transcript to be made was named a pri-microRNA. The later, shortened form and precursor of the mature form was named the pre-microRNA. Additional features included a species identifier and an arm identifier (see **Figure 2.1B**). Finally, any confusion between microRNAs and the endogenous short interfering RNAs (siRNA) of the RNAi pathway was clarified. While they entered a similar pathway and did similar things, such as functioning as ~22 nucleotides and repressing target mRNAs bearing complementary sequences, distinctions were clear. MicroRNAs and endogenous siRNAs came from different sites in the genome and varied in the types of target they acted on. The siRNAs usually came from the same loci as the RNAs they target, were less conserved between organisms, varied in precursor structures and worked differently, as duplexes vs single strands. In early 2004, we still had very few functional insights into what individual microRNAs did in animals and only about a dozen mRNA targets of human microRNAs had been convincingly validated. The amount of gene repression by individual microRNAs on their targets was uncertain. The algorithms made a lot of wrong guesses, and just because a microRNA could align with an mRNA did not mean that they interacted in nature because they could be expressed in different cells or at different times. But, altogether, this was a breathtaking achievement: a new field of biology, born and matured in record time. The discoveries had a profound gravitational effect, drawing in researchers from other fields, with labs redirecting their resources to try to scoop up the prize of the next breakthrough. And many important discoveries were still to come.

Technology Helps Solve the Numbers Problem

One of the big uncertainties during the early years was around how many targets a microRNA actually has in a cell. Put another way, how many of the expressed genes in a given cell are regulated by microRNAs? By the mid-2000s, it was known that a seed match of only seven nucleotides was needed for a microRNA:target match-up. With 3 billion bases to choose from, it is not unlikely that you come across seven nucleotides in a row for a microRNA. In principle, the numbers of predicted targets of some microRNAs ran into the hundreds. In order to prove whether multi-targeting actually occurred in nature, researchers would need ways to simultaneously measure every gene at once. Large-scale mRNA and large-scale protein screening was needed. New technology arrived in the nick of time. New microchip-like devices called microarrays had been developed that were coated with short segments of nucleotides complementary to any gene. To measure the amount of any expressed genes, you extracted RNA, converted it to DNA fragments using the reverse transcription reaction, labelled them with a dye and added them to the plate. The labelled fragments stuck to specific sites on the chip. This is called hybridisation and the usual Watson-Crick base-pairing principles apply. More copies of gene transcripts give a stronger signal, which is read and interpreted by a slide scanner and computer program. In 2005, microarray technology was applied by a commercial entity called Rosetta Inpharmatics in partnership with Bartel at MIT, to answer the question of how many genes are really controlled by microRNAs in human cells.[35] This led to three important discoveries. First, microRNAs indeed controlled the expression of large numbers of genes. Second, microRNAs didn't just reduce translation but could directly lower levels of their mRNA targets. Third, microRNAs were very powerful sculptors of cell type. That is, microRNAs alone could make a cell one type or another.

The central experiment was elegant and simple. Take HeLa cells, add in a microRNA unique to a tissue or cell type, then measure what happens to levels of all the mRNAs in the cell. What was added to HeLa cells was miR-124, a microRNA that Tuschl's lab had reported as brain-enriched. The effect was remarkable. More than 170 mRNAs were down-regulated by this single microRNA. When the list of genes down-regulated by miR-124 was compared to the genes normally present in the human brain, they found that these were all genes normally expressed at low levels in the brain. This implied that the job of miR-124 was to maintain low levels of non-brain genes, preventing non-brain cell proteins from being made in brain cells. Introducing miR-124 into HeLa cells had coaxed them into a more brain-like cell, at least from a molecular perspective. No one actually tested whether the cells acquired specific brain cell properties such as the ability to make and release neurotransmitters. To prove this wasn't unique to this particular microRNA; the experiment was repeated using miR-1, a heart-enriched microRNA. Now the HeLa cells developed a molecular profile more like heart or muscle.

A key job for microRNAs had been added to the list. Prior to this, it wasn't clear why microRNAs like miR-124 and miR-1 continued to be made in mature cells at such high levels. Here was an answer. Steady-state microRNAs work to ensure that the gene pro-grammes that make a cell one type or another *remain that way*. They enforce the appropriate gene landscape for specific cells and, by doing so, ensure that the functional properties of cell types stay the way they should. One further issue was worth checking. Did the gene transcripts that were down-regulated by the microRNAs really contain binding sites for these microRNAs in their 3' UTRs, the non-coding portion of the mRNA transcript? Or could the microRNAs be acting in different way? Perhaps they altered the activity of just one or two transcription factors. By reducing a key driver of gene expression, a bit like turning off the gene tap, the end result would be similar. But this wasn't what was happening. Most of the down-regulated gene transcripts contained 3' UTRs with sites for miR-124. Multi-targeting effects were a property of microRNAs. A further experiment helped improve our understanding of the importance of those first nucleotides of a microRNA, at positions 2 to 8. When certain nucleotides in the miR-124 sequence were replaced, switching out nucleo-tides 5 and 6, the HeLa-to-brain effect of miR-124 was lost. That is, introducing the mutant version of miR-124 to HeLa cells failed to convert them to the brain cell gene profile. In contrast, if the mutated nucleotides were outside the seed, at positions 9 to 10, the brain cell–converting effect of miR-124 remained. The positions 2 to 8 seed region was really critical for the effects of the microRNA.

Now, there are limitations with using microarray technology to determine the effects of microRNAs on their targets. Chief among these is that microarrays only measure mRNA levels. Ultimately, we want to know if a microRNA affects the amount of a protein. But also, if a microRNA blocks translation without affecting levels of the mRNA target, a microarray experiment would give the appearance of the microRNA not regulating the target. Recording the complete effects of microRNAs in cells needs a way to analyse protein levels, ideally together with analysing mRNA. Developments in the field of quantitative mass spectrometry would come to the rescue, helping to clarify how much of an effect a microRNA has on the protein levels of its target(s). Mass spectrometry had been around for some time, but it was getting better and better at precisely measuring proteins in biological samples. While there are different instruments and techniques, the basic principle is the same. Take a sample containing a mix of proteins, fragment and ionise them using a spray of electrons, then accelerate them along a tube to a detector. The mass and charge ratios are deconstructed to yield identifiable proteins and an estimation of their abundance.

The year 2008 saw the first evaluation of the effect of a microRNA on the complete proteome,[36] a term referring to the totality of all the proteins in the cell. This also came from Bartel's group and the core experiment was a similar design to the previous one using microarrays to measure the totality of mRNA changes. Take a typical or plain cell, introduce or remove a microRNA, wait a while, then extract all the proteins and measure them. However, standard mass spectrometry was not sensitive enough to pick out small differences in the abundance of many proteins, so they used a modified mass spectrometry technique called stable isotope labelling by amino acids in cell culture (SILAC). Starting with two plates of cultured cells, one is then fed with amino acids that have been labelled with a heavy form of a carbon atom. For example, one of the amino acids is labelled with carbon-13 (C^{13}) instead of carbon-12 (C^{12}). As new proteins are made, the 'heavy' amino acids get incorporated, which makes the resulting protein a tiny amount heavier. The heavy proteins are extracted and mixed together with the non-labelled cell version of the proteins, chopped up and ionised, and it all gets run on a mass spectrometer. For a given peptide, the detector sees two nearly identical fragments and, based on the intensities of one versus the other, enables a determination as to the difference in abundance. By measuring the abundance of different fragments of the same original protein, you build up a highly accurate picture of how much there is in a sample. If a microRNA is blocking production of proteins, you can now spot that change and accurately measure the effect size.

The proteomic analysis used HeLa cells treated with miR-124. More than 1,500 proteins were accurately detected by mass spectrometry. Introduction of the non-native (ectopic) microRNA resulted, as expected, in lower levels of dozens of proteins. When the mRNA sequences for these changed proteins were searched, one sequence was far more abundant than any other in the 3' UTRs: GUGCCUU, a '7-mer' sequence. This aligned to positions 2 to 8 from the 5' end of miR-124. It was an exact match for the 5' seed binding site. Put another way, the transcripts for the proteins that were down-regulated by the introduction of miR-124 contained a site that could base-pair to miR-124. When an A was in position 1 of the microRNA, a 7-mer-A1 match, the effect on protein levels was strongest. This was not unique to miR-124; repeating the experiments using miR-1, the heart-specific microRNA, or miR-181, another brain-expressed microRNA, produced equivalent results, albeit affecting a different set of proteins whose transcripts bore seed binding sites for those microRNAs.

This was the best evidence yet that a single microRNA can down-regulate large numbers of proteins that bear specific seed sites in the 3' UTRs of their transcripts. But perhaps adding a 'foreign' microRNA into HeLa cells, a cell type to which the microRNA is not normally hosted, is not physiologically relevant? Or maybe too much microRNA was being added? To guard against these concerns, a further SILAC experiment was run, in which an endogenous microRNA was deleted. This created a complementary test to determine how many proteins were under the control of that microRNA, with the expectation that higher protein levels would be found for any target directly controlled by the deleted microRNA.

The chosen microRNA was miR-223, a microRNA enriched in neutrophils, an abundant class of white blood cell. The team obtained neutrophils from mice genetically engineered to lack miR-223 and then ran a SILAC study comparing the protein levels in these cells against normal mouse neutrophils. The results were highly complementary to what happened when the microRNA was added. A large set of proteins were more abundant in the cells that lacked miR-223. The transcripts of those proteins that increased contained 7-mer or 8-mer sites in their 3' UTRs for miR-223, and proteins whose mRNA transcripts contained only six nucleotide matches did not change.

The application of proteomics not only proved how broad an effect a microRNA can have on gene expression but sharpened understanding of the seed. First, the number of nucleotides that were needed to base-pair. Whereas substantial numbers of proteins were down-regulated if their corresponding message contained a 7-mer site match to the 5' end of the microRNA, any mRNAs that contained only a 6-mer match did not show significant reductions in their corresponding proteins. So, microRNA targeting produced more effective changes when there was at least a seven-nucleotide match to the target's 3' UTR site. An 8-mer match also worked very nicely. The experiments also weighed in on the issue of whether potential seeds outside the 3' UTR of transcripts were important. Poring over the proteomic data found little evidence that sites in coding regions of mRNAs were being targeted or effective at reducing protein production. The proteomic work also allowed scientists to check the validity of some of the algorithms that had slightly different weighting systems for predicting targets. Targetscan was one of the winners, having been based on species-conserved 3' UTRs containing at least 7- to 8-mer sites. Large-scale protein studies had proven that the seed length and where it resides within the mRNA are critical for the effects of microRNAs. By digging a bit deeper into the data, one or two other important findings were made. The mRNA levels, which were also measured during the SILAC studies, generally tracked closely with the protein level, going up or down upon microRNA manipulation. But protein-mRNA correlations differed in some cases enough to conclude that some targets of microRNAs change only at a protein level. That is, some microRNA interactions block translation while leaving the mRNA alone. However, the mRNA was always altered anytime a microRNA changed the protein level by 50 per cent or more. The strongest suppressive effects of microRNAs were accompanied by changes to both mRNA and protein. So, while modest effects of microRNAs on proteins can occur via translation repression alone, the more important biological effects of microRNA targeting involved destabilisation of mRNA.

These large-scale studies measuring mRNA and protein answered important questions. However, the methods had manipulated one microRNA at a time. When you add together *all* the microRNAs in a cell, what is the effect on their targets? How many of the ~20,000 genes in our genomes contained sequences in their 3' UTRs that would place them under microRNA control? One approach to the answer was a comparative analysis, aligning and comparing the 3' UTRs of large numbers of mammalian genomes and searching for the conserved microRNA sites (e.g. the 7- or 8-mer matches). Estimates as early as 2005 suggested that one-third of all protein-coding transcripts in humans bore sites suitable for control by microRNAs. Later estimates, using further algorithms that better integrated real-world data coming out of experiments with microarrays and proteomics, put the estimate above 50 per cent. A remarkable 45,000+ microRNA sites were found to be conserved in the 3' UTRs of more than 10,000 genes.[37] It was correct to say that a majority of protein-coding genes in humans were controlled by microRNAs.

Competition by the Numbers

In order to understand how microRNAs work, we must consider their abundance relative to their targets. They bind in a one-to-one manner with target mRNAs. The more abundant a microRNA, the more repression it can produce. In a hypothetical scenario, if there are 100 targets for one microRNA in a cell then it will take 100 copies of that microRNA to occupy all the available sites. If there are only 50 copies of the microRNA in that cell then half of its targets will go unregulated. The ratio of microRNA to mRNA is therefore important. And the ratio is normally heavily tipped in favour of the targets. That is, there are always more microRNA binding sites than there are microRNA molecules that match. Many of the conserved microRNAs in human cells have been found to have hundreds of target sites. Some mRNAs are targeted more than once by the same microRNA – that is, the target has multiple sites for the same microRNA. This is the case even for highly abundant microRNAs. Studies show that even in the case of a microRNA that is present at more than 100,000 copies per cell, and this is the case for miR-122 in liver cells, the number of target sites still exceeds this number. This means that microRNA binding sites are normally not saturated. That is, there is spare capacity for microRNA binding sites on target mRNAs. This creates a sensitivity to increased abundance of microRNAs. With free sites available on targets, a sharp rise in microRNAs can quickly translate to biologically meaningful changes to the protein levels of the target mRNAs that house sites for the microRNA. This relationship will flux as transcription of target and microRNA change. For those microRNAs that derive from introns of protein-coding genes, the transcription of the host gene will be closely matched by increased levels of the microRNA contained within an intron. But many microRNAs do not reside within shared transcriptional units. In those cases, expression of targets and microRNAs may not track together. If microRNA levels rise without a corresponding increase in mRNA targets, then the effects of that microRNA on its target pool will be increased and more repression will occur. **Figure 2.2** highlights how, in some cases, a single microRNA can act on hundreds of transcripts, although the effect is generally mild, but multiple microRNAs can also act on the same transcript.

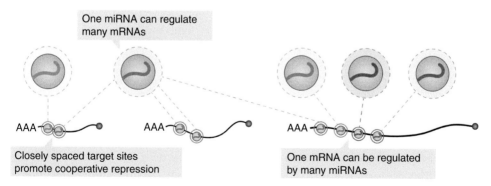

Figure 2.2 Single and multi-targeting effects of microRNAs

Schematic shows how microRNAs work to regulate mRNA transcripts. One microRNA can target many different microRNAs. Equally, one mRNA can be regulated by several different microRNAs. Cooperative and thus stronger repression is achieved when binding is to closely spaced target sites. Combined, the two mechanisms enable microRNAs to exert regulatory control on complex gene networks.

Source: Reprinted with permission from Gebert & MacRae, *Nature Reviews Molecular Cell Biology*, vol. 20, pp. 21–37 (2019).[38]

There is a further and important implication of the gap in abundance between microRNAs and targets. It undermines the biological importance of the lowest expressed microRNAs. Since there is always an over-abundance of targets for microRNAs in cells, a rise in levels of a low-expressed microRNA, effectively the addition of a few copies of microRNA per cell, will have a negligible effect on targets because so many sites remain unoccupied. This has implications for a proposed mechanism of cell-to-cell communication via the packaging and shuttling of small numbers of microRNA copies. We will meet this in more detail later in the book. For now, we can see that the absorbance by a cell of a package containing just a few copies of a microRNA is unlikely to have a biologically meaningful impact on the recipient cell's vast target pool for that microRNA. We could imagine, however, potential scenarios where this would not apply. For example, if the incoming microRNA encounters a low-expressed target within a discrete sub-domain of the cell separate from the main target pool, then additional microRNA molecules, even if few in number, might make a difference.

Why We Need MicroRNAs

This is a suitable moment to ask a simple question. Why do we need microRNAs at all? What is it about gene expression that demands a system for the later correction of protein levels? Why hasn't nature been able to simply get it right the first time, producing the right amount of mRNA and protein needed in a given cell at a specific moment in time? Is that so hard? Why the extra step with microRNAs? Let's start with an indirect but powerful argument for the fundamental need for a microRNA system for life, the observation that the system has independently evolved multiple different times in different branches of life. This is an example of convergent evolution. Genetic studies show that distinct but similar microRNA systems evolved in animals, plants, slime moulds, sponges and algae (in fact, chlorophyte green and brown algae have distinct systems). So, nature keeps findings ways to evolve a microRNA system. Why? The answer is that gene expression is intrinsically noisy. Gene expression varies a lot between individual cells, having a surprisingly large degree of randomness. Gene expression is *stochastic*. This was known as early as the 1950s, but to be properly studied it required further developments in molecular biology, which became available in the 1990s. Without the right controls – with 'just' genes and transcription factors – the programmes that control organisms are unstable. This problem is not exclusive to what has evolved naturally. Studies in the field of synthetic biology found exactly the same issue with their 'designed' genomes. Noise and randomness in gene expression are funda-mental not only to natural but also to artificial life.[39] It was studies in synthetic biology that would show that having a negative regulator of gene expression reduced the variability in gene expression between individual cells.

One source of this noise is intrinsic, meaning that it arises from bursting behaviour during transcription and randomness and variability in the cell's gene expression machin-ery. The other is extrinsic, involving factors from outside the cell that influence the rates of transcription. Not all genes are as noisy as others. Those that respond to stressors tend to be noisier than habitually active ones. Higher rates of transcription are associated with lower levels of variability in gene expression. Notably, these discoveries came around the time in the early 2000s when microRNAs were found to be widespread in the living world. Later research showed that cell-to-cell fluctuations in gene expression can be higher in more complex organisms. This is partly owing to additional layers of control on genome accessibility, including open and closed segments of chromatin. But transcription rates are not the only source of noise. Several other steps affect noise, including rates of translation. Experiments and modelling show that if you marry a higher transcription rate with measures that limit translation, then you have lower fluctuation. That is, more stable gene expression. This negative regulation of translation is what microRNAs do and, together, this helps explain the key properties of microRNAs and the advantages they confer on biological systems.[40] The point at which microRNAs act along the gene pathway also confers a specific advantage. By acting at a late stage, in the cytoplasm at the point of translation, there is an opportunity to correct earlier variation or excess. This also offers efficiencies compared to intervening later, after energy and resources have been expended building a protein. Complementing this late moment to intervene, microRNAs also get distributed to specific corners of the cell to locally regulate translation. This places them right at the site of action of proteins whose translation is coupled to incoming signals, ensuring localised fine-tuning of protein levels. Some of the best examples of this happening are found in the brain. Gene noise, although common to life, is rarely useful and must be overcome. And the problem of stabilising gene expression between cells becomes much larger for more complex organisms, so noise resistance measures are essential. MicroRNAs are one of nature's favourite solutions, a genomic revolution that has provided ways for organisms to become increasingly more complex. Being small and having relatively simple sequence and structural needs, with light-touch impact on existing gene networks, they were an ideal fix.

Resilience: MicroRNAs Confer Robustness to Biological Systems

There are several ways in which microRNAs can act to contribute to stabilising gene expression and thus improving cell and organism performance. A common mechanism by which they act is to tune gene expression, setting the level of a gene in a cell at a given time. They also act to buffer gene activity, reducing the amount of variation in transcript levels. And they stabilise gene expression against external stressors. This creates robustness, an ability to endure and maintain a cell or tissue phenotype in the face of intrinsic and extrinsic pressures. This has been experimentally observed many times when microRNAs have been blocked or deleted from genomes. There follows an increase in phenotype variability. One example is loss of miR-9, which controls the development of sense organs such as eyes in D. melanogaster. Without sharp control of gene expression, the miR-9-lacking flies develop extra sense organs.[41] The ability to reduce variation in traits is called canalisation. Organism complexity increases as a function of an increasing number of traits; highly heritable traits are more responsive to natural selection. MicroRNAs increase the heritability of phenotypes and traits. The activity of the microRNA system during development is strongly conserved, ensuring minimal variation in the phenotype of the organism despite variation in the external and internal environments in which the organism is developing. As an underlying mechanism of canalisation, microRNAs are de facto important drivers of natural selection towards more complex organisms.[42]

So, microRNAs confer robustness, the ability of a biological system to function in the face of perturbations. This property of resilience means that they can carry on despite a change in conditions or when one part fails. The survival advantage of robustness for organisms covers a broad sway, from the level of an individual signalling pathway where microRNAs adjust gene dose, through to enforcing patterns of gene expression that establish cellular identities within a developing tissue, all the way up to a whole organism level, providing resilience to external perturbations such as injuries, infections and other threats to survival. It is achieved by feedback systems and redundancy in systems. During development, microRNAs sharpen transitions from one stage to another by eliminating residual transcripts that were required at earlier stages. This works a little like a sieve, removing residual copies of gene transcripts that are no longer needed for the next step in tissue development. As organisms develop and tissue complexity increases, we see a corresponding increase in the diversity of the expressed microRNAs. But we also know that microRNAs help retain cell identity once the final features of a cell are reached. So, our system needs to account for both processes, sharpening gene expression during transition phases as well as sustaining or setting long-lasting patterns of gene expression once the cell has reached its terminal differentiated state.

Studies of microRNA expression during animal development and computer modelling have uncovered how this works (see **Figure 2.3**). Let's start with microRNAs as part of a simple negative feedback loop. Hypothetical component A activates component B, which is a microRNA, which inhibits component A. Examples of this are known. The MECP2 protein, the gene which is often lost in the rare neurodevelopmental disorder Rett syndrome, promotes transcription of miR-132, which in turns targets the *MECP2* transcript. If levels of MECP2 rise then this is accompanied by more microRNA targeting *MECP2*, creating a stable loop that prevents overproduction of MECP2.

Another example is what is called a coherent feedforward loop. Hypothetical component A activates component B, a microRNA, which inhibits component C, which is also inhibited by component A. Temporary loss of component A is compensated by component B. Using a real-world example, there is a coherent feedforward loop in which the transcription factor C/EBPα inhibits the transcription factor E2F1, which regulates steps during the production of white blood cells. Further, C/EBPα also switches on expression of miR-223, which has binding sites in the *E2F1* transcript. This loop has a feedback option, too: E2F1 inhibits production of miR-223. This type of loop is widespread among microRNA gene networks. Combinations of microRNA-embedded feedforward and feedback loops better allow for what needs to be transiently controlled versus more stably expressed (**Figure 2.3**).

Incoherent feedforward loops also exist which help reduce variation in protein levels owing to unwarranted transcription factor activation. In that loop, the transcription factor increases levels of a microRNA as well as its target gene(s). Researchers in my lab found an example of one such loop in studies on a microRNA that limits inflammation in the brain (see Chapter 6). The microRNA targets the transcript up-regulated by the transcription factor. Excess transcription factor activity is curbed by the production of the microRNA. If the transcription factor activity drops then so too does the microRNA level, enabling a rise in the level or translation of the transcription factor's generated protein-coding transcript. These are simple examples and more complex relationships are present in most systems. For example, it is common that pathways feature regulation of a component by multiple microRNAs. This both ensures redundancy, an important safety mechanism, and can amplify the strength of the microRNA control. In the event that the microRNA targets a transcriptional repressor, stronger microRNA control can promote more complete pathway switch-off or pathway activation. And many genes are controlled by multiple transcription factors, acting coherently with other signals and not in isolation. Modelling these loops using computer simulations backs up what nature created. The microRNA system is more effective and efficient than a system that relies only on transcriptional repressors and

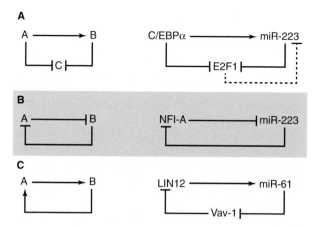

Figure 2.3 Feedforward and other loops by which microRNAs operate to stabilise gene expression

The figure shows examples of the feedforward and other loops within which microRNAs operate to stabilise gene expression.

Panel A shows a coherent feedforward loop. In the example on the right, this both directly and indirectly inhibits the cell cycle regulator E2F1 during the production of granulocytes. Note, this feedforward loop is interlocked with a feedback loop via E2F1 inhibiting production of miR-223.

Panel B shows a mutual negative feedback loop. In the example on the right, this contributes to bi-stability between myeloid precursors and granulocytes, helping avoid cells returning to a precursor state.

Panel C is a positive feedback loop. In the example on the right, this enforces lineage commitment of nematode '2 degrees' vulval cells. LIN12 directly activates transcription of miR-61, which then represses a negative regulator of LIN12 called Vav-1.

Key: C/EBPα, CCAAT-enhancer-binding protein alpha; NFI-A, nuclear factor 1A; Vav-1, Vav Guanine Nucleotide Exchange Factor 1.

Source: Adapted with permission from Ebert & Sharp, *Cell*, vol. 149, pp. 515–24 (2012).[40]

activators. The microRNA system is better at buffering molecular noise and curtailing fluctuations in gene expression. And no other system of transcriptional control has been found that matches the ability of the microRNA–mRNA system to fine-tune gene expression. But no system is completely foolproof, either. If we remove a microRNA from a loop with limited redundancy of microRNAs, we can generate an unchecked system. A similar effect could be achieved if we lose the long 3' UTRs that harbour multiple microRNA sites. Both actions would leave components unrestrained. If that component is lost from a microRNA shut-down loop in the cell cycle then this can give rise to unrestrained cell division, a hallmark of cancer.

The Evolution of MicroRNAs and How MicroRNAs Helped Us Evolve

Let us now dip into the origins and evolution of microRNAs in the animal kingdom. The *let-7* discovery revealed microRNAs to be evolutionarily ancient, present in the last common ancestor we share with sea urchins. Was *let-7* the founder microRNA? Or are there more-ancient microRNAs? How far back along the branches of the tree of life do we find them? When did they first appear in organisms and which form of life was the first or simplest to have a microRNA? How do new microRNA genes emerge and what is the driving force? Is there evidence that they have been important for human evolution? Are we finished with microRNA evolution or is there more to come? Our ability to discover new microRNAs and to look back in time at the organisms and their ancestors from where they evolved was facilitated by two key research tools. First, advances in sequencing technology, meaning that the genomes and the RNAs produced by any organism could be mapped, at manageable cost, in fine detail. Second, the computer algorithms that had been refined to know precisely what features to look for, such as the hairpin-containing precursor molecules and the ability to align and look for seed sequences.

Finding the *let-7* gene in the sea urchin genome set the clock of microRNA origins to at least half a billion years ago. This coincided with an important time in the diversification of animal body plans, a time when some of the most fundamental differences between major animal groups emerged. In fact, sets of microRNAs appear at several key transition points in the animal kingdom. A large set of microRNAs was conserved between two major groupings, or clades, in the animal kingdom: protostomes and deuterostomes. This was after the earlier emergence of bilateral animals, animals with bilateral symmetry and usually a head, tail, front and back (humans are members of bilateria). The protostomes and the deuterostomes shared a common ancestor more than 600 million years ago. The protostomes are considered the much more successful of these two, giving rise to more than a million different species alive today. Additional expansions of the microRNA gene pool coincide with the start of the vertebrate lineage, during the Cambrian explosion just over 500 million years ago. This was still well before animals developed jaws. Another expansion of microRNA genes occurred in the ancestors and lineage that led to placental mammals. So, microRNA gene expansion coincides with major transition events in the animal kingdom. **Figure 2.4** shows the relationship between key branches of the animal kingdom and the expansion of microRNA genes.

Given what we know of their role in organism development and the specification of tissues and different cell types, it seems likely that microRNA were critical to evolutionary change, including events that would eventually lead to us, *Homo sapiens*. This leads us to an important observation, something fundamental about microRNAs and the living world. There is a correlation between the number of microRNAs and morphological complexity. That is, the more complex an organism is, with higher numbers of systems, organs, tissues and cell types within those tissues, the higher the number of microRNAs in its genome. Hydrazoa, a simple animal related to jellyfish, has fewer than 20 microRNA genes. But *C. elegans*, the roundworm, has more than 100 microRNA genes. Insects including the fly *D. Melanogaster* have slightly more than 200. Sequencing the microRNAs of the lizard *Anolis carolinensis*, a reptile, found about 300. Moving up, we find about 1,000 microRNAs in a bird such as *Gallus gallus* (chicken) and, on to mammals, more than 700 in mice. Humans have more than 2,000 microRNAs, although this number is still a moving target. That estimate is based on miRBase and a 2019 study by a highly reputable group using widely agreed criteria.[44] But a 2015 study in the journal *Proceedings of the National Academy of Sciences of the United States of America* that sequenced multiple different human tissues put the number of human microRNAs up by another 3,700.[45] Some of the discrepancies are likely because precursor transcripts can give rise to more than one detectable mature microRNA. Regardless, this relationship is not seen for protein-coding genes. Higher numbers of protein-coding genes do not track with organism complexity. *Arabidopsis*, the model plant we met earlier, and *Daphnia*, a water flea, both have more protein-coding genes than humans. There are more chromosomes in the potato genome than in the human genome. But there is a linear increase

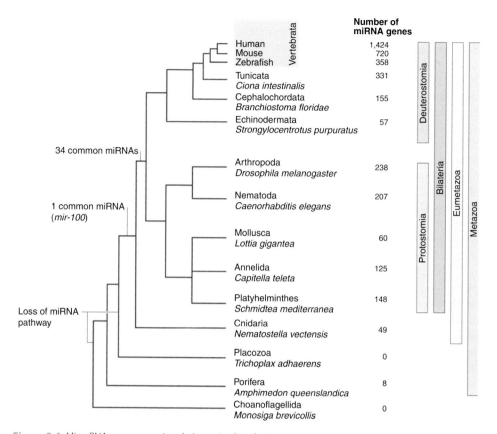

Figure 2.4 MicroRNA gene expansion during animal evolution

The figure is a cladogram showing numbers of microRNA genes present in key animal groups. Analysis has revealed that microRNAs were present at the dawn of metazoan evolution. Also notable are the bursts of microRNA numbers at key branches during animal evolution including at the base of the vertebrate lineage. Branch lengths in the cladogram are not to scale.

Updated microRNA gene numbers provided by Albert Sanfeliu using miRBase v22 are as follows: *Monosiga brevicollis* (Choanoflagellida) (0), *Amphimedon queenslandica* (Porifera) (8), *Trichoplax adhaerens* (Placozoa) (0), *Nematostella vectensis* (Cnidaria) (141), *Schmidtea mediterranea* (Platythelminthes) (148), *Capitella teleta* (Annelida) (129), *Lottia gigantea* (Mollusca) (59), *Caenorhabditis elegans* (Nematoda) (253), *Drosophila melanogaster* (Arthropoda) (258), *Strongylocentrotus purpuratus* (Echinodermata) (63), *Branchiostoma floridae* (Cephalocordata) (156), *Ciona intestinalis* (Tunicata) (348), zebrafish (355), mouse (1234), human (1917).

Source: Adapted with permission from Berezikov, *Nature Reviews Genetics*, vol. 12, pp. 846–60 (2011).[43]

in the number of microRNA genes as we go up in organism complexity. This discovery helped resolve what is called the C/G-value paradox in biology, that is, the disconnect between the number of genes in an organism and the complexity of that organism. This was being puzzled as far back as the 1950s. MicroRNAs were the solution to one of biology's mysteries, how it is not necessarily the amount of DNA or the number of protein-coding genes that explains organism complexity but the number of microRNAs. They give rise to and contribute to the complexity of life.

Another piece of evidence for the importance of microRNAs in driving new branches of animal life is that once they appear in a particular lineage, they rarely disappear. That is, they are passed on to descendants. This implies important and necessary functions. If not, mutation errors, which naturally occur with regularity, would accumulate and inactivate them, leaving behind a non-productive gene. As an example, many species, including ours, acquired mutations in the enzyme that makes vitamin C, presumably because the dietary availability was so high that there was no natural selection pressure to keep it working.[46] Errors accumulated without affecting reproductive success. The fact that many microRNA genes, once present in the genome, remain implies that they are necessary for reproductive success. Nature plays a hard game of use it or lose it.

Can we go further back? How ancient are microRNAs? All three major branches of life have small RNAs or microRNAs specifically encoded in their genomes which they use to regulate gene expression. That includes the prokaryotes bacteria and archaea (also single-cell organisms, but a fully separate branch of life with fundamentally different chemistry from bacteria), and eukaryotes, organisms made up of more than one cell, which includes plants, fungi and animals. Precise timelines in the animal kingdom are difficult, but at least one microRNA is shared with animals of the sub-kingdom eumetazoans that evolved as far back as 600 million years ago, of which we humans share a common ancestor. Nevertheless, there are examples of animals which appear to lack a microRNA system. The Ctenophores are jellyfish, simple marine animals, whose lineage is possibly the oldest in the animal kingdom, dating back to around 600 million years ago. An analysis of genomes reported in *Nature* in 2014 found no evidence for the enzymes that produce microRNAs in Ctenophores.[47] Since these animals possess nervous and digestive systems, albeit very simple ones, this implies that complex multicellular life is possible without a microRNA system. But other small RNAs are present in Ctenophores.[48] It remains possible that another short RNA-based system functions in these animals, but awaits proper characterisation.

Some viruses can make microRNAs, but viruses are not technically a branch of life because they lack various features of being alive. They do not grow, move, sense, have needs of nutrition or produce waste. The discovery of viral microRNAs is a powerful indicator of the importance of microRNAs. What is so remarkable about virally encoded microRNA? Two things. First, viruses are tiny. Genomic real estate is at a premium. Whatever is encoded in their genome is put to good use. There is tremendous selection pressure on viral genomes to be as compact as possible. They have no room for unnecessary parts. A great example of this is the genome of the hepatitis C virus. Everything it needs to replicate is transcribed as a single long RNA molecule which is then chopped up, each segment encoding proteins and other 'tools' the virus uses to make more copies of itself. The second interesting consideration is that the virus uses a microRNA rather than another tool to get the job done. MicroRNAs have versatility and strengths, as we have seen and will be obvious later in the book. Some viruses deploy microRNAs to shut down the machinery that the infected cells would otherwise use to mount a counter-attack. Since microRNAs can be multi-targeting, this is an efficient way to deal with the problem of host cells that, if one pathway is evaded, may switch to another. The virus may not be able to fully shut down a system with a microRNA, but it can blunt multiple attacks this way. An evolutionary arms race is underway in organisms between viruses and their hosts, and using microRNAs encoded in a viral genome is a neat way to win.[49] The evolution of viruses dates back to the last universal common ancestor (LUCA), that is, the population from which all organisms now living on Earth descended. So, microRNAs or microRNA-like molecules may well date back to some of the earliest molecular events in life on Earth.

Pushing for More MicroRNAs

What was the driving force for microRNA-like regulators to evolve and what was the first proto-microRNA? Current thinking is that the system emerged in lower, single-celled organisms as a form of defence. Versions of key genes that make and use microRNAs in animals are present in the genomes of bacteria. Their job is to generate short RNAs that are then used to inactivate foreign RNA during infection. They defend the host organism against hostile takeover. It is notable that mitochondria, which have their own genome and were once free-living bacteria-like organisms before being subsumed into the ancestor of all eukaryotic cells through the process of endosymbiosis, contain microRNAs. Thus, eukaryotic and later complex multicellular life may owe a debt of gratitude to an ancient bacterium for evolving microRNAs in the first place.

How do new microRNA genes emerge? First, we need a sequence that is transcribed and from which a hairpin or fold-back RNA structure can result, enabling it to be recognised and enter the microRNA pathway. This is not such a stringent requirement as RNAs readily form loops and three-dimensional shapes. Indeed, that property is at the heart of the various RNA machines in our cells, such as ribosomes. From there, there are several ways microRNA genes can evolve. The main driver of new microRNAs is duplication of existing microRNAs. About a third of human microRNA genes are grouped into families and arose from duplication of founder microRNA genes. The microRNA copy may remain in the same originating locus or appear elsewhere, including on different chromosomes. The origin of many younger, species-specific microRNAs is from introns of protein-coding genes, whereas exons are not sources of novel microRNAs. Introns are ripe for new microRNA generation, being already transcribed as a co-product of the host protein-coding gene. This repurposing of a sequence, from intron to microRNA, is an example of a process known as exaptation. Some intron-lurking microRNAs appear to then later evolve independent transcriptional control, separating them from any dependence on the host gene. A third driver of new microRNAs is by the actions of transposable elements. We met these already; they're sections of genetic material that can cut and paste into genomes. Like intron-derived microRNAs, these are more common in species-specific microRNAs.

So, how do microRNAs know to stop evolving? MicroRNA sequences will vary until a pressure upon them causes that to be fixed. The pressure is probably the point when a sufficiently large or important set of targets is under control. At that point, the sequence of the microRNA becomes fixed. What was so remarkable about *let-7* was that the entire 21-nucleotide sequence is conserved across such a long period of evolutionary time. It's remarkable because only the seed region, nucleotides 2 to 8, was thought to be important for the targeting event. Selective pressure to retain that sequence is understandable, but if other regions do not contribute significantly to function, they would be expected to vary over such a long period of natural history. Perhaps sequences outside the seed were important after all? This would turn out to be the case. Sites outside the seed are important for microRNA function, not directly by binding to the mRNA but because of interactions with proteins along the way from biogenesis to the matching of seed to mRNA. That is, evolutionary pressure existed on other regions of the microRNA sequence, but for different reasons than selective pressure on the seed to remain the same. What also emerged through studies of microRNA evolution is that while the microRNA sequence may become fixed, the target pool remains flexible. The system remains adaptable such that the same microRNA can regulate new targets during animal evolution.[43]

The conservation of microRNA sequences is markedly different from what is seen for endogenous siRNAs. The principles behind this were already understood 20 years ago.

Because the endogenous siRNAs come from the same section of the genome they target, any mutations would tend to change both the target and the siRNA. A switch of a C to an A, for example, in both is tolerated. This lowers pressure on sequence conservation. Over time, as mutations accumulate, the sequences of both would diverge in an organism. This neatly accounts for why endogenous siRNAs are highly variable between species. In contrast, because microRNAs originate from genes that specify the targeting of very different and sometimes distant genes, selection pressure is very high to keep the microRNA sequence. That is, a mutation in the microRNA would be very unlikely to be accompanied by the same mutation in a target of the microRNA. Thus, evolutionary pressure will conserve the microRNA sequence. Another way for microRNAs to evolve is called arm switching. This is where the passenger strand (microRNA*) becomes the more dominant species taken up and used as the guide to target an mRNA. There are also examples of the two arms being used in different tissues. There are clear advantages to the existence of microRNA families, where microRNA seeds may differ by only a single nucleotide. In the event that a sequence change arises in the 3' UTR of one or more target mRNAs, an alternate member of the microRNA family will have that 'covered'. This may maintain targeting of key transcripts despite the appearance of new sequences.

Current models of how microRNAs evolve see them initially as low-expressed transcripts restricted to specific cell lineages.[43] The level and the range of cell types and tissues in which the microRNA is expressed increase over time, with a weeding-out of any deleterious targeting. Consistent with this, conserved microRNAs that are 'older' tend to be expressed at higher levels and in more tissues than newer-evolved microRNAs. MicroRNAs can continue to evolve, however, picking up changes in sequences, including within the seed. If a change bestows a survival advantage or is neutral, it will be passed on. It is not only microRNA sequences that have evolved. There is an ongoing molecular arms race between protein-coding genes and microRNAs, each of which sometimes vies for control over the other. The genes that underlie highly specialised cell types such as neurones display long 3' UTRs, endowing them with sensitivity to the actions of various microRNAs. In contrast, housekeeping genes, the levels of which are normally similar between cell types, display short 3' UTRs, thus taking them outside of microRNA control. The differing lengths of 3' UTRs are likely a result of microRNA target co-evolution. Studies of the genomes of cichlid fish, a common model for studying how different species emerge, found that target sites for microRNAs are among key elements in the genomes that drive speciation.[50, 51] That is, changes to the target sites of microRNAs, as well as the microRNAs themselves, help shape evolution and the emergence of new species.

Plant MicroRNAs

As we have seen, microRNA systems are present in all major branches of eukaryotic life. While this book focusses on their role in animals, the discoveries made about microRNAs in plants are worthy of a mention. Notably, post-transcriptional gene silencing by RNAs was known about a decade before the first microRNA was identified in plants. Studies in the late 1980s and early 1990s had shown that introducing RNAs into plants with sequence complementarity to endogenous genes resulted in silencing of gene expression. Shortly after Fire and colleagues' 1998 *Nature* paper on RNAi in *C. elegans*, studies followed in plants that demonstrated the existence of an RNAi system which appeared to function primarily to protect plants against viruses.[8]

As with their animal counterparts, the discovery of microRNAs encoded in the genomes of plants in the early 2000s triggered a wave of interest from the plant molecular biology community. There followed intensive searches for microRNA sequences in the genomes of model plants and other species, tracking down the biochemical pathway by which they were made, their rules of engagement with targets and their evolutionary origins. The same tools used to discover animal microRNAs such as gene alignment algorithms also helped plant scientists on their quest to understand microRNAs. The plant microRNA system shares similarities with that of animals, with the mature form of a microRNA being 21 to 24 nucleotides in length and processed from longer precursor RNAs that possess hairpin-like fold-back structures. After processing to the final length, they are brought into contact with targets as part of a silencing complex. Plant microRNAs, like animal microRNAs, recognise mRNA targets with imperfect sequence complementarity, and the effect of the microRNA attaching is down-regulation of the protein, via a mixture of target degradation and translational inhibition. However, much longer stretches of microRNA:target sequence matching are found in plants compared to animals. One other difference is the proportion of the expressed genes that are directly controlled by microRNAs. It appears that only a few per cent of protein-coding transcripts in plants are subject to microRNA control, compared to ~60 per cent in humans. So, why so few and what makes those few genes that are subject to microRNA control so special? In plants, the targets are predominantly transcription factors. This means that a little goes a long way. By controlling only a few transcription factors, plant microRNAs are still able to regulate a large swathe of the protein-coding landscape.

The range of functions regulated by plant microRNAs is extensive. The most heavily regulated processes are leaf and root development. Plant microRNAs also function in resistance to drought and salinity, respond to nutrient deprivation and seasonal temperature change, and defend against pests.[52] The experiments that underpin these findings include work comparing the microRNA profile of resistant vs susceptible species and the effects of introduced or deleted microRNAs on plant function. Not surprisingly, microRNAs have been a subject of interest because of the economics of horticulture – fruit and vegetable crops. The microRNA system is being looked at as a target for bioengineering.[53] The idea is to improve crop yield, selectively enhance features such as colour, taste, flavour and shape, and mitigate against the impacts of climate change.

The evolution of plant microRNAs is very well understood.[54–56] Going back in time, many microRNA families present in modern plants can be traced to an ancestral embryophyte, the land or terrestrial plants. These emerged half a billion years ago. A further set of microRNAs trace their ancestry to the first spermatophyte, the seed-bearing plants that include flowering plants and trees. The timing of this branching of the plant kingdom is during the mid-Devonian period or about 385 million years ago. Different branches of the plant kingdom show variation in the diversity of microRNA families, although there is some sampling bias. The highest number of microRNA families is found in *Arabidopsis*, the plant equivalent of *C. elegans*, but if similar efforts were applied to other species of plant, the winner by microRNA numbers might be different. Studies on plant microRNA evolution suggest that, similar to animals, there have been distinct periods of microRNA expansion that coincide with important physiological change and adaptation. However, a causal role in events such as the emergence of flowering plants is unproven. Also, there is counterintuitive evidence that the overall rate of microRNA evolution may be relatively constant. When two species separated by half a billion years of evolution were compared, they were found to have evolved almost identical numbers of unique microRNAs, 67 and 66 in the moss *Physcomitrella patens* vs *Arabidopsis thaliana*. This suggests that microRNA evolution in plants may be quite steady and a kind of molecular clock. More extensive sampling and deep sequencing across the plant kingdom are needed. As with the animal kingdom, once evolved, plant microRNA genes are rarely lost. The mechanisms by which new microRNAs evolve in plants are not fully understood. One proposed mechanism is by an inverted duplication of the target gene. Transcription of this produces hairpin RNAs with initially complementary sequences to the originating gene; however, genetic drift and accumulation of errors reduce the complementarity. Retention or loss of this new microRNA gene would then depend on whether there was an advantage and natural selection pressure to conserve.

One of the most exciting discoveries to emerge from studies of plant microRNAs is a role in cell-to-cell and even organism-to-organism exchange of information.[57, 58] That post-transcriptional silencing could spread from a point of introduction in an organism is not new per se. Studies in the late 1990s in *C. elegans* and plants found that introduced double-stranded RNA, used to trigger RNAi, could spread from the start or introduction point to have effects throughout an organism. Analysis of plant phloem, the vascular system that transports nutrients, revealed the presence of various microRNAs and shoot-to-root trafficking of microRNAs has been reported. It is well demonstrated for microRNAs involved in plant root development where the mature form of certain microRNAs is in cells remote from the source of their production. This helps create gradients of transcription factor activity that drive root tissue specialisation. The mechanism of this transfer is interesting and a cause of some controversy. A proposed packaging mechanism is within tiny vesicles called exosomes. The problem, as outlined earlier, is that the number of copies of a microRNA in some of the information packets is extremely low. Too low, some argue, to mediate biological effects on pathways in recipient cells. But transmission of small RNAs in plants may allow for more substantial cell-to-cell communication and amplification of the signal. Some of the biochemical details of the signal amplification process are understood, although the structures, cell-to-cell movement and transmission through the plant vascular system, as well as the distance over which such signals can pass, remain a matter of ongoing investigation. The trafficking of microRNAs around plants has been implicated in development and stress responses. However, inter-species trafficking of microRNA has been recently discovered. That is, one plant communicating with another via exchange of microRNAs. In one case, microRNAs expressed by a parasitic plant were found to suppress host genes in the attacked plant. There are also examples of inter-kingdom microRNA transfer. Plant microRNAs have been detected in fungal pathogens, where they are thought to represent a form of plant-based host defence. In plants, specific microRNAs switch on that target genes involved in fungal replication. We will return at the end of the book to these still-controversial ideas about microRNAs and long-distance signalling. Regardless, microRNAs serve roles in almost every aspect of plant development, survival and reproduction. They share most core aspects in common with animal microRNAs, while bearing the hallmarks of a uniquely evolved system that functions to serve in ways best suited to the challenges of plants.

MicroRNAs That Make Us 'Us'

Much of what makes us human has arisen from tinkering with pre-existing parts of the genome – placing pre-existing genes under new management – and from microRNA evolution. Evolving new microRNAs is a whole lot simpler, as well as faster and more efficient, than evolving completely new protein-coding genes. As we have seen already, humans have an abundance of microRNAs that are not present in lower mammals. Some of these are specific to the primate lineage and some are unique to *Homo sapiens*. Given what we know about the relationship between microRNA diversity and organism complexity, we can already predict that human-specific microRNAs probably underlie human-specific traits. Is there evidence for that? The brain is a good place to focus when addressing what human-specific microRNAs do, since that is an organ which displays considerable additional complexity over other mammals, including our primate cousins.[59] It is early days in running experiments that prove that a human-specific microRNA produces specific traits. And it is difficult to see how some experiments will ever be possible. A certain amount can be gleaned from comparing human brain samples, available following brain surgery or donated after death, to other primates, although the availability of non-human primate and great ape brain tissue for comparative analysis of microRNAs remains a barrier. Studying microRNAs in human brain cell models is possible and the recent ability to generate 3D human 'organoids' by culturing cells in certain ways may get us very close to having models that can directly test whether or not a specific microRNA controls a uniquely human feature. It is also possible to humanise other organisms, for example inserting a human-specific microRNA into, say, the mouse genome and tracking the effects on development and physiology.

If we take brain size as a rough measure of complexity, a simplification that will suffice here, analysis of hominin skull cases indicates that brain size doubled sometime between 2 million and 700,000 years ago. Further expansion occurred between 500,000 and 300,000 years ago to reach the size in modern humans (~1,350 cm^3). That is a threefold increase in the past 4 million years, prior to which there was little change in the previous 80 million years of primate evolution. Modern human brains show a massive increase in surface area, expansions in regions that provide fine motor control, planning and execution, and language. The density of wiring patterns indicates greater computational capacity, that is, more processing power. There is also a prominent increase in the diversity of brain cell types in humans over lower primates, and cell specification is a favourite marker of the actions of microRNAs. If we look under a microscope, we can see enhanced complexity at the level of individual brain cells. A key driver of the additional brain cell number comes from events in a part of the brain called the outer subventricular zone (OSVZ). This region of brain tissue is known to facilitate a much longer period of the birthing, or neurogenesis, of new cells in the human brain. This is where we find stem cells, which are primordial cells that are capable of repeatedly dividing; this, given the right combination of active transcription factors, directs the daughter cells to become one of the multiple different cell types in the brain. The OSVZ tissue is enriched in primate-specific microRNAs. Their targets include transcripts that encode the protein regulators of cell division. Levels of these transcripts differ in this part of the brain in humans compared to non-human primates during brain development. But it isn't cell numbers alone that distinguish the human brain. The diversity of brain cell types is greater in the human brain than in the brains of lower primates; we have a richer repertoire than any other mammals. This is thought to enable more-complex information to be encoded and interpreted as signals pass around the brain. This diversity comes from new combinations of transcription factors and patterns of gene expression and here again is where microRNAs have been busy, shaping new cell types by providing new patterns of control on networks of genes.

So, it appears likely that primate and human-specific microRNAs arose that helped drive this phenomenal expansion ability and cell type specialisations, contributing to the power of our brain. By some estimates, the brains of humans and other primates show differences in the expression of about 40 per cent of microRNAs in one or more brain region. More than 200 microRNAs show either higher or lower expression in the human brain compared to chimpanzee and macaque brains. Human-specific microRNA expansion is broadly divided into new (*de novo*) microRNAs and expansions of existing microRNA families. An example of a *de novo* human-specific microRNA is miR-941. This was discovered in a 2012 study that searched for microRNAs that were present in humans but not in a list of 10 other animal groups.[60] This led to the identification of 10 new microRNAs that are specific to humans. Most were expressed at extremely low levels, with one exception, miR-941. This was highly abundant in the human brain but absent from the brains of other primates. Introns are a melting pot for microRNA evolution and the new human microRNA was buried in the intron of a gene that encodes a protein chaperone. The function of the protein is to direct other proteins and protein-RNA complexes to the correct place in a cell. Maybe that sounds a bit 'so what?' unimportant, but mutations and loss of the functions of the host gene lead to a number of human diseases, including progressive loss of brain function. A remarkable seven copies of the gene for miR-941 were found in the human genome, all containing suitable hairpin precursor structures. The team were able to determine when the sequence evolved, finding it present in the genome of Denisovans, an extinct hominid lineage that diverged from our ancestors about half a million years ago. The number of copies of miR-941 also varied in modern humans, indicating possibly ongoing or active evolution. The study also identified some of the genes controlled by miR-941. This was achieved by adding the microRNA to a variety of human cell types and measuring changes to mRNAs. One of the pathways with the most genes altered by miR-941 controlled development, specifically the ability to generate new cells. This is consistent with miR-941 being one of the group of microRNAs driving the larger size or cell density in the human brain. The study also found that potential sites for miR-941 were also lost in humans. That is, sites in 3' UTRs for this microRNA were present in some non-human primates but missing in humans. This perhaps counter-intuitive finding is consistent with evolutionary theory, which states that when a microRNA first emerges it can have deleterious effects by targeting essential genes. These sites are then selected out, leaving behind those targets that confer beneficial regulatory effects. This is not the only example of a human-specific microRNA that is linked to helping us evolve bigger brains. A University of California team in 2018 reported that miR-2115, a great ape–specific microRNA, is enriched in germinal zones, that is, sites generating new cells, in the developing human brain.[61] The microRNA appears to sustain replication states of cells, allowing cell division to continue longer, and packing more cells into the human brain.

The human-specific microRNA landscape is more than just new microRNAs. A second important source of human-specific microRNAs is sequence and copy variation in con-served microRNAs. Comparing the genomes of humans and non-human primates reveals microRNAs that differ in sequence or copy number from other mammals. An example here is members of the miR-320 family.[62] In humans, this is a set of eight genes representing five different but closely related microRNAs. Humans express a complement of 1 × miR-320a, 2 × miR-320b, 2 × miR-320c, 2 × miR-320d and 1 × miR-320e. Each member differs by a single nucleotide. The first, miR-320a, is present in all primates, whereas various numbers of the other members are found in other apes and Old World monkeys, those native to Africa and Asia, which includes baboons. Notably, targets of this microRNA also include regulators of brain development. Altered levels of some of these microRNAs have been detected in brains from people with Alzheimer's disease and psychosis.

A third mechanism of human-specific microRNA evolution is to change the timing, the on/off, of conserved microRNAs. By changing the control switches, a microRNA can be active at a different moment, bringing it into contact with new targets and changing gene expression. This has been observed for miR-92, which is highly conserved in mammals but displays a unique pattern of on/off in humans compared to other primates. Thus, when and where a microRNA is used is a potent force for adaptation. A fourth mechanism of human-specific microRNA evolution occurs through changes in the target sites in human genes. That is, the gain and loss of microRNA target sites in 3' UTRs. This can cause genes to fall under new control or to break free of previous microRNA control. Related to this, changes to the microRNA sequence outside the seed may also adjust patterns of expression. A confirmed example of this is miR-299, which has a different pattern of expression in humans compared to other primates, although the seed sequence is the same.

While the complete picture continues to unfold, microRNA and target co-evolution appears to be a key driver of human evolution and the traits that make us unique. Innovations in the human genome, including the emergence of new microRNAs and changes to the sequences of shared microRNAs, their transcriptional control and their targeting sites, have significantly expanded the complexity of human cells, tissues and organs. The microRNAs unique to us hold a special place in the history of human evolution and are certain to continue to drive our species changes, whatever those might be, into the future.

Reflections

This chapter began with a key moment in the history of microRNA science: the moment when it became clear that microRNAs were not limited to worms but were fundamental to animal life. MicroRNAs emerged with the dawn of animals and probably all forms of complex life. They are a remarkable example of convergent evolution. For those branches of life that lack the microRNA system, similar solutions were achieved. They are an important biological answer to the inherent problem of the randomness of gene expression, conferring on cells the resilience they need in the face of hostile forces from outside and within. They enable higher organisms to continue to generate ever-increasing complexity and specialisation. They appear to have been instrumental in the biological processes that led to us – *Homo sapiens* – and some of our specialist adaptations.

Now that we know which organisms make microRNAs and why they need them, let us begin the next part of our journey into the microRNA world. How are microRNAs made? How do they do what they do? What experiments and discoveries led us to this understanding?

Chapter 3

Epic Journey
From Biogenesis to Extinction

Of the Golden Fleece in Argo the ship at a King's grim hest.
Of a surety ye be: my soul hath knowledge of everything.

From The Tale of the Argonauts by Apollonius of Rhodes, *translated by Arthur Sanders Way*
(J. M. Dent & Co., 1901, p. 55, ll. 211–12)

In the epic Greek poem *Argonautica* by Apollonius Rhodius, the hero – Jason, in search of the Golden Fleece – was helped on his journey by a crew of 49 sailors aboard the ship *Argo*. They were known as the Argonauts. Their quest set them among the very bravest and finest heroes in Greek mythology. Argonaute is the name of a family of proteins that are at the very heart of how microRNAs work. The mature and functional microRNA sits within a groove inside an Argonaute protein. Once in place, the Argonaute begins its own quest, trafficking along the lengths of mRNAs until it finds a site of suitable complementarity to the microRNA within its care. It then locks down and either the mRNA is degraded or translation of the mRNA into a protein is blocked. In many ways, Argonaute is the centrepiece of the whole microRNA show.

The name Argonaute was coined in a 1998 paper in the *EMBO (European Molecular Biology Organization) Journal* on the development of leaves of *Arabidopsis thaliana*, the plant used extensively to understand genetics in a way that is similar to the use of *C. elegans* to understand animals.[63] The team used a chemical called ethyl methanesulfonate to mutate the plant's DNA. Treated seeds were planted and then the plants that grew from them were examined for features of leaf malformation, the thinking being that the mutagen will inactivate genes, some of which will be crucial to how the leaf normally develops. Find the mutant leaf and then search the DNA for the damaged gene. Similar approaches underpinned the *C. elegans* discoveries of the first microRNAs. One of the plant mutants displayed an unusual leaf shape that the authors felt resembled a small squid (**Figure 3.1**). They named the mutant 'Argonaute'. Homologues of the gene exist in animals – elongation initiation factors such as *EIF2C2*. In humans we have four versions of the Argonaute genes – *AGO1–4*.

In this chapter we will encounter Argonautes and the other structural proteins and enzyme companions that accompany microRNAs on their epic journeys. We understand the biochemical pathway of microRNAs in significant depth, beginning deep within the nucleus where transcription of the RNA occurs, all the way to the end and the final destiny of the microRNA. It has been gleaned from more than 25 years of research – a journey much longer than that of Jason and his Argonauts. And it is no less full of [scientific] heroes, achieved by teams across the world, often working together, using combinations of methods spanning genetics, biochemistry, molecular biology, structural biology and

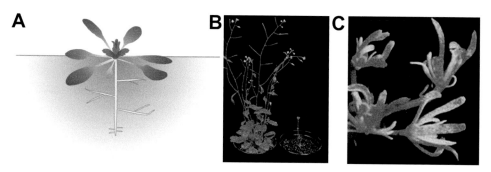

Figure 3.1 Coining of the Argonaute name

Panel A is a drawing of the normal *Arabidopsis thaliana* (note the leaf shape).

Panel B is a six-week-old wild-type plant and (right lower corner) the ago mutant.

Panel C is the inflorescence (complete flower head) of a six-week old 'ago' mutant.

Source: Panel A image from clipart.org. Panels B and C reprinted with permission from Bohmert et al., *EMBO Journal*, vol. 17, pp. 170–80 (1998).[63]

molecular imaging. By bringing these various research tools to bear, we have a deep understanding of the microRNA biogenesis process from start to finish. It is by the actions of proteins – enzymes and RBPs – that this occurs. Most of the core components are found in all animals. Indeed, many of the discoveries of the pathway were first made using lower model organisms, before later being teased apart in mammalian cells and tissues. Our story is thus built using knowledge from various animal species. We will zoom in on where this is important for understanding human differences in the pathway. Otherwise, the pathway will be described generally with references to the specific species in which the discovery was made only where important for context or history.

Unlike Jason's journey, we are not yet finished. We may never be fully satisfied that we know *everything* about the microRNA pathway. New and often unexpected findings regularly appear in journals. Some of the knowledge gaps will be pointed out along the way. As researchers dig ever deeper, they uncover more details, a more sophisticated understanding, particularly of how specific reactions are controlled and regulated and what directs specific actions to occur at a given moment. We are getting closer to full atomic-level detail of certain events, understanding which atoms of the microRNA interact with atoms within the proteins and RNA complexes in which they work. As technology becomes ever better, it has been used to explore the processes in ways not possible previously. Indeed, there is a kind of productive arms race with technologies being developed that allow new questions to be asked that drive further work in a reinforcing cycle that continues to deepen our knowledge and toolkit.

Figure 3.2 provides a simple overview of the basic steps involved in microRNA biogenesis as a primer for the chapter as a whole. It shows a multi-step process. The life of a microRNA begins with the reading of the DNA code and generation of an RNA molecule. This molecule, a long series of As, Cs, Gs and Us (not Ts), is then processed into smaller and smaller parts, in different compartments of the cell, until we finally have our mature microRNA. The microRNA is then ready to begin its job. The discovery of this elegant and highly conserved pathway will be covered in this chapter, and for key events we will go into some depth, including the initial transcription, key processing events and

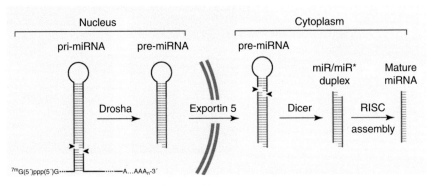

Figure 3.2 The basic steps in microRNA biogenesis

MicroRNAs are transcribed as long primary structures (pri-miRNAs; the letters on the base of the structure are the cap and poly-A tail). Drosha cleaves the flanks of pri-miRNAs to liberate ~70 nucleotide stem-loop structures called pre-miRNAs. These contain the ~22 nucleotide mature microRNA in either the 5' or the 3' half of their stem and the pair of cuts made by Drosha (Pasha in flies) establishes either the 5' or the 3' end of the mature microRNA. Pre-miRNAs are moved from the nucleus to the cytoplasm by Exportin 5. In the cytoplasm, Dicer makes the pair of cuts that defines the other end of the microRNA, generating a duplex. One strand is then taken up by an AGO protein to assemble the RNA-induced silencing complex (RISC), completing the basic process of microRNA biogenesis.

Source: Reprinted with permission from Tomari & Zamore, *Current Biology*, vol. 15, pp. 61–4 (2005).[64]

how, by working with Argonaute (AGO) proteins, the microRNA does its job. As before, we will review some of the actual experiments that were performed that led us to this understanding. The description of the pathway in this chapter is still a bit of a moving target, however. New discoveries are continuously being made, and some of the very latest will be covered in Chapter 9. Now, let's begin the voyage.

Genomic Location

As mentioned in Chapter 2, and accepting the final number is not yet agreed, the human genome contains about 2,000 microRNA genes. Some microRNAs exist in the genome as discrete genes. These are the *intergenic* microRNAs. These are separate, individual and independent microRNAs, transcription units existing within the genome separate from other microRNAs or the genes they regulate. They are autonomous, with on/off switches built in upstream that respond to signals. This is DNA that, when transcribed, generates a distinct, independent microRNA, albeit contained within a longer precursor molecule. An example of one of these is miR-7. But a sizeable number, about half of all microRNAs, come from within the gene sequences of protein-coding genes, specifically the introns that are part of the initially transcribed RNA. Where microRNAs are found in introns, the introns tend to be larger than normal and the microRNA sequences tend to lie more or less in the middle. However, the introns that harbour microRNA sequences tend not to be those that are important for alternative splicing, a process where different combinations of segments of a mRNA are chosen, producing proteins of different size and in some cases function. Because these microRNAs are derived from protein-coding genes, albeit the 'unwanted' parts, they are transcriptionally dependent on their hosts. They usually cannot independently switch on and off, so if the host gene gets transcribed then so do they.

While some microRNAs are singletons, other microRNAs are bundled together in a multi-pack called a poly- or a multi-cistronic unit. This is a series of microRNAs, one after the other, that come from the same original long RNA molecule but as the processing of the RNA occurs a series of individual microRNAs spill out. Some of the microRNAs from the same polycistronic unit share targets, enabling microRNAs from the same locus to exert synergistic effects on a pathway. In some cases, one of the microRNAs targets one set of mRNAs while another takes on a different set. We sometimes also see that microRNAs transcribed together have targets that are functional opposites. Where one microRNA blocks an activator pathway, the other blocks the inhibitor pathway. This produces balance and nuance, avoiding excessive suppressive effects on a given pathway or process and avoiding over-targeting of a cellular process.

Biogenesis

Transcription of most microRNAs involves the same process we covered in Chapter 1 that creates the mRNAs for protein-coding genes. An RNA polymerase is brought to a particular site in the genome where chromatin is open and where it can access the DNA code. The RNA polymerase multi-protein complex unzips and separates or 'melts' the DNA double-helix and, using the template strand, starts transcribing and building the RNA molecule. The polymerase subsequently gets free of the promoter and transcription factor complexes and then things ramp up faster. It goes into full production mode, synthesizing a long RNA molecule based on the read DNA code, the process of elongation. The growing RNA strand exits one end of the polymerase while the DNA template exits another and re-seals with the other DNA strand. Finally, specific sequences in the DNA cause this process to halt or terminate and the polymerase then drops off. The identification of the polymerase that generates most microRNA sequences came in 2004.[65] This was actually after the discovery of how precursor microRNAs were cut down to the right size. Transcription generates the precursor molecule called a primary or pri-microRNA. This RNA sequence can be more than 1,000 nucleotides (1 kilobase [kb]) in length. Thus, the mature microRNA can comprise as little as ~2 per cent of the original RNA sequence. A pri-microRNA contains a hairpin structure, a region of RNA nucleotides that has folded back on itself, one section base-pairing with a section of RNA from the same strand. This forms a distinctive loop of ~33–35 nucleotides. The mature microRNA lies within this structure, on either the 3' or the 5' side of the stem.

The enzyme responsible for transcribing most mammalian microRNAs is called RNA polymerase II (RNAP II or Pol II for short – the naming convention dates to classic experiments in the 1960s; Pol II was the middle of three enzymes discovered with RNA synthesis activity). Pol II is a huge enzyme made by combining a dozen smaller protein subunits, each encoded by specific genes. Its best-studied role is as the transcriber of protein-coding genes (i.e. mRNAs). Pol I transcribes the RNA that forms the parts of the ribosome, and Pol III transcribes other small non-coding RNAs. Pol III was initially the prime suspect as the microRNA-transcribing enzyme because it was known to transcribe small RNAs. But a few things didn't add up. Pol III cannot make very long RNA molecules and dislikes rows of consecutive Us; both are features found in many pri-microRNA transcripts. Also, many microRNAs display stark developmental regulation, appearing and disappearing at very specific moments in organism development. This was a feature of many Pol II transcripts but not the ones made by Pol III. And one other detail about microRNA sequences and chemical features didn't make sense if Pol III was generating them. Many pri-microRNA transcripts contained a cap structure at their 5' end; this is a feature of all mRNAs that are generated by Pol II but not Pol III activity. The cap serves a couple of purposes, including protecting the RNA from being digested and directing it to be sent out of the nucleus.

The race to identify the main transcriber of microRNAs was won by Narry Kim's team based at the Seoul National University in Korea (they win another key race – see later). After noting the presence of the cap, a telltale sign of Pol II activity, they looked at the other end of the pri-microRNA and found that most had a poly-A tail. This also had the hallmarks of Pol II's work because mRNAs are all poly-A tailed. They then measured what happened to pri-microRNAs when they treated cells with a chemical known to selectively block Pol II. When used at low doses, α-amanitin, a chemical from *Amanita phalloides* or 'death cap' mushroom, is relatively selective to block Pol II (α-amanitin can also be derived from the even more poisonous-sounding 'destroying angel' mushroom). Treating cells with α-amanitin caused pri-microRNA levels to drop, whereas levels of RNAs known to be produced by Pol I and Pol III remained unchanged. This was evidence that Pol II was the enzyme making microRNAs and was further cemented by experiments that physically demonstrated that Pol II was bound to microRNA promoter sites on DNA.

'On' Signals for MicroRNA Transcription

While some genes are transcribed at steady rates, many switch on for specific periods of time. Some genes are expressed in all tissues, while others are expressed only in certain places, such as the brain, or in specific cells within a tissue or organ, such as a neurone. We even have genes that are only expressed within subtypes of cells. For example, the gene encoding the neuroactive peptide substance P, which acts to limit excessive brain activity, is made in a subset of neurones. The control of microRNA transcription is handled by transcription factors that bind upstream to specific sequences in the DNA. In the case of those microRNA genes embedded within introns of protein-coding genes, the transcription factors are those which drive the host gene. Stand-alone microRNAs have their own regulatory elements that link to the pathways they act within. Through intrinsic and extrinsic signals, the transcription factors determine which microRNA is made and when.

The first study to link a specific transcription factor to the control of microRNAs in humans appeared in *Nature* in 2005, by Joshua Mendell's team at Johns Hopkins University in the USA.[66] The transcription factor was a protein called c-Myc. Named owing to a similarity to a virus that caused cancer in birds, c-Myc can control more than 1 in 10 human genes. The transcription factor lies downstream of the signalling pathways that tell cells to replicate. Once made, c-Myc produces biological effects by activating the genes needed for cell growth and division. It is a very well-studied transcription factor with the functions of its domains understood and its preference for particular DNA sequences known, including CACGTG, known as an E box sequence. But c-Myc also has a darker side. If its expression becomes persistent, locked in an 'on' state, it can drive excess growth and cell division leading to certain cancers. Mendell's study showed that when c-Myc is activated, it binds to the DNA promoter sites of three major microRNA clusters, resulting in a large set of microRNAs being transcribed. This included the miR-17~92 cluster, a set of six microRNAs, where they found that a c-Myc binding sequence lay 1,480 nucleotides upstream.

Another big advance came in a series of papers published in 2007 that revealed that protein p53 was a microRNA transcription factor.[67-69] At the time, p53 was known to be critical for responding to cancer-forming signals, triggering cells to die in the event of, say, DNA damage. A year earlier, a study had mapped more than 500 sites in the human genome where p53 can bind and regulate transcription (i.e. p53 target genes). The identification of the DNA sequences that p53 was attracted to also enabled the team to predict additional targets of p53. Returning to the 2007 studies, researchers found that a set of microRNAs called miR-34s were directly controlled by p53. When cells were exposed to agents that caused DNA damage, a known trigger for p53 to begin its work, there was an increase in levels of the microRNAs. Their functions included shutting off survival genes, thus enabling cell death – a desired outcome to avoid risk of an out-of-control dividing cell. As a brief aside, the same year saw a key advance, published in the journal *Cell*, that would herald a new era in how researchers would discover and measure microRNAs: *small RNA sequencing*.[70] Many of the techniques used up to this point either were laborious and required very specialised molecular biology skills, or involved chips coated with pre-designed detectors for each microRNA based on their known sequences. While this could tell you how much of a microRNA you had in your sample, it couldn't discover new ones. But RNA sequencing was easier than many of the earlier methods and didn't require a priori knowledge of what microRNAs were present in a sample. It just told you what was there and how much of it. The new method began with extracting and purifying RNA from a sample. Individual RNA strands were then 'bookended' by synthetic nucleotide sequences called adaptors, one added (ligated) to the 5' end and one to the 3' end of every strand. These were then reverse transcribed to generate complementary DNA sequences that can be read on a sequencer. Billions of RNA molecules could now be measured and identified in a few days. The era of sequencing of small RNAs would propel forward the discovery of new microRNAs. The *Cell* paper surveyed which microRNAs were made in which tissues in mice and humans. There was now an atlas of microRNA expression in a variety of tissues. If you wanted to know where your microRNA was made and how abundant it was, you could now look it up.

Returning to the transcription factors that promote microRNA expression, one further example is Mef2, which controls expression of the miR-379~410 cluster of around 50 different microRNAs. These are uniquely expressed in the brain and control various aspects of how neurones develop and function. The Mef2 transcription factor responds to elevations in brain activity, meaning that the transcription of microRNAs links to the behaviour of neurones. One of the microRNAs in this cluster, miR-134, will feature heavily in later chapters. A team led by Gerhard Schratt, at the time based at the University of Heidelberg in Germany, searched upstream of the cluster, whose genomic location was already known, for possible sequences where transcription factors might bind.[71] Ten favourable sites were found for just one transcription factor, myocyte enhancer factor 2, or Mef2, named originally for its role in controlling genes that produce muscle. The transcription factor contains two domains that it uses to bind to promoter regions of genes. The team proved that Mef2 was attached to the promoter region of the miR-379~410 cluster and showed that when Mef2 was blocked, the microRNA levels no longer changed in response to neuronal activity.

'Off' signals are also important. The function of many microRNAs is to shape protein levels at distinct moments in a cell's life. Stopping production at the right time is critical for properly timed control of gene expression. We are learning more about the signals that keep microRNAs from being transcribed. One of the signals that switch microRNAs off is methylation of DNA. This is a widely used *epigenetic* mark, the addition of CH_3, usually onto a C base in the DNA that encodes the gene. This does not change the DNA code but causes a shift to a closed state, preventing whatever carries the mark from being transcribed by restricting access to transcription and enhancer elements in the DNA. A number of microRNAs can be switched off by such epigenetic marks. My own group found that the amount of miR-27a present in brain tissue was strongly linked to whether or not the DNA was methylated. We were able to map this to a site within the pre-microRNA sequence and show that a gradient existed with higher amounts of miR-27a present in brain samples with low methylation and vice versa.[72] We found another 12 microRNAs where the amount of methylation was inversely correlated with expression of the microRNA. Other mechanisms of transcriptional repression of microRNAs have been identified. These include proteins that dock onto the promoter sites of the microRNAs and either physically block transcription or call in the machinery to methylate the gene.

A Role for Pol III?

The evidence that Pol II transcribes most microRNAs became further settled in subsequent years. But Pol III was not done yet. It came back into focus in 2006 as a study from a team at the University of Iowa, reported in *Nature Structural and Molecular Biology*, argued that it could transcribe some microRNAs.[73] The researchers looked at a subset of microRNAs that were close to repetitive elements in the genome. This includes something called an Alu element. Repetitive elements are sequences of DNA that got embedded in the genomes of our ancestors more than 100 million years ago and that we, modern humans, continue to deal with. Each stretch is around 300 base pairs long so they do not code for proteins, and there are more than a million of these in our genome. They cannot be deleted, but many are silenced by specific enzymes that search for these and coat the segments with a methyl tag that prevents their transcription. Some do influence expression of nearby genes, however, and many Alu elements contain promoter sequences that attract Pol III to transcribe them. The Iowa team looked at a cluster of 46 microRNA genes called C19MC. This is particularly interesting because it is found only in the primate lineage. They found that these microRNA genes lay within genomic regions that are rich in repetitive elements. Moreover, they found Pol III docked at Alu sites upstream of the sequences that encoded the microRNAs. In the years since, however, the uniqueness of Pol III to transcribe these microRNAs was challenged. Experiments showed that the microRNAs in the C19MC cluster could also be transcribed by Pol II. This included showing that Pol II could dock onto the genomic site and that transcription of the microRNAs was sensitive to a low dose of α-amanitin. Thus, Pol II continues to be regarded as the principal means by which microRNAs are expressed, which leaves open the possibility that Pol III might transcribe some microRNAs under certain conditions.

The First Cut Is the Deepest

With transcription over, the precursor RNA or pri-microRNA begins the next stage of its journey to becoming a mature microRNA. Next up, it gets significantly shortened. This happens by the actions of enzymes called ribonucleases. These are enzymes that digest or cut long RNAs into smaller pieces. This is standard practice during the normal pathway from DNA to protein for traditional genes. The RNA is transcribed from the DNA template, but it contains introns that must be cut out. The remaining parts, exons, then get spliced together. There are several ribonucleases in the human genome, organised into subfamilies that share preferences for features of RNA to work on. The ribonucleases that process the precursor forms of microRNAs are RNase IIIs and are examples of *endoribonuclease*. This means that they cut the RNA within the main or central part of the molecule, rather than starting at one end or the other. The RNase IIIs work on RNA molecules that contain double-stranded RNA, which includes the precursors of microRNA on account of their hairpin structure. That is, they contain RNA that is folded back on itself, creating a segment that is double-stranded. The first RNase III to be identified was found in *E. coli*, the model organism for bacteria, in the late 1960s. There are several other members of the endoribonuclease family, each with different roles. For example, RNase A is made in the pancreas and works to digest RNA in the gut.

While still in the nucleus of the cell, the pri-microRNA sequence is cut substantially. Indeed, as much as 90 per cent of the original length is lost, with the trimming leaving behind an RNA molecule of typically ~70 nucleotides in length. The resulting RNA molecule still contains the hairpin loop wherein the microRNA lies. The enzyme that cuts the pri-microRNA is called Drosha. The name was coined in 2000;[74] the gene was identified in studies on the model fly *D. melanogaster*. Drosha is a member of the class II type of RNase IIIs and contains two catalytic sites for cutting RNA in a special domain of the protein (the class I versions contain only one of these). The proof that it was the enzyme that processed pri-microRNA was made by Kim's team at the Seoul National University in Korea, in a landmark paper in *Nature* in 2003.[25] This was the same team that a year later would demonstrate that Pol II was responsible for transcribing most microRNAs. Interestingly, the enzyme that processed the later step, cleaving the pre-microRNA to form the final mature microRNA, had already been discovered, details of which are coming up shortly. The Korean team had suspicions that Drosha might act on pri-microRNAs because pre-microRNAs contained a distinctive di (or '2') nucleotide overhang characteristic of the actions of the RNase III family. It was known that enzymes like Drosha, when they cut RNA, left behind this telltale biochemical mark. As we will see, this then serves as a mark for the next enzyme to get to work. The researchers also used knowledge of the whereabouts of different RNase III enzymes to argue the case for Drosha. While the pre-microRNA was found in the cytoplasm of cells, the longer pri- sequence was found only in the nucleus. The enzyme that performed the first stage of processing microRNAs had to be a nuclear-localised RNase III. One of the potential candidates, an enzyme called Dicer, was therefore ruled out because it was known to be in the cytoplasm. Armed with these insights, they began their search for the enzyme that processes pri-microRNA. They began by extracting the intact Drosha enzyme from a commonly used lab cell line. This can be done using an antibody to stick onto the protein, weighing it down, after which you can purify the antibody-bound protein and finally wash off the antibody, leaving behind your ready-to-use protein. They mixed the Drosha with primary microRNA sequences and then measured the lengths of the resulting RNA fragments. The reaction produced RNA molecules of the exact size of pre-microRNAs, 60–70 nucleotides. To complement this finding, they reduced levels of Drosha in cells and noted that this resulted in the accumulation of pri-microRNAs. A major step in the process was now known. Drosha performed the cut to the pri-microRNA. The discovery drove detailed follow-on work that has led to a deep understanding of the cutting process at atomic-scale resolution. Different parts of the Drosha protein have been studied to drill down on exactly how it works.[75] We know which atoms within the catalytic site do what and how other parts of the protein help hold and fold the RNA molecule. The site where the cleavage occurs is mapped to an action on both strands of the stem, at a site near the base of the primary loop. One RNase III-capable region cuts the 3' strand of the pri-microRNA leaving a dinucleotide overhang, while a second domain capable of cutting RNA then strikes at the 5' strand. The key machinery for binding to nucleotides and cutting RNA lies at one end, the C-terminal of Drosha, while the other end (N-terminal) is required for Drosha to stay localised inside the nucleus.

Fine-Tuning the Fine-Tuners

It didn't take long before more complexity was to emerge. Researchers knew there had to be more to the story because recombinant Drosha, the pure enzyme and nothing else, had RNA-cutting activity but lacked much specificity. The Drosha cut is critical because it defines the end of what will become part of the real microRNA. Alone, Drosha didn't produce the highly specific ends characteristic of pre-microRNAs. The answer came a year later in *Nature*.[76] Researchers revealed that a second protein, not an enzyme that cuts RNA but a co-factor, conferred the missing specificity. That protein, specialised in binding to double-stranded RNA, was called DGCR8. Working in partnership with Drosha, this created the *microprocessor*. The name DGCR8 comes from a syndrome first described by an American doctor called Angelo DiGeorge. Patients with the disease had heart problems, distinct facial features and neurodevelopmental problems. The cause was traced to deletions or mutations in chromosome 22. Several genes were missing from this region in the patients, so were named as a series 'DiGeorge Syndrome Critical Region . . .' plus a number. The protein encoded by *DGCR8* was linked to microRNA processing by experiments that started by looking for partners for Drosha. They extracted Drosha from human cells and then separately identified the proteins stuck to it using mass spectrometry. As we covered earlier, proteins are chopped into tiny pieces and their masses measured and then, using knowledge of the weights of different amino acids, you can reconstruct whatever was the original protein. They were able to identify several proteins with known ability to bind to RNA. When they looked for the simplest combination of Drosha with a single partner, they found that it was DGCR8. The two proteins together had the full pri-microRNA processing activity. When DGCR8 was removed from cells, the production of mature microRNAs ceased in a way similar to losing Drosha. That is, the two together were *necessary* and *sufficient*. The approximately 20 other proteins that could stick to Drosha in cells were found not to be critical for the main activity, meaning that they must serve other functions or were non-specific interactions. This work was performed using human cells, but it was quickly confirmed that this tandem protein complex was the very same in other animals. The fly *D. Melanogaster* and the worm *C. elegans* use an identical system. This provided strong evidence of highly conserved and ancient evolutionary origins for this first step in microRNA maturation.

In the years since, details of how the microprocessor works, how it recognises the right RNA to cut, what different parts of the internal structure do, how it cuts, and the surface topology and molecular features whereby Drosha and DGCR8 interact have all been resolved to a large extent (see **Figure 3.3**). The activity and the specificity of the microprocessor are critical because most mature microRNAs come through this pathway. Any drop in its efficiency would impair overall microRNA levels in cells and, in turn, lose a critical layer controlling gene expression. Details of how the system works at atomic resolution regularly emerge. This includes mapping key amino acids in the protein and

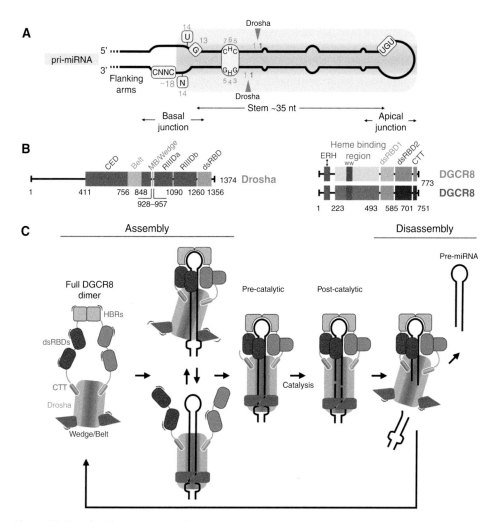

Figure 3.3 How the microprocessor works

Panel A shows a pri-microRNA and nucleotide sequences which are important for recognition by Drosha. The sites where Drosha cuts are indicated with arrows. The relative nucleotide position from Drosha cleavage sites is indicated with numbers.

Panel B shows the basic domain organisation of Drosha and DGCR8. Numbers indicate positions of amino acids.

Key: CTT, C terminal tail; CED, conserved central domain; dsRBD, double-stranded RNA binding domain; dsRNA, double-stranded RNA; HBR, haem-binding region; RIIID, RNase III domain.

Panel C shows the proposed model based on cryo-electron microscopy for how Drosha and DGCR8 assemble and disassemble during cutting for a single pri-microRNA (the hairpin structure is shown in black). The HBRs and the dsRBDs of the DGCR8 and Drosha Belt/Wedge areas are flexible when RNA is not bound. Further, DGCR8 recognises specific features in the pri-microRNA structure. The pri-microRNA affects whether it is DGCR8 or Drosha that drives the assembly of the microprocessor. After cropping, Drosha is most likely to dissemble first.

Source: Reprinted with permission from Ruiz-Arroyo & Nam, *Current Opinion in Structural Biology*, vol. 76, 102442 (2022).[75]

nucleotide motifs, short sequences of two or three bases, that the microprocessor uses to recognise the pri-microRNA. In technical terms, DGCR8's role is to recognise the junction between the single-stranded part of the pri-microRNA and the double-stranded region, along with holding the stem region. It is thought that the structure that the pri-microRNA has is also important for the recognition process. There is much diversity among pri-microRNAs; not all contain the same recognition elements and the minimal requirements continue to be explored. A big jump forward came when parts of the microprocessor were crystallised, enabling full structure–function studies to be performed. By crystallising a molecule and then firing X-rays and analysing the patterns of these, crystallography can produce views in three dimensions, often with the protein of interest in contact with its substrates such as other proteins or nucleic acids. Appearing in 2016 in the journal *Cell*, the crystal structures uncovered more details of structure–function relationships for human Drosha.[77] Ever more advanced techniques of imaging the microprocessor in action have clarified further points.[78] They reveal, for example, that the process of contacting a pri-microRNA molecule physically changes the shape of Drosha. It wraps around the RNA, in a sort of four-finger grasp. Further parts of Drosha called 'Belt' and 'Wedge' are required for arranging the RNA correctly. Then, DGCR8's role includes physically shifting parts of the Drosha enzyme. Another discovery was that DGCR8 actually works as a dimer, as two molecules together. One part, called a haem binding domain, forms a seat for the loop of the stem to lie against. Then, RNA binding domains on DGCR8 wrap around the next segment, holding it in place. The contact with Drosha ultimately brings the two cut sites into alignment with the jaws and the RNA strands are cut.

Before we leave the microprocessor and move on, a few final points of note. As befits the epic *Argo* journey that began this chapter, Drosha does not float aimlessly in the nucleus sea, awaiting a pri-microRNA to randomly pass by before landing its catch. In 2008, teams at the Universities of Oxford and Rome revealed that Drosha in fact sits adjacent to sites of transcription, right at the heart of the action where recently generated pri-microRNAs can be immediately worked on.[79] Drosha attaches to the sites of chromatin bearing microRNAs, getting recruited to where chromatin is in an open state, with active transcription of pri-microRNAs by Pol II. This occurs for both intergenic stand-alone microRNA genes, and intronic microRNAs. Efforts to time this event indicated that recruitment followed shortly after the beginning of transcription. This co-location at sites of transcription also benefited from the presence of DGCR8, the loss of which reduced the amount of Drosha at these sites. In the case of intronic microRNAs, Drosha begins its cutting even before the intron that contains the microRNA precursor has been cut from the protein-coding transcript. How impatient of Drosha!

The functions of other proteins that bind to Drosha and DGCR8 are not fully understood, but progress is being made.[80, 81] Some of the interactions are important for stability and localisation of the complex, making sure it is in the correct orientation and in the right place inside the cell. The surface of the microprocessor can be chemically modified by the actions of other enzymes. For example, the addition of a phosphate molecule (PO_4) helps keep it localised to the nucleus. Other chemical modifications are being found with regularity. Roles beyond microRNA processing have also emerged for Drosha. Drosha also cuts mRNAs, including the mRNA for its partner DGRC8. This is thought to destabilise the mRNA and may serve a feedback function to maintain microprocessor activity within the correct range. This is not the only mRNA that can be targeted by Drosha. Several other mRNAs that code for proteins during development are also substrates. Drosha seems to select these through similar rules because hairpin loop-like structures are a common feature, albeit not ones that can generate functional microRNAs.

Relocation to Cytoplasm

We now have a pre-microRNA (not to be confused with pri-microRNA). It is not ready to target mRNAs, however, still being a longer precursor, and it must change its location. The site of most microRNA-mediated actions is out in the cytoplasm where the mRNA is to be translated by ribosomes. This is where the pre-microRNA gets sent when it leaves the nucleus for the final stage of cutting that will yield the mature and final microRNA. Like most trafficking between the cytoplasm and the nucleus, this process is heavily regulated. The nucleus has its own membrane, which acts as a barrier to the movement of any large molecules. A passageway is needed, a pore or gap through which the pre-microRNA can pass. This is called the nuclear pore complex. Two families of proteins are the gatekeepers of this trans-membrane trafficking. One allows movement of molecules into the nucleus while the other facilitates movement out of the nucleus. The former are aptly called Importins, the latter being Exportins. One of these, Exportin-5, handles the movement of pre-microRNAs from the nucleus out to the cytoplasm.[26, 82] The protein looks for specific features in the RNAs it carries, recognising double-stranded RNA of a certain length and the two nucleotide overhang at the 3' end of the RNA, the feature left by the cuts of Drosha. This takes effort and requires energy to drive it. Exportin gets the driving force it needs from a Ran protein, also located within the nucleus. Ran carries a molecule of guanine triphosphate (GTP). This is a chemical cousin of the more common energy currency ATP and used to drive the process. So, together with Ran-GTP, Exportin-5 carries the pre-microRNA out of the nucleus and into the cytoplasm all ready for the final stage in the maturation of the microRNA. Once it has passed through the pore, the GTP is broken down and the grip on the pre-microRNA is released.

Dicer and the Final Cut

The pre-microRNA, now in the cytoplasm, still contains the loop structure that was part of the original pri-microRNA. Before it can function, a final cut is needed. This is achieved by the actions of another RNase III enzyme, Dicer. A molecule of Dicer is a little larger than Drosha. In three dimensions, it has a slight 'L' or hatchet shape. The features that allow it to do what it does are highly conserved. If you lined up the fly, the worm and the human Dicer, you couldn't really tell them apart. The papers that identified Dicer as the enzyme responsible for the final step in generating the mature microRNA appeared in 2001. At the time, the teams that would make the discovery were based at Cold Spring Harbor, where James Watson of DNA fame was then president, as well as the Universities of Massachusetts, Harvard and Utah in the USA and the Max-Planck Institute in Göttingen, Germany. All were trying to tease out the mechanisms of RNAi, the pathway discovered in 1998. In 2000, the team led by Gregory Hannon at the Cold Spring Harbor laboratory had isolated an enzyme that carried out the cutting of the mRNA in the RNAi pathway.[83] That enzyme was Argonaute 2 or AGO2. The discovery of Dicer would reveal that the main events in RNAi occurred via two distinct and separate actions. One enzyme produced the short RNAs and then AGO2 used the short RNA as the guide to line up and cut or slice the target mRNA, resulting in gene silencing. Published in *Nature* in the January of 2001, Hannon's team identified Dicer.[84] When fed double-stranded RNAs, the enzyme generated the telltale 22-nucleotide RNA fragments that were the hallmark of the RNAi pathway for gene silencing in *Drosophila*. Although Hannon's team coined the name 'Dicer', the enzyme was already known (as 'CG4792'), and it was known to have a preference for acting on double-stranded RNA. The team were able to demonstrate that Dicer had the exact biochemical features to explain production of these short RNAs and they showed that removing Dicer from *Drosophila* prevented RNAi. They were also able to show that Dicer required ATP for the reaction. This was not the case for Drosha, which helped distinguish otherwise similar properties of the two enzymes in some experiments. But they did not specifically link Dicer to the final step in the maturation of microRNAs. That came later that year, with a paper from Craig Mello, a later Nobel prize winner, in *Cell* and two more papers in *Science* from other teams, each paper coming a month apart. Although they all came to the same conclusion, namely that Dicer was generating mature microRNAs, each came about this through slightly different approaches. For example, Mello's team knocked out Dicer in *C. elegans* and showed that this impaired production of mature *let-7*, the microRNA we met in Chapter 2, and caused build-up of the ~70 nucleotide precursor forms of microRNAs in the animals.[16] Phillip Zamore's team, also working on *C. elegans* and based at the University of Massachusetts, performed similar experiments in human cells and came to the same conclusions.[85] They showed that reducing the amount of Dicer in HeLa cells led to accumulation of the longer, precursor form of *let-7*, while the mature form could no longer be detected. Thus, Dicer was also required for microRNA maturation in human cells. This study also clarified that two different outcomes were possible through the same enzymes. When the short RNA generated by Dicer was fully complementary to a target mRNA, you got degradation, the slicing action of RNAi. When it was only partially complementary, as with *let-7*'s target, you saw only a reduction in translation of the mRNA into protein, the feature of microRNA.

The last of the three key papers, from a team at Utah, produced genetic evidence that Dicer was required for microRNA maturation.[86] This was important and something the authors of the earlier work had called for to be definitive. The way the other teams had proven that Dicer was involved in microRNA maturation was by reducing its levels using the tricks of RNAi. They designed double-stranded RNAs that would be complementary to the *Dicer* mRNA and fed them to cells, resulting in lower Dicer levels. They then monitored for changes to precursor and mature forms of the *let-7* microRNA. The Utah team's work used a genetic mutant of *C. elegans* to prove that Dicer generated the final mature microRNA. Their ability to do this was a result of a research community effect that had developed over the years. At the time, a group of laboratories that all worked on *C. elegans* were sharing worm mutants, animals with natural or artificially mutated segments of DNA. The consortium had a mutant that lacked a 2,470-nucleotide section of DNA in the *dcr-1* gene that encoded the *C. elegans* version of Dicer. The team could now learn about Dicer in an animal carrying a genetic mutation. The animals lacked the ability to perform RNAi. Injecting the mutant worms with a double-stranded RNA targeting certain genes produced no knock-down of the intended protein. The team did not look for impairments in *let-7* processing. They did, however, observe that the worms lacking *dcr-1* had a feature strikingly similar to worms with a mutation in *let-7*. They guessed, correctly it turned out, that DCR-1 could also generate other small RNAs.

Work to understand how Dicer does its job has been going on ever since it was first found to be the enzyme that performed the final cut to generate the mature microRNA.[80, 81, 87] This has involved many of the techniques we have seen for other components, including mutating or removing key parts of the enzyme and creating crystals with and without its pre-microRNA cargo. At one end of Dicer, the C-terminal, we have the 'bite' of the enzyme, the RNA-cutting core. There are two parts to this, which work together a bit like jaws. This part of Dicer shares some similarities with the region of Drosha that does its cutting. At the other end, we have a domain known as the helicase, specialised to recognise the loop feature of the pre-microRNA. The two ends of the pre-microRNA bind to a region of Dicer called PAZ – named after domains found in three other proteins: Piwi, Argonaute and Zwille – which has a pocket for each. This is possible for the PAZ domain only because of the overhang at the 3' end. It seems that the gap between the PAZ domain and the cutting function of the two RNase domains works as a molecular ruler. The 5' end of the pre-microRNA binds to Dicer in a way that places the cut point 21–25 nucleotides from the end of the pre-microRNA; hence, most microRNAs are of ~22 nucleotides in length. A major early advance in our atomic-level understanding of how Dicer worked came from the University of California at Berkeley. This was not human Dicer but Dicer from a species of parasitic worm. Owing to the high sequence conservation, the findings were likely to extrapolate to mammalian and human forms. Ian MacRae was the first author, reporting the crystal structure of the main part of the Dicer enzyme in *Science*.[88] The 2006 paper featured a last author called Jennifer Doudna who would later win a Nobel prize for discoveries on CRISPR (short for 'clustered regularly interspaced short palindromic repeats'), an enzyme system from bacteria that provides virtually limitless possibilities to edit the genome. The PAZ region, which is where the 3' overhang of the pre-microRNA sits, formed the 'handle' of the hatchet-shaped structure with the RNase III cutting domains where the blade would be. An α helix, the twisted protein structure, connects the two. The two RNase III domains are further connected around the back by another helical structure. They could then measure the distance between the end of the pre-microRNA and the cutting point. This was 65 angstroms (an angstrom is a 10 billionth of a metre), the length of about 25 base pairs or a typical mature microRNA. Analysis of the structure also revealed how it cuts. The enzyme uses two metal ions for the catalytic reaction that cleaves the bonds of the RNA (see **Figure 3.4**).

A Partner for Dicer Is Found

Like Drosha, Dicer has an important co-factor, an RNA binding protein called TRBP (TAR-RNA binding protein). That discovery was made in 2005 by a team at the Wistar Institute in Philadelphia.[89] The group tagged Dicer in HEK293 cells, another popular human cell line, and then used it to trawl for anything else stuck to it. What they found was a protein they identified as TRBP. Further experiments using proteins purified in the lab confirmed that the two proteins could bind together. But their experiments showed that mixing in some TRBP made no difference to the efficiency of Dicer in processing pre-microRNAs. If TRBP was not required for pre-microRNA processing, what was it doing? The team went on to discover that TRBP acts as a bridge to AGO proteins. It forms a type of scaffold, a trimer, that brings together Dicer and AGO, which do not directly interact. As a result, the generated mature microRNA can pass directly into the arms of the protein it needs for mRNA targeting. Since then, TRBP has been found to have additional functions in the microRNA pathway. Dicer processes different pre-microRNAs at different rates owing to variations in the 'stickiness' of the RNA-protein interaction. One of the properties of TRBP is to enhance some of the processing rates, changing the dicing kinetics. Pre-microRNAs get turned into mature microRNAs more quickly when TRBP is stuck to Dicer. This is because TRBP actually alters both the binding of pre-microRNA to Dicer and the release of the processed microRNA after dicing. Interestingly, TRBP doesn't always speed things up; in fact it slows down the processing of some pre-microRNAs, those that contain certain features around the stem. This means that TRBP's actions depend on the structure of the double-stranded RNA being processed at the time. Another important function of TRBP is a role in producing *isomirs*. These are variants of a microRNA that differ from the encoded sequence. Often, they have one additional nucleotide, but they can have more. This can be important because if the additional nucleotide is on the 5' end of the microRNA, it changes the seed sequence; if that changes, the target pool will also change. Experiments have shown that TRBP can alter the position of the loaded pre-microRNA in Dicer, making it more likely to generate an isomiR. Altogether, TRBP is important not only in bringing together the machinery for microRNA function but also in adjusting the chemistry of the microRNA and its effects in the cell.

The activity of Dicer is also regulated in other ways. One mechanism is by a microRNA-regulated feedback loop. The mRNA that encodes Dicer contains binding sites for microRNAs. This is thought to ensure stable and appropriate levels of Dicer in cells. The Dicer protein is also littered with sites where post-translational modifications can be made: amino acids can be acted upon by enzymes that deposit chemical marks such as phosphates. These can drive up or down the enzyme's activity, adjust how it binds to its RNA substrates or even act as a signal for it to be degraded. **Figure 3.4** provides an overview of the basic organisation of the enzyme and how it works with TRBP to cut pre-microRNAs.

The end-product of the actions of Dicer is a duplex: two RNA molecules of approximately 22 nucleotides in length without the loop domain connecting them. For most microRNAs, one of these strands is always the one that becomes the functioning microRNA, with the other cast aside and dismantled. Sometimes it is the 5' end of the original pre-microRNA structure (indicated by the ending -5p) and sometimes the 3' end (-3p). The selection process is based on thermodynamic stability. The protein into which the mature microRNA gets loaded is AGO. Before we get to that step, and the essence of how the microRNA aligns with and targets mRNA, a final point of note. Why the separate cutting tools, Drosha then Dicer? Why not simply have Dicer? The step-wise processing with Drosha followed by Dicer is thought to benefit cells by enhancing the efficiency and the accuracy of processing. It also allows compartmentalisation of the whole process, which might have benefits for robustness and fine regulation of microRNA maturation.

Rule-Breakers

What is described so far is the standard or 'canonical' pathway for microRNA biogenesis. Another pathway exists by which microRNAs can be generated, called the *non-canonical* pathway. This route skips either the Drosha or the Dicer processing steps. One sub-family of microRNAs called *mirtrons* has been discovered that does not require Drosha during maturation. These mirtrons were first identified in 2007, reported in a set of three papers

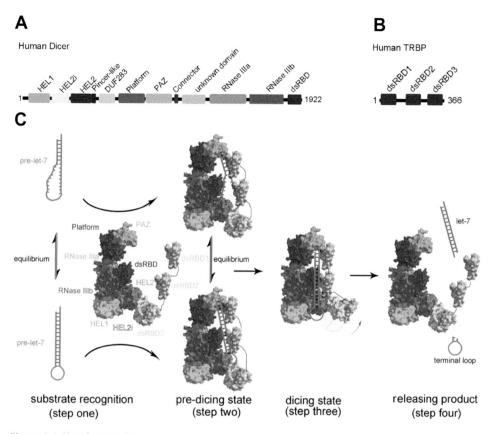

Figure 3.4 How Dicer works

Panel A is a schematic of the functional domains of Dicer.

Panel B shows the functional domains of TRBP. Numbers indicate amino acid positions.

Key: DUF, domain of unknown function; dsRBD, double-stranded RNA Binding Domain; HEL, helicase; PAZ, Piwi, Argonaute and Zwille.

Panel C shows a model of pre-microRNA processing by human Dicer based on cryo-electron microscopy. In the example, Dicer recruits pre-let-7 with the aid of TRBP. The pre-let-7 is loaded into Dicer's processing centre for precise dicing reaction. After dicing, the cleaved products are released from the complex.

Source: Reprinted with permission from Liu et al., *Cell*, vol. 173, pp. 1191–1203 (2018).[90]

within a few months of each other.[91-93] Mirtrons come from introns during the processing of protein-coding mRNAs. They contain a hairpin feature, although not the same as the ones in the canonical pathway of microRNA precursors, and the pathway is highly conserved, being found in worms, flies and mammals. MicroRNAs have also been found to be generated when Pol II terminates prematurely during transcription of protein-coding genes. Certain half-finished RNAs can fold back on themselves and can then be exported, albeit by a different Exportin, followed by recognition and processing by Dicer. MicroRNAs can also derive from other small non-coding RNAs, but there is still limited evidence for whether and how these work as bona fide microRNAs. For now, these remain potential microRNAs; they could simply be molecular noise, although we must be cautious in this assumption – a lot of small RNAs were once thought to be such.

There is a rare instance of a microRNA that becomes functional without Dicer. This is miR-451 and it was found by one of the same teams that first linked Dicer to the maturation of short RNAs for RNAi.[94] The 2010 study in *Nature* came across this unusual microRNA maturation event as part of a study looking at the effects of loss of AGO2 on mouse development. One of the most striking features in new-born mice lacking the *Ago2* gene was anaemia. While the mouse embryo was still developing, there was a dramatic failure of red blood cell production. This prompted a search for changes to microRNAs in the mice deficient in AGO2. They found reduced levels of mature miR-451, one of the most abundant microRNAs found in red blood cells. All other microRNAs reached their mature form in the *Ago2* mutants. Analysis of the precursor structure revealed that miR-451's mature sequence extended around the loop region and had features meaning that Dicer would be unable to process it. Indeed, blocking Dicer had no effect on levels of mature miR-451. Further experiments showed that AGO2 itself cleaves the precursor to form the mature miR-451. This appears to be the only example and it has been speculated to act as an evolutionary protective layer that maintains a catalytically active AGO2, preventing the accumulation of variants in the *Ago2* gene that inactivate its slicer activity, essential for RNAi, in mammals.

Molecular Diplomacy: Argonaute Introduces MicroRNAs to Their Targets

We have nearly reached the moment when the mature microRNA carries out its principal function of gene silencing. To recap the multi-step biogenesis process, the transcribed pri-microRNA molecule has been cut twice and we now have a duplex comprising two strands lying opposite each other, still connected via base-pairing. The next step is for one of the two strands to get passed to an AGO protein. Only one strand is taken up. The strand that makes it into the grasp of AGO is called the *guide*. The other is referred to as the *passenger* strand. Which strand gets picked? It is usually a winner-takes-all situation. That is, either the 3' or the 5' strand is selected as the guide, depending on the microRNA, and only one or the other is found loaded into AGOs. It is rarely a mix with some AGOs holding the 3' and others the 5'. The reason for the asymmetry, the fact that the two strands are not equally likely to end up being picked for the microRNA 'team', was partly unravelled and the rules established in a *Cell* paper from Zamore's team in 2003.[95] If you recall, any individual RNA strand by default has both a 3' and a 5' end. They noted that the strand that was always selected was the one whose 5' end is less tightly bound to its RNA strand partner. Put another way, the end that is relatively easier to unravel or 'fray' at the 5' end gets chosen. An A:U Watson-Crick match is less strong than a G:C, even though both sets of bases pair (look again at **Figure 1.2**). This is because there are three hydrogen bonds holding the GC pair together and only two hydrogen bonds between the A and the U. This renders the A:U pairing less thermodynamically stable and 'easier' to separate. Zamore's team made artificial duplexes which had A:U matches at the 5' end of one strand and a G:C match at the 5' end of the other strand. They found that the AGO complex always contained the strand that had the A:U match. When they designed both strands to end with G:C matches, this resulted in similar amounts of both strands being loaded.

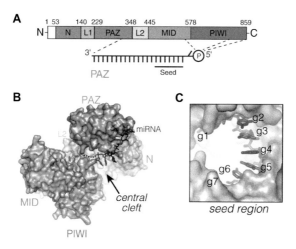

Figure 3.5 How Argonaute works

Panel A is a schematic of the functional domains of Argonaute. Numbers correspond to amino acids in human AGO2. The regions that contact the 5' and the 3' ends of the microRNA guide are indicated.

Panel B is a surface representation of human AGO2 bound to a microRNA. Note the arrangement of the major domains.

Panel C shows an enlarged view of where the guide nucleotides lie within Argonaute. Note that only guide nucleotides g2–g4 are fully available for initiating interactions with target mRNAs.

Source: Reprinted with permission from Sheu-Gruttadauria and MacRae, *Journal of Molecular Biology*, vol. 429, pp. 2619–39 (2017).[96]

Much work has since confirmed the rules and further probed the mechanisms that underlie strand choice for AGO loading. But the principles of the 2003 paper hold up. That is, strand selection comes down to the 'flavour' of the nucleotides at the 5' end (Us and As, not Gs or Cs) and their thermodynamic pairing stability compared to the other strand, with weaker pairing favouring selection. We have also learnt that the same rules apply for all four of the mammalian AGOs: AGO2 is no different from AGOs 1, 3 and 4, despite having the additional slicing function. Researchers have been able to map the physical features on the AGO protein that implement the rules to a part called the MID (middle) domain (see **Figure 3.5**). This includes two sensors formed by amino acids in the protein which contact the 5' end of prospective guide strands and direct selection.

Once loaded to AGO, we have our targeting module. An RNA-induced silencing complex, or RISC, which goes on to promote degradation of mRNAs that contain suitably complementary matches to the microRNA or puts a brake on translation. In the next section, we will see some of the major features of this event, the properties of AGO and how the microRNA-loaded module works.

As we have seen with the descriptions of the microRNA processing steps, structure gives rise to function. We have gained a good understanding of AGO's structure–function relationship using the tools we met before. Molecular biology tells us what the main subparts probably do, followed by changing bits of the protein and seeing the effect of this on AGO's actions, and X-ray crystallography gives us our 3D view of the enzyme in action. **Figure 3.5** provides an overview of the key features of Argonautes, using the example of human AGO2.

The AGO protein acts as a singleton, with two main lobes with two each of the four key subparts in each lobe. Each lobe provides a specific function. The PIWI, at the far end or C terminal of the AGO protein, and the MID domain hold the 5' end of the microRNA while stretching it across a central groove to the 3' end, which rests within the PAZ domain. Other studies showed that AGO proteins can all equally collect and perform microRNA-mediated actions. Because most mature microRNAs can associate with any of the four human AGO proteins, the process will be described for all, but with some AGO2-specific features called out.

Rules of Engagement

The basic pairing rules of microRNAs and their targets were covered in Chapter 2. The preferred and strongest site for a microRNA on its target is a stretch of at least six nucleotides that match to positions 2 through 8 on the microRNA and have an A opposite the first nucleotide of the microRNA from its 5' end. An mRNA target can still pair with a microRNA if it has complementary matches only at positions 3 to 8 or 2 to 7 of the microRNA, but the suppressive effect on the target is likely to be weaker (**Figure 3.6A**). The target recognition event is a two-stage process. Much of the detail was worked out in elegant experiments by MacRae's team, then at Scripps in California, in a landmark paper published in *Cell* in 2015.[97] In order to understand how the microRNA-loaded AGO finds and settles on specific regions of mRNAs, which can be very long and contain one, many or no sites for a given microRNA, they devised experiments to actually *watch* AGO. They worked out a way to study the behaviour of a microRNA-loaded AGO 'live', tracking it as it moved along mRNAs. To do this they used a microscopic technique called single-molecule fluorescence resonance energy transfer (FRET). The method places fluorescent dyes on the two objects of interest and powerful microscopes are used that can both light up the dye and then detect changes to the direction and the wavelengths of light that return when the two molecules interact closely. They staked out mRNA targets modified with one dye on a glass slide. They then fed a microRNA labelled with another dye to an AGO2 protein and placed the two close together, following the movement of AGO2. The signal changes could be traced in space and time, telling them if the AGO2 was moving and how fast. Because they knew the sequence of the target, they could also determine which nucleotide sequences caused the movement to slow down or speed up.

When the target had a complementary seed for the microRNA, a pulse of light occurred, signalling that the AGO2 had docked with the target. Each time the docking occurred, the AGO2 sat there for a certain amount of time. This dwelling only happened when the target had a seed for the microRNA. It occurred with as few as three complementary sites. The AGO2 complex never docked to RNA targets that lacked sequence complementarity with its loaded microRNA. Almost like it knew a potential target when it saw it. And it sat for longer if the complementarity of the sequence was greater. For a three to five nucleotide match, they measured the dwell time at 1 second. This doubled when it was a six-nucleotide match. More matches than that, seven or longer, and AGO2 never disengaged. It stuck fast. This backed up results of other experiments that predicted there would be strong binding if there was a match between the target and the two to eight nucleotides of the 5' end of the microRNA. **Figure 3.6B** provides an overview of the model of the AGO2 search process.

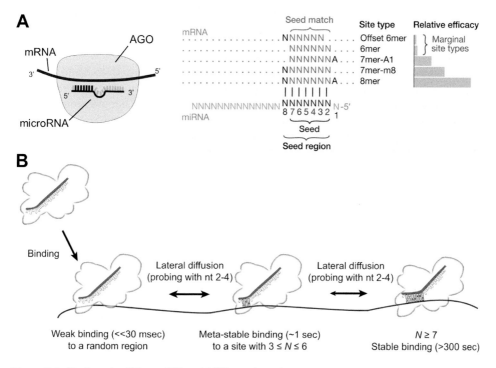

Figure 3.6 Aligning microRNA to mRNA and AGO's search mode

Panel A shows an AGO-bound microRNA brought to alignment with a mRNA target and the relative strength of suppression based on the number of base-pairing sites. The most effective are 7–8 nt sites that match the microRNA seed (positions 2–7).

Key: N, any nucleotide.

Panel B is a model for the proposed steps in target recognition by a microRNA-loaded AGO2. The AGO2-microRNA complex binds the target RNA and diffuses along rapidly, sliding over 69 nucleotides (the length of the target construct in the experiment) in less than 100 milliseconds. Complementary sites of three or more nucleotides cause the complex to pause and remain meta-stably bound on the order of 1 second. When site complementarity extends to the full length of the seed (nucleotides 2–8) or longer, the complex remains bound stably for extended times (over 300 seconds).

Source: Panel A box schematic cropped and reprinted with permission from Bartel, *Cell*, vol. 173, pp. 20–51 (2018).[98] Panel B reprinted with permission from Chandradoss et al., *Cell*, vol. 162, pp. 96–107 (2015).[97]

The next experiments revealed that the AGO2 complex spends more time on a target when there is more than one set of complementary sites. Two sites increased the dwell time further. Finally, they explored how the different domains of AGO2 were working during this process. The microRNA is held by the MID and PIWI domains in a way that exposes nucleotides two to four so they can probe for sites of complementarity. Nucleotides two to four of the microRNA protrude slightly and are used in search mode, allowing AGO2 to rapidly scan for potential sites of complementarity, sacrificing specificity for the fluid and more rapid mobility afforded by few and lighter target binding. More extensive pairing comes later and results in a firm lock. We therefore have a good understanding of the behaviour of a microRNA-loaded AGO protein. The complex is attracted to sites with some complementarity. This type of docking is fast, but it lifts off again or moves further along the RNA when the complementarity is limited. Where it encounters sites of high complementarity, the complex locks on. The team also found regions outside the seed of the microRNA that influenced binding and the strength of actions, at the other end of the microRNA, particularly nucleotides 13 to 16. Binding in this supplementary region explained some of the differences in the effects of microRNAs that share the same seed.

As we have seen earlier, understanding how a component of the microRNA machinery works takes time and different complementary approaches. The generation of crystals of AGO alone and in combination with RNAs has, once again, helped explain what parts of AGO do what during the targeting process. We know this in some cases at the resolution of the individual atom. The first structural analysis of a crystal of AGO2 came in 2012,[99] with a later paper by the same team, led by MacRae, in 2014,[100] both in *Science*. The later study incorporated a target RNA in the crystal and had other improvements over the earlier effort. You may have noticed the chronology here, with the AGO crystal structure work coming later than that resolved for Dicer and Drosha. This was mainly owing to specific technical issues with 'stickiness' that made isolating and crystalising AGO without other molecules difficult. Challenge solved, the crystal was made and studied. The analysis revealed that parts of AGO2 open to create a groove shape that can accommodate a target containing a seed match. The microRNA seed, nucleotides two to eight, now forming a duplex, then lies within a central cleft of AGO2. A key anchoring mechanism is for the first adenine base of the target into a narrow pocket formed by two domains of AGO2, MID and a linker structure. But mostly it is the physical shape of AGO2, formed by the sub-domains and how they fold and interact, that dictates how the microRNA and the target are co-recognised. Grooves lined by certain amino acids interact with the duplex through different types and strengths of electrical charges and atomic bonds. When we get beyond the seed region, things change. The complex lacks space to accommodate nucleotides beyond the ninth position. That is, the groove cannot hold more of the RNA duplex without a change in shape of the AGO2. This helped explain the biochemical experiments and computer-based predictions that features beyond the seed are less important for AGO2-mediated effects. But there is contact between AGO2 and the parts of the microRNA outside the seed. As the microRNA exits the seed cleft, it wraps over the surface of the PAZ domain. This appears to permit the 3' end of the microRNA to make further contacts, where there are complementary nucleotides, with the target. This is so-called supplemental pairing, the importance of which is not fully understood. The crystal structure of AGO2 also allowed some speculation as to how and when the slicing action of AGO2, reserved for those instances where there is extensive complementarity, is brought to bear. It involves an additional position, with repositioning of a metal ion in the active site of AGO2.

Research continues to generate insights into the various outcomes of microRNA–target pairing and how additional complementarity beyond the seed works.[38] There are also examples of microRNAs with less than perfect seeds that nevertheless have potent actions on targets. The chief suspect in those circumstances is supplementary base-pairing, those sequences adjacent to but beyond the seed. And more mysteries remain to be solved. Analysis of RNAs bound within AGO frequently includes regions of the protein-coding sequence (CDS) instead of the 3' UTR of the target mRNA. This is not where AGO is thought to do its work and the segments of RNA stuck to AGO often lack the right seed or lack any apparent effect of being in the AGO. That is, the protein encoded by the mRNA does not appear to be blocked. So, some of the rules are still not fully understood and there may be another class of microRNA recognition element we need to learn about.

Decision Time: Translational Block or mRNA Decay?

We now reach the next important stage of the journey. The microRNA is docked with its target within the grasp of an AGO. What happens next? How do we get from here to 'gene silencing'? There are two mechanisms. One is translational repression. In other words, the translation of the mRNA to protein is reduced or fully prevented. The other is mRNA decay. This is not the same as cleavage of the mRNA – at least not initially. Let us take these in turn. The first mechanism is simple enough. The locked-on AGO complex physically impedes the reading of the mRNA. It's like a large knot in the middle of your shoelace that prevents you lacing up a boot; you can feed the first part of the lace through, but at some point it gets blocked. With the AGO-microRNA complex latched on, the target mRNA simply cannot be fed through the ribosome to allow translation. Using the same analogy helps explain why there are stronger effects when several microRNAs target the same transcript. Multiple knots in the shoelace make it even harder to thread it through. A docked AGO-microRNA will also displace some of the machinery for translation. It basically elbows out of the way some of the other factors, called eukaryotic initiation factors, that an mRNA needs to be bound to in order to be read by the ribosome.

Now the second mechanism, decay of the mRNA. This is more complex and comprises a series of steps. Step 1 is for an AGO to recruit a scaffolding protein called trinucleotide repeat containing adaptor 6 (TNRC6 or GW182 in flies). Step 2 is for this protein to interact with another protein called poly A binding protein cytoplasmic (PABPC). This begins the process of dismantling the mRNA. That begins with removal of the poly-A tail. A further two sets of proteins come to the growing complex, including enzymes specialized at removing A nucleotides. Next, we lose the cap. A special enzyme complex performs this de-capping reaction. Without the cap, the mRNA is stripped of its 'don't eat me' signal and is now vulnerable to digestion. The enzyme exoribonuclease 1 (XRN1), which we will meet again shortly in the context of how microRNAs are eventually disposed of, will now digest the mRNA, starting at the 5' end. The two modes of action are complementary and likely interconnected. Their contributions are not, however, equal. The decay process dominates in most contexts, with studies estimating that this accounts for 66 per cent to 90 per cent of the silencing by microRNAs. Only in early embryonic development do we see the translational suppression effect as the dominant consequence of microRNA actions. There are also additional regulatory layers on the processes described earlier. Much of this is still being worked out and the influence of individual changes and the context within which these occur remain poorly understood: AGO and the proteins that carry out the events downstream of microRNA–target binding can each be regulated in different ways. Chemical modifications of their surfaces, including the addition of phosphates mediated by enzymes, change their activity levels. **Figure 3.7** provides an overview of the two processes.

Long-Distance Voyages and the Whereabouts of MicroRNAs

The biogenesis of a microRNA features molecular travel across a vast expanse of physical space within the cell. It is a journey that starts in the nucleus and ends up out in the cytoplasm. In fact, if you consider that the signals to switch on a microRNA often

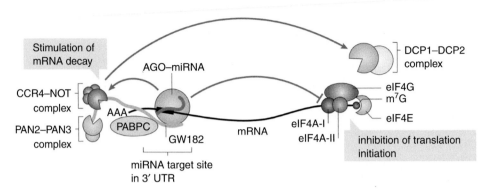

Figure 3.7 How microRNAs silence gene expression

There are two main ways that microRNAs bring about gene silencing. In the first, microRNAs inhibit translation at the initiation step, likely through release of proteins within the complex such as eukaryotic initiation factor 4A-I (eIF4A-I) and eIF4A-II. The second process is by mediating mRNA decay through interactions with GW182 proteins: GW182 binds the polyadenylate-binding protein (PABPC) and the deadenylation complexes poly(A)-nuclease deadenylation complex subunit 2 (PAN2)–PAN3 and carbon catabolite repressor protein 4 (CCR4)–NOT. Deadenylation is followed by de-capping by the complex mRNA–de-capping enzyme subunit 1 (DCP1)–DCP2 and 5'–3' mRNA degradation (not shown).

Source: Reprinted with permission from Gebert & MacRae, *Nature Reviews Molecular Cell Biology*, vol. 20, pp. 21–37 (2019).[38]

originate from the surface of the cell, you could say that the journey starts all the way out there. For a molecule the size of a microRNA, these are sizeable distances. A typical human cell is perhaps 20 micrometres across (or 0.02 mm). This is about 3,000 times the length of a typical microRNA, based on the 65 angstroms length of a microRNA sitting in the molecular ruler of Dicer. As we will see in Chapter 5, the physical distances are often staggering. Certain brain cells stretch one metre in distance and we can detect microRNAs and the machinery distributed from one end to the other. That's 10 thousand million angstroms. If you were to travel that far from Earth in kilometres, you would pass Neptune before being halfway done. Quite the journey compared to Jason and his Argonauts navigating a few islands around Greece. And it is not only the microRNA making the journey; microRNAs are chaperoned along the way, never left alone to find their own way as they would be quickly destroyed by the various nucleases in our cells if separated from their protein protectors.

It is simplistic to view the microRNA journey as only from the nucleus to the cytoplasm. This has undergone significant revision over time as more and more compartments of the cell have been probed for components of the microRNA pathway.[101, 102] Studies exploring the cellular whereabouts of microRNAs have led to the conclusion that the proper co-location of the microRNA machines, the microRNA itself and the targets is an additional layer of regulation that shapes how microRNAs shape the gene expression landscape. These components are not floating aimlessly in the cystolic sea but clump together and lie within specialised domains inside the cell. One of the sites where components such as AGO and proteins that assist with the breakdown of the target mRNA are found is called a P (for 'processing') body. These are found in the cytoplasm and have an appearance a bit like granules. They lack a membrane and their function can be thought of as forming a physical scaffold or platform upon which the various proteins can congregate and assemble. They appear to form as a consequence, rather than a cause, of microRNA activity. Further, P bodies may represent a storage mechanism for blocked but potentially recoverable mRNAs. Their importance for microRNA function, and the context in which they form inside cells, are poorly understood and the rules governing entering and whether exiting is possible continue to be studied.

Components of the later stages of the microRNA pathway are also found near or resting on the surface of various organelles, including the nucleus. After going to so much trouble to get the microRNA outside and functional in the cytoplasm, a portion of AGO and the machinery that assembles to carry out translational repression and mRNA decay is also found back inside the nucleus. This is not by chance, with sequences that mark them for nuclear entry facilitated by import proteins. Within the nucleus, some of the work done is traditional microRNA-mediated gene silencing. Many of the targets have roles in gene activity, suggesting that this function may have evolved to bring microRNA control closer to the point of transcription. If we go deeper, there is more. Components such as AGO have even been found to rest on chromatin itself, the very structure of our genomes. What it is doing there is not altogether clear, but it may involve effects on gene transcription.

Another site is the endoplasmic reticulum, a network of sacs for protein transport. Part of this organelle resides immediately outside the nucleus and is coated with the machinery for translation of mRNA, namely ribosomes. These are a fitting venue for microRNAs, and components of the machinery for biogenesis and microRNA loading have been detected at these sites. Components of the pathway have also been found farther out still, adjacent to or within other cell organelles, including the Golgi apparatus, which is involved in packaging proteins for transport around and outside the cell. It is essentially unknown what microRNA functions occur there and the presence may relate to late-stage events such as recycling of the microRNA machinery. More is known about microRNAs and mitochondria. MicroRNAs have been found inside these organelles. Some are microRNAs encoded in the cell's main genome, but others are actually encoded in the mitochondria's own DNA (mitochondria contain DNA and instructions for making some of the proteins they use; these are remnants of their ancient origins as independent organisms). The levels of some of the nucleus-encoded microRNAs found inside mitochondria are often higher than outside, implying that an active import process has occurred, leading to their accumulation. Their presence implies that microRNAs impose some control over the genes that support energy generation in the cell.

MicroRNAs are also found outside the cell where they are referred to as extracellular microRNAs. These observations date to the early days of microRNA studies. Researchers noticed that their cell culture solutions and media around the cells contained microRNAs. This could have simply been owing to leak from dead cells, but could also indicate active trafficking of them outside the cell. Chapter 8 will go into how this finding could be exploited for diagnostic tests for various human diseases. Where present outside cells, microRNAs could be detected inside tiny secreted, membrane-enclosed spheroids that also contained other proteins and RNAs. Researchers latched onto the idea that these microRNAs might be internalised by other cells and, if so, could potentially be a form of cell-to-cell messaging system. Some of the microRNAs most often found packaged in vesicles contain a common nucleotide sequence, suggesting that there are package-me-for-export signals encoded in the microRNA genes. This idea is not without controversy. The techniques for isolating pure vesicles and removing surface RNAs are technically difficult, whereas the methods for detecting microRNAs are exquisitely sensitive; even the faintest trace of a microRNA not washed off the surface could give the impression of it being inside a vesicle. Some of the vesicles are also of similar size to the spherical vesicles that form when cells undergo programmed cell death, a form of cell suicide. Therefore, they could be remnants of dead cells, like the ejected contents of a dying star. It has also been difficult to show that there are enough microRNAs inside to significantly change a biological process in a recipient cell. We will return to this idea in Chapter 8. As our understanding of the varied distribution of the components improves, more questions arise. What are the signals that direct components to different sites and what regulates those decisions? What is the impact of the components in these unusual locations relative to traditional sites of action in the cell?

Extinguishing MicroRNAs: The End of the Journey

We come now to the end of the microRNA journey. What happens to the microRNA once its job is finished? All regulatory systems in cells need ways to switch off. We need a proper ending just as much as a start and a middle. The existence of machinery for microRNA degradation makes sense. The involvement of microRNAs in cell functions that occur very quickly or drive transitions between cell states would necessitate systems that turn off as quickly as they turn on. Let us start with what signals the end of the show. Before we see how this is done for microRNAs, how does it work for other molecules? Let's use the example of proteins. The way cells turn over their proteins is by digesting them back to their constituent parts – amino acids. One of the molecular garbage disposal systems in our cells is the ubiquitin-protease system (UPS). The breakdown process begins with adding an 'eat-me' signal to the protein, that is, tagging the target protein or substrate with a peptide called ubiquitin, a chain of 76 amino acids. The ubiquitin tag gets glued onto a lysine, one of the target's amino acids. The reaction requires an enzyme called an E3 ligase, which acts as a bridge between an E2 ligase, which carries the ubiquitin tag, and the target or substrate protein. Once the tag is attached, and often more than one gets attached, the protein is recognised and gets drawn into the UPS. The protein goes in one end and is digested; amino acids come out the other end, after which they may go on to be assembled into a new protein. There are around 600 of these E3 ligases in the human genome, each having specificity for one or more protein targets. A fully functioning UPS is important for the health of the cell. If it fails, proteins accumulate to toxic levels. Several years ago, my colleagues Robert Meller and Roger Simon in Portland, Oregon, found that the UPS is activated in brain cells by the low oxygen levels that occur when someone has a stroke. The neurones used the UPS to adapt to this stress by removing key proteins from synapses, the contact points between neurones in the brain.[103] This had the effect of dampening communication routes between brain cells, at least temporarily, and helped them survive. But there is also another side to the UPS. My colleague Tobias Engel observed that neurones in areas of the brain with lower activity of the UPS survived better in models of severe epilepsy.[104] Modelling this finding by treating mice with a drug that blocked the UPS had the effect of protecting brain tissue against the harm caused by long-lasting seizures. So, the UPS can serve different purposes depending on context. Controlling the UPS is an active area of drug development, with a UPS inhibitor, bortezomib, now used to treat certain cancers.

We also have systems to get rid of RNAs using RNases, and the microRNA system has an end-of-life plan.[105-107] The steps involved were rather overlooked for a while, with more attention paid to the phases of biosynthesis and targeting. But the termination of a microRNA, the degradation of the mature, functional microRNA, is becoming a larger focus in molecular biology labs and progress is being made. How this process is controlled is important for understanding microRNA function in health and disease. How long does a typical microRNA last once it has been made? Early assessments of the longevity of individual microRNA species suggested half-lives, the time it takes for levels to drop by half or 50 per cent of their starting quantity, in the region of half a day or longer. This is quite stable relative to other RNAs. Experiments show that once loaded into an AGO, microRNAs are well-protected, tucked in and away from the enzymes that could degrade them by domains of AGO that effectively shield them from the teeth of RNA-degrading enzymes. But evidence would emerge showing that turnover of microRNAs could be rapid. How do we study this process? One approach is called a pulse-chase experiment. A label (e.g. a radioactive atom) is introduced to newly synthesized RNA followed by sampling over time to monitor for disappearance. Another common tactic is to block new RNA transcription. This can be done using actinomycin D, a compound isolated from *Streptomyces* bacteria and an effective antibiotic. Add actinomycin D to your cells and then measure the declining levels of the precursor and the mature forms of RNA in your system. Another approach is to block the ability of the cell to make new mature microRNAs by eliminating Dicer followed by monitoring the decline in microRNAs. In early experiments, microRNAs could be detected long after the new transcription or biogenesis had been blocked. When researchers measured the level of a given microRNA at one time point and checked back a day later, and despite no new precursor microRNA being made, mature levels were much the same as before. But researchers soon found some microRNAs that flouted these rules. Their levels fluctuated dynamically, particularly in dividing and developing cells and organisms. This tipped them off that there was an active process for lowering microRNA levels. It was also clear that this was microRNA-specific. Some microRNAs showed rapid turnover, while others remained quite stable over time. Other clues were the finding that there could be stable levels of precursor microRNAs, pre- and pri- forms, whereas simultaneous measurement of the mature form would show rapid flux. Unsurprisingly, such rapid turnover was found in the setting of cell division at different phases of the cycle. But rapid microRNA turnover also occurred in certain neurones that are mainly non-dividing and designed to live very long lives. In 2010, a team at the Friedrich Miescher Institute in Basel, Switzerland, led by Witold Filipowicz, identified a large set of microRNAs that rapidly came and went in light-sensitive cells of the retina, at the back of the eye.[108] During dark-adaptation, a process during which the pigment in light-sensitive cells (photoreceptors) is being regenerated and light sensitivity becomes greatest, levels of monitored microRNAs declined rapidly. The estimated half-lives were just 90 minutes and levels of several microRNAs were even shorter, dropping significantly within 30 minutes. Other cell types in the eye, including Müller cells, a support cell, showed no such microRNA turnover. Rapid microRNA turnover was also found for certain microRNAs in structures deep within the brain. While decreased biogenesis was involved, there was also clear evidence for active degradation processes. The study also gave some of the earliest clues that microRNA turnover was linked to cellular activity. For example, immature neurones that did not display the normal patterns of electrical activity lacked the rapid turnover feature. Somehow, the machinery to break down microRNAs was monitoring and reacting to the behaviour of brain cells.

Biochemical Features That Signal MicroRNA Demise

This all pointed to cells having ways to pick out different microRNAs for quick turnover, making choices about the molecular lives of microRNAs. Who lives and who doesn't. The factors and rules that govern microRNA decay are complex and still not fully understood.

However, they include both sequence and context elements. Early experiments found that nucleotides at the 3' end of the microRNA were important for determining whether a microRNA cycled faster. We have learnt since that one element is the binding and the degree of complementarity between the microRNA and its target. There is some evidence that how and to what a microRNA binds (i.e. the target mRNA) can influence the stability of the microRNA. This is called target-directed microRNA degradation (TDMD). More extensive complementarity between the microRNA and its target seems to favour microRNA turnover. How much this occurs in nature is not yet known because many experiments are performed using reconstituted systems and synthetic RNAs. But the number of examples is growing and this seems to be a broad mechanism influencing microRNA degradation. Certain viruses have evolved to exploit the system, encoding RNAs that have extensive complementarity to critical microRNAs that would otherwise interfere with their stability or replication. In Chapter 7, we will meet the hepatitis C virus that exploits a microRNA during its life cycle. This type of sequence-related microRNA turnover can work in both directions, with evidence that target binding opposes as well as promotes microRNA degradation. Research continues to understand the context and the precise sequence rules by which TDMD works.

Nucleotide changes are the other major determinant in microRNA degradation. This is called tailing and trimming and occurs at the 3' end of the microRNA. Additions or removals of nucleotides influence stability and attract complexes that perform the degradation process. In animals, a number of enzymes have been identified that add nucleotides to the 3' ends of microRNAs. These include terminal uridyl transferases (TUTs), which apply uridines (uracil attached to a ribose) to the end of the RNA. Another family of enzymes can add adenosines (adenine attached to a ribose) to the ends of a microRNA. The importance of these additions remains slightly unclear because interference experiments, where the modifying enzymes are removed or blocked, do not universally extend the lives of microRNAs as would be expected if they simply signalled the microRNA for destruction. This could be because the 3' end of a microRNA remains sheltered by its AGO. We know this because experiments that removed the PAZ part of the AGO protein that shields 3' microRNA ends results in extensive nucleotide additions and susceptibility to degradation. It is likely that while these are independent processes, it is a combination of TDMD and tailing and possibly other regulatory factors that affects AGO stability, that together influences the selection of microRNAs for degradation.

The Enzymes Involved in MicroRNA Degradation

Straying briefly from the focus on animal microRNAs, let me note that studies in the *Arabidopsis* plant were the first to isolate an enzyme with the ability to specifically degrade mature microRNAs. That study,[109] reported by a team from the University of California at Riverside in *Science* in 2008, discovered that a family of exonucleases termed small RNA-degrading nucleases (SDNs) could degrade microRNAs, working from one end of the microRNA to generate breakdown products of around eight to nine nucleotides in length. The team also showed that loss of the enzymes impaired plant development, indicating microRNA degradation is important. Since then, other enzymes have been identified that can degrade mature microRNAs, now referred to broadly as 'miRNAses'. All are exonucleases: they digest starting at one end or the other of the RNA molecule and work their way along, with some preferring to run 3' to 5' while others run 5' to 3'. This includes XRN-1, which is one of the best-studied in mammalian cells. Other organisms have versions of other enzymes that possess miRNAse activity.

Many of the details of the process remain to be clarified. This includes the features of the microRNA and presumably its targets that direct the machinery of degradation and even the choice of the degradation machinery that is brought to bear upon the microRNA. When and where to act upon a specific microRNA is not well understood. There are also other ways by which microRNA degradation occurs in a more global way. One of these is by degradation of AGO. The AGO protein can itself be tagged for destruction. Any microRNAs riding inside get released and, now unprotected, suffer the same fate as their host – destruction. Mendell's team recently identified an E3 ligase called ZSWIM8 that tags AGO with ubiquitin for destruction by the UPS.[110] Experiments blocking ZSWIM8 stabilized cellular levels of microRNAs that were known to be degraded through the TDMD process. Additions of nucleotides to the microRNA 3' end made no difference. They were also able to identify the specific lysine amino acid on AGO2 where ZSWIM8 added the ubiquitin tag. This adds more detail to our understanding of the sequence of events, at least in the context of TDMD, which ends the lives of microRNAs.

Reflections

We have come to the end of the fantastic journey and life cycle of microRNAs. We have seen how they begin life, their biogenesis and how, through binding to AGO proteins, they carry out their search and destroy functions. And we have seen how their actions are terminated, setting the stage for new rounds of transcription and target engagements. This part of the voyage is complete. While there was no Golden Fleece for our AGO protein, the cargo it carries and the journey it makes in every cell at every moment are absolutely precious.

Opening Act
Fine-Tuning During Development

All of the processes of neural development . . . – patterning, proliferation, differentiation, cell migration, axon guidance, synapse formation – rely on differential gene expression . . . [E]ach . . . is subject to noise.

From Innate: How the Wiring of Our Brains Shapes Who We Are, *by Kevin J. Mitchell (Princeton University Press, 2018, p. 69)*

What would you say is the most important moment in your life? The birth of a child? The death of a parent? Graduation? The answer to this depends, of course, on who you ask. But if you pose that sort of question to a developmental biologist or geneticist, they might respond that the most important moments are really the earliest in your life, during embryo formation, growth and the first days, weeks and months of postnatal life. Trillions of molecular and cellular interactions that influence whether and who you will be. When it comes to microRNAs, when are their effects felt the most? What happens if we lack a functioning microRNA gene or the enzymes that make it? Do we really need microRNAs at all?

This chapter will focus on two key aspects. First, the research that has informed our views of how fundamental microRNAs are to organisms. Here we begin broadly, looking at the effects of general disruption to microRNA production and function and then looking at specific microRNAs and how changes to these affect different systems in the body. Second, we will take some examples of microRNAs critical to organism development and explore what cellular processes and decisions they are influencing and how this shapes events such as cell division and differentiation.

One of the experiments scientists often try when a new gene or biological process gets discovered is to remove it, to 'knock out' the gene in question and see what happens. This is often done in model organisms such as *C. elegans*, *D. melanogaster* or mice. We've seen a couple of examples already. Thanks to new technologies such as CRISPR, we can do this more accurately than ever as well as more cheaply, including in human cells and animal models. The approach can tell us something about the overall importance of the gene and what it does. Of course, removing a gene and observing a change in how an organism develops, survives or behaves does not tell us as much as we'd like to think. Removing a component can cause the tissue or organ to fail, but we don't always learn much about why it went wrong or what it would have been doing otherwise. A useful way to think about this is found in Kevin Mitchell's book *Innate* on how gene variation affects brain development; it concerns how combustion engine cars work. Removing the spark plugs from a car will stop a car from going. But spark plugs alone do not confer an ability to move/drive; the capability of a car to move also requires many components besides spark plugs. This should be kept in mind in how we interpret the results of microRNA 'knockout' studies. It is the rule rather than the exception that a protein performs functions in more than one pathway. This is true of the enzymes that generate microRNAs and support their function; AGO2 and Dicer are also the machinery that carries out RNAi in cells. So, we must bear in mind that deleting genes within this pathway not only interferes with microRNA actions but also impairs the RNAi pathway. Knockout studies are a useful tool in the scientific arsenal, but these caveats should be kept in mind and results from other types of experiment are needed to build the full picture. Bearing this in mind, what happens when we disrupt components of the microRNA biogenesis pathway? What happens if they are removed at different times or from only certain systems in an organism?

As we saw in Chapter 3, the number of genes involved in microRNA function is quite large, so we'll be selective and focus on a few of the most important ones. Let's start with Dicer, the enzyme that completes the final step in generating the mature microRNA. As is common, efforts to delete the enzyme began in simple organisms such as *C. elegans*. The first study to report what happened when the *Dicer* gene was deleted in a mammal, in this case a mouse, came from Hannon's lab, working at the Cold Spring Harbor Laboratory.[111] The study, published in *Nature Genetics* in 2003, saw the team generate mice lacking one or both copies of *Dicer* (full knockouts lack both copies of the gene, whereas heterozygotes or 'hets' have one normal copy of a gene and one absent or mutant version). This was achieved by splicing a foreign piece of DNA into a section of the *Dicer* gene, exon 21, that codes for the first RNase III domain. While Dicer protein could still be made from the gene, the resulting enzyme lacked the ability to produce mature microRNAs. They now bred male and female mice, each carrying one mutant copy of *Dicer*. Basic genetics predict that the matings will result in three types of offspring: wild-type animals born that carry two copies of the normal *Dicer*, mice with one copy of the normal and one copy of the mutant *Dicer* (hets) and mice carrying two copies of the mutant *Dicer* (knockouts). Offspring carrying two copies of the mutant *Dicer* were never found in the litters. That is, embryos that carried two mutant *Dicer* copies, and were thus incapable of maturing microRNAs, failed to develop. The team traced this failure to the first week of embryonic life. Some likely failed at an even earlier stage. The team were able to recover some early mutant embryos and when they checked they found that the embryos lacked the normal number of stem cells. This strongly suggested that microRNAs were required very early in vertebrate development and were fundamental to self-renewing cells.

Let's look next at deletions of AGOs. We've already come across one study where *Ago2* was deleted, which led to the identification of the Dicer-independent pathway for maturation of miR-451. The genetic deletion of *Ago2* and its effects in mice was first performed by Hannon's team and published in *Science* a year after their Dicer study.[112] The approach was similar. They first generated mice lacking one copy of *Ago2* (written as $Ago2^{+/-}$). When these were bred with other mice also lacking a copy, they found only litters of mice that contained either two normal versions of *Ago2* or one with the mutant copy. But a quarter of the offspring should have been full knockouts ($Ago2^{-/-}$ or 'null'). The fact that these embryos were absent meant that they were unviable, a so-called embryonic lethal event. Therefore AGO2, like Dicer, was essential for key aspects of the early development of the mouse embryo. When they looked at where *Ago2* was expressed in the embryo during development, they found that the densest region was in the brain. Consistent with this, embryonic development in mice lacking *Ago2* began to fail as early as nine days post-fertilisation, with defects in the closure of the neural tube, one of the key structures to form. The heart also failed to develop properly, with embryos displaying signs of cardiac failure. Biochemical studies confirmed that cells from *Ago2*-null cells could not perform RNAi. The findings contrasted with earlier studies that had found loss of some of the other AGO members to be well tolerated. This indicated that AGO2's special slicer activity, which sets AGO2 apart from AGO 1, 3 and 4, was essential for organism development.

What happens when the microprocessor is knocked out? Experiments to delete *Dgcr8* from mice were reported in *Nature Genetics* in 2007.[113] It might seem more important to focus on knocking out Drosha, but this was actually a clever approach. Drosha has a role in non-microRNA pathways, generating the RNAs that form part of the ribosome engine for protein synthesis, whereas DGCR8 seemed specific to microRNAs. It's a slightly cleaner experiment therefore to go after DGCR8 if we want to know how fundamentally important the generation of microRNAs is for organism development. The cells of mouse embryos lacking both copies of *Dgcr8* had no pre- or mature microRNAs, confirming that the DGCR8 protein was essential for microRNA biogenesis and, by inference, no other gene can substitute. Cells with one healthy copy of *Dgcr8* could still produce pre- and mature microRNAs, but the levels were lower than normal. No mice were born when both copies of *Dgcr8* were missing, with most embryos failing to develop at an early stage. Without microRNAs, cells could not differentiate; they could not form different cell types. Together, the studies deleting *Dicer*, *Ago2* and *Dgcr8* in mice proved that general microRNA production and function are critical to exiting from the early embryonic stage to begin to produce the various specialised tissues and cells of the body.

While effective at proving the importance of microRNAs in early development, the early lethality of full knockouts made studies on later, postnatal development impossible. Subsequently, these global approaches of fully knocking out biogenesis genes gave way to more refined strategies. Researchers wanted to ask questions such as what happens if I knock individual genes such as *Dicer* out of just one organ during development? Or what if I leave the animal to develop normally and then knock out the gene in the adult? Technologies are available that allow both types of experiment to be performed. It is even possible to toggle between these, knocking it out and then putting it back in. One of the most popular ways to do this is using the cyclic recombinase (Cre) system. This is an enzyme borrowed from a P1 bacteriophage, a virus that infects bacteria. The Cre enzyme can cut DNA. To know where to do this, it needs specific signals. Short DNA sequences called loxP sites are an 8-base pair spacer central region flanked by two 13-base pair sequences. These must be placed at either end of the DNA segment to be altered. This natural system has been co-opted by researchers for genome editing and works as follows. First, the gene to be targeted must be engineered to be flanked by two loxP sites. The Cre enzyme must also be coaxed into being made by the host organism, tissue or cell, or it can be delivered separately. A common way to deliver Cre into the organism is by packing it into a virus. Upon finding loxP sites in the genome, the Cre enzyme cuts the DNA and this results in the gene being deleted. The system is sophisticated and you can often disrupt a gene by just deleting a small part. Gene excision can now be controlled at specific moments. Activate the Cre, and the gene is excised. Thus, researchers can assess the effects of interrupting microRNA biogenesis or the production of specific microRNAs during later stages or even after development is complete. This can be useful in learning whether microRNAs are still needed in the adult organism. We can go further, however. By placing Cre under the control of a gene promoter that is active in only one tissue or cell type, it can now be switched on in a specific tissue *and* at a specific time. This allows researchers to block microRNAs at just one place and time in the body. With these tools, various teams have looked at what happens when microRNA actions are prevented in different tissues and at different times. These more selective approaches were being applied as early as 2005 and have now been widely used to study what happens when you block microRNA biogenesis in different systems in the body.

While the *Ago2*-null embryo studies in 2004 had observed that microRNA machinery was highly active during early mouse brain development, it wasn't clear if microRNA biogenesis remained as important after development was complete. Working at the Rockefeller University in the lab of Nobel prize winner Paul Greengard, Anne Schaefer used the Cre system to learn what happened when *Dicer* was deleted in the cerebellum.[114] The cerebellum is a large brain structure that resides at the back or 'hind' brain. Among its various functions, it helps coordinate movements and balance. The cells in the cerebellum are neatly organised and their connections are well-known. To knock out *Dicer* in the cerebellum, the team bred two different mice together. One mouse had the loxP tags surrounding the *Dicer* gene and the other mouse made the Cre enzyme just in the Purkinje cells of the cerebellum. These are huge neurones that carry out the main work of that part of the brain. A Purkinje cell–specific promoter had been discovered previously, meaning that the gene encoding Cre could be placed under the control of that promoter, resulting in it being switched on only in those cells in the cerebellum. The mating of the two mouse lines would result in offspring that lacked microRNAs just in specific cells in the cerebellum. Better still, the promoter controlling Cre was active only after the cerebellum had formed. This made it possible to block microRNA production after development of the cerebellum was complete. So, what happened? The team estimated that Dicer was no longer working in these cells by the time the mice were four weeks old. A check at 10 weeks showed nothing unusual. But then it all changed. Brains from 13-week-old mice that had no Dicer in their Purkinje cells were changing. The parts of the cell that receive signals from other cells began to retract and disappear. Another month later and they started to find dead neurones in the cerebellum. The cause of this death was unknown and at the time the team speculated that it might be from accumulation of proteins or RNA, either because proteins were free from their microRNA control to be more abundant or because too much pre-microRNA was building up in the cells, unable to be processed to mature microRNA. The death of brain cells coincided with other changes in the mice. They began to walk differently, had poor grip strength and displayed a tremor, a regular shaking motion of the body. The study confirmed for the first time that microRNAs were needed in the mature brain and that without them the brain would degenerate.

With the broad availability of such genetic tools, other teams began to investigate what happened when microRNA production was blocked in other parts of the brain and other organs. A year later, in 2008, teams showed that when *Dicer* was deleted from the neurones that respond to the neurotransmitter dopamine, multiple changes followed in mouse movement.[115] These included poor coordination. Notably, dopamine is the neurotransmitter that is depleted in people with Parkinson's disease. Unlike the Purkinje cells, the dopamine-responsive neurones didn't die after *Dicer* was deleted. The consequences of blocking maturation of microRNAs in the developed brain depended, therefore, on the specific *cell type*. This meant that, at least in terms of survival, microRNAs were more essential for some neurones than others.

Neurones are not the only cell type in the brain, however. Interestingly, blocking microRNAs in the support cells for neurones, called glia, also had catastrophic effects on the brain.[116] In 2011, a team made up of scientists at the University of California, Los

Angeles and Shanghai investigated what happened when *Dicer* was deleted from cells in the brain called astrocytes ('astro' because they look a bit like stars). Astrocytes are one of the most abundant cell types in the brain and they perform many roles. These include supplying neurones with the chemical building blocks for making neurotransmitters and responding to injury by coordinating repair processes. There are promoters for astrocyte genes and these were exploited to make a Cre system that switched on only in astrocytes. The team used the Cre system to knock *Dicer* out just from astrocytes within a few days of the mice being born. Just like the Schaefer study, the mice behaved normally for the first few weeks. However, the researchers then started to observe changes, initially in how the mice walked and moved. Occasionally the mice would have a convulsion, the hallmark of the brain disease epilepsy. By eight or nine weeks of age, the mice lacking *Dicer* in astrocytes had become immobile. The speed and the severity of the effect of losing *Dicer* in this brain cell type was unexpected. The study demonstrated a broad need for ongoing microRNA activity in the developed brain even in the support cell populations. **Figure 4.1** shows some of the

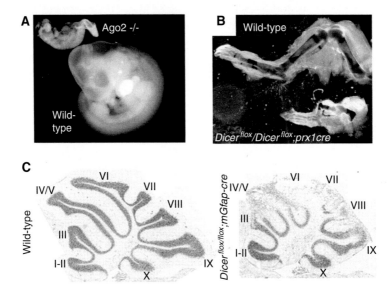

Figure 4.1 Phenotypes in mice lacking components of the microRNA biogenesis pathway

Panel A shows a photograph of two 10.5-day mouse embryos, comparing an *Ago2*-null embryo (top) to a wild-type mouse embryo.

Panel B shows a skeletal preparation of a forelimb from a wild-type mouse (top) and a mouse in which *Dicer* was deleted specifically from cells in which the Prx1 homeobox domain transcription factor is active during limb development (*Dicer*^flox/*Dicer*^flox;*prx1cre*). Note the small size of the limb although the major bones such as scapula and humerus are present.

Panel C shows histological images of the cerebellum of the mouse (nissl staining – cells appear as dark spots). The left image is from a normal mouse. The right image is from a mouse in which *Dicer* was deleted in postnatal astrocytes. Note the extensive neurodegeneration (loss of nissl staining). The Roman numerals identify the different lobes of the brain structure.

Source: Panel A reprinted with permission from Liu et al., *Science*, vol. 305, pp. 1437–41 (2004).[112] Panel B reprinted with permission from Harfe et al., *Proceedings of the National Academy of Sciences of the United States of America*, vol. 102, pp. 10898–903 (2004).[117] © National Academy of Sciences, U.S.A. 2005. Panel C reprinted with permission from Tao et al., *Journal of Neuroscience*, vol. 31, pp. 8306–19 (2011).[116]

examples of features (phenotypes) that appear during mouse development or later in life when components of the microRNA biogenesis pathway are deleted either from all cells or from specific cell types.

Other Ways of Knowing We Need MicroRNAs

The knockout of biogenesis components tells us broadly that organisms need microRNAs to develop and continue to need them afterwards. Collapsing parts of the microRNA pathway has severe effects on developing and mature organs, tissues and cells. But the approach taken, deleting the genes of biogenesis, has its limitations. As discussed, the biogenesis enzymes have some microRNA-independent functions. Some of the effects of removing a gene will be unrelated to microRNA maturation and function. Even DGCR8, which was initially thought to be unique to microRNA biogenesis, has subsequently been found to act in other ways, maturing RNAs besides microRNAs and other functions.[118] A second issue is the longevity of microRNAs. Some microRNAs persist in cells long after new synthesis is blocked. Some of the microRNAs produced in non-dividing and long-living cells last the longest. The microRNAs in the heart ('myo-mirs') are particularly persistent. Studies in lab mice, which have lifespans of two to three years, have tracked microRNAs in cells more than a year after microRNA biogenesis was blocked. This makes it very difficult to conclude, having disrupted Dicer and seen that a particular function is normal, that microRNAs are not important. MicroRNAs may still be there doing their jobs. Another consideration is that some microRNAs bypass the canonical biogenesis pathway. Last, many of the approaches to knocking out biogenesis components are non-reversible. The gene is gone and not coming back. Experiments that go on to show that reintroduction or restoration of microRNA function rescues the phenotype, putting things back to how they were, close the loop and offer more complete evidence.

These concerns have prompted researchers to look for other ways besides knocking out biogenesis components to study what happens when you shut down microRNA function. One such alternate approach was described in a study in the journal *eLife* in 2021 by a team led by Andrea Ventura based at the Memorial Sloan Kettering Cancer Center in New York.[119] They developed a method to disrupt, in a reversible manner, the complex that docks with AGO to perform the degradation of targeted mRNAs. This involved borrowing a segment of the TNRC6 protein. We met this in Chapter 3. The TNRC6 protein binds to AGO and brings together the required machinery for dismantling the targeted mRNA, the de-capping and de-adenylation steps. The part of the protein that physically links TNRC6 to AGO has been mapped and is called T6B. When separated from the other parts of the TNRC6 protein, the T6B peptide can act as a blocker of microRNA-mediated target degradation. It jams the system. The team took advantage of this, further engineering the T6B to include an on/off switch controlled by the chemical doxycycline. When cells were exposed to doxycycline, the T6B peptide would start to be made. If the doxycycline was discontinued, T6B production quickly ceased. When they tested this in cells, they showed that when T6B production was switched on, the complex to degrade the targeted mRNAs didn't form and targets of microRNAs began to accumulate in cells. The team made several further checks. The peptide had no effect on microRNAs getting into the RISC and did not affect the RNAi pathway that uses AGO2 to cut RNAs and does not rely on the TNRC6-related complex. After proving that their method to block microRNA function worked in cells, they moved to mice, generating animals in which the T6B peptide was made under the control of doxycycline. When mice were fed doxycycline, the T6B peptide could be detected just a day later in cells. When doxycycline treatment stopped, it disappeared within four days. It was quick and reversible. Using this system for blocking microRNA function, but not microRNA production, they were able to record broad increases in gene expression when T6B was switched on. They also confirmed some of the key findings from knockout studies. For example, if T6B was switched on early enough, embryos did not develop. Switching T6B on later, mid-gestation, had less-severe effects, but surviving mice still appeared smaller and underdeveloped. When T6B was switched on even later, once the mice were adults, the animals appeared outwardly healthy. On closer inspection, however, they found differences: a slight anaemia owing to lower red blood cell production and some missing white blood cells. The experiments implied that microRNA function could be suppressed in adults without severe consequences. However, the effect of T6B, and thus blocking microRNA function, became much more obvious when the mice encountered a stress. For example, adult mice with blocked microRNA function could not recover from colitis, an inflammation of the intestine. When they modelled the effects of chemotherapy on bone marrow, the T6B-producing mice could not recover their blood cell production. So, while a reduction of microRNA function could be tolerated in many parts of the body in an unstressed, healthy adult animal, microRNAs were essential for adults to survive stress and repair damaged systems. There were further important findings. A lack of microRNA function had strong effects on the heart and skeletal muscle. Mice fed doxycycline and making T6B showed a decline in muscle mass along with signs of heart failure. Since this was in the absence of any external or internal stress, it suggested that these tissues require microRNAs for *normal function*. So, while some adult tissues and organs can carry out functions without a working pool of microRNAs, other tissues could not, requiring active microRNA function in normal as well as stressed conditions. The study was important in one further aspect. It confirmed some of the reservations about the knockout approach to learn about microRNA function. When Dicer is knocked out in later life, the heart and the skeletal muscles of mice remain normal, presumably because of the long-lasting nature of the muscle microRNAs. The T6B system allowed rapid block of microRNA function and revealed that microRNA function was indeed important in those systems. We must remember, of course, that the T6B peptide could have had interactions with components of pathways beyond the microRNA system. Also, some microRNA actions escaped the effect of the T6B peptide. In particular, the team were not able to get the T6B system to work in the brain. Finally, the studies were in mice and findings may be different in other organisms.

Missing Individual MicroRNAs

It is estimated that each of the core microRNA families, 90 that we share all the way back to our last common ancestor with fish, has more than 400 conserved human mRNA targets. That is consistent with estimates that more than 60 per cent of human mRNAs are under microRNA control. It is likely that no developmental or physiological process in our cells occurs without microRNA influence. But how important are specific, individual microRNAs? What happens if you delete just one, leaving the others working just fine? Does this have any measurable effect? If so, loss of which microRNA produces an effect? Under what conditions? Targeting individual microRNAs has been tried in various species, including the common model organisms. The earliest work was performed in *C. elegans*. Some of the leading groups that discovered how microRNAs function and the biogenesis pathway in *C. elegans* also led efforts to systematically delete microRNAs from *C. elegans* and record the results. They found that many microRNAs could be disrupted without obvious effects on the worms. In contrast, deleting individual and families of microRNAs in flies produced harmful outcomes much more often. Harmful effects of deleting microRNA families also emerge in mammals. A majority of the 90 core microRNA families have now been targeted in mice.[98] Detrimental effects of knocking out a microRNA family have been reported for more than half of those tested. That is, under normal lab conditions, the deletion of a microRNA produces animals that do not appear normal. In some cases, the abnormalities are severe, with reduced lifespans or severely disrupted functions of the nervous system and cancers. Deletion of others results in animals that develop and function and are indistinguishable from their microRNA-intact littermates. This suggests that there is redundancy among microRNAs or that some systems are more tolerant than others of losing their microRNAs. Other microRNAs, or indeed other regulatory systems entirely, may compensate owing to overlapping functions, buffering the molecular pathway in the absence of a microRNA. Phenotypes appear more often, however, when microRNA-deficient animals are stressed. That is, push the system and weaknesses and failings begin to emerge. In some contexts, compensation is not possible.

We must be slightly careful in extrapolating the mouse findings to humans. The mature microRNA may be identical in mice and humans, but the target site of a microRNA on the 3' UTR may not be identical. A mouse microRNA may regulate slightly different genes from its human equivalent. Another factor to bear in mind is the difference between knockout, where both copies of the gene are removed, and heterozygosity, where one copy remains. In most cases, a microRNA phenotype is observed only when a full knockout is made. With one copy remaining, phenotypes are less common. Thus, even if it is half the normal level, some expression of a microRNA can be enough to manage the particular actions on targets without noticeable problems.

We will not go through all the results of knocking out different microRNAs in mice. A very brief scan-through shows multiple systems and developmental impacts. For simplicity, I have not indicated whether this is a single microRNA or a family of microRNAs. Some microRNAs appear multiple times. Infertility occurs in mice if we knock out the genes for miR-7, miR-9, miR-34 or miR-200; mice display heart defects after removal of miR-1, miR-133 or miR-145, altered liver function following knockout of miR-122 or miR-429, altered pancreas function with loss of miR-7, miR-184 or miR-375, abnormal brain development with loss of miR-9 and miR-199, immune and blood system failings (knockout of miR-29, miR-31, miR-125, miR-150, miR-223, miR-451 and many others) and sensory impairments (loss of miR-211). Several knockouts result in lethal phenotypes, either pre- or postnatal. This includes removal of miR-9, miR-19, miR-34, miR-92, miR-124, miR-126, miR-137, miR-181, miR-218 and miR-219.[98]

Heart of the Matter

As a general rule, the severity of the phenotype increases when more than one member of a microRNA family is disrupted. What were some of the most interesting results of these systematic efforts to look at microRNA gene knockouts? Let's start with miR-1. This is the most abundant microRNA that can be detected in the heart. Another important cardiac microRNA is miR-206, which shares the same seed region and thus its targets overlap with miR-1. Humans and mice actually have two different genomic loci with a gene for miR-1.

They are generated along with another, miR-133a, which is important for gene programmes in striated (voluntary) muscle. In line with the naming conventions we met in Chapter 1, these are miR-1-1 and miR-1-2. The mature forms are identical and arose because of a duplication event in the genome. Presumably there was sufficient evolutionary pressure to keep both. The double miR-1 gene complicates experiments, however, because if you want to know what happens if you are completely missing miR-1, you actually have to knock out two genes. As a result, the first effort to knock out miR-1 led by a team at the University of California, San Francisco, in 2007, removed only one of the two, miR-1-2.[120] This was picked as it showed a slightly earlier switch-on during embryo development. Fully deleting miR-1-2 resulted in a 50 per cent reduction in overall miR-1 levels. This reduction was sufficient, however, to produce various cardiac problems in the mice, including holes in the heart called a ventricular septal defect. Although many mice did not survive, some did. Echocardiography on the survivors, an ultrasound technique used to look at the heart in action, appeared normal in the survivor mice. But the survivors, managing with just miR-1-1, had electrical conduction faults and thicker heart walls and the mice often died suddenly, in episodes akin to heart attacks. The team also looked into what happened to gene expression in mice lacking miR-1-2. A large set of transcription factors and cell cycle regulators were found to be increased, which may have destabilised gene programmes in the heart and contributed to the abnormalities. **Figure 4.2** shows examples of the findings in the mice lacking miR-1-2 in the heart.

In a subsequent effort, the same team investigated the effect of removing miR-1-1.[121] This produced similar outcomes as were seen in the miR-1-2 knockouts, including cardiac conduction defects. They then bred these mice with the mice lacking miR-1-2, creating full miR-1 knockouts. None of the double-miR-1-deficient mice survived beyond 10 days after birth. Heart defects in the complete miR-1-null mice were more severe than in either of the single-miR-1 knockout mice. This included more obvious structural defects in the heart walls and a much more disorganised electrical rhythm by electrocardiogram (EKG). Delving into what was happening at the level of individual heart cells, they found that they did not display the correct organisation of the contractile proteins that are part of the mechanism to

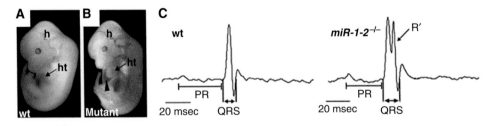

Figure 4.2 Cardiac phenotypes in mice lacking miR-1

Panels A and B show a wild-type embryo at day 12.5 and an embryo from a mouse in which miR-1-2 was specifically deleted from the heart (using a Cre recombinase under the control of the Nkx2.5 gene, which is active early in cardiac progenitor cells). Note the developmental delay and the pericardial oedema (arrowhead).

Key: ht, heart; h, head.

Panel C shows examples of electrocardiograms. The second peak in the QRS complex (R') is observed in more than half of mutant mice.

Source: Reprinted with permission from Zhao et al., *Cell*, vol. 129, pp. 303–17 (2007).[120]

change length. This could be partly rescued by injecting heart cells with copies of miR-1. One of the targets of miR-1 found was a smooth muscle protein called Telokin. A key function of Telokin is to keep smooth muscles in a less contractile state. Without miR-1, levels of Telokin were higher than normal, contributing to the poor contractile properties of the miR-1-deficient hearts. Put another way, a key job for miR-1 is ensuring that heart muscle has the correct properties by preventing expression of genes that define the properties of other muscle types. Thus, miR-1 has an essential role in the development and contractility of the mammalian heart.

The Blinding Effects of MicroRNA Loss

In any system where a microRNA is enriched or particularly abundant, there is often a phenotype when that microRNA is deleted, whether a change when the system is first forming, an altered function in adulthood, or an incomplete or failed response to a stress or insult. Let us zoom in on one other interesting example in relation to the importance of microRNAs in the visual system. Your visual system has two main parts: the sensory organ itself, the eye, and the wiring system that takes the information on what you have seen and processes it to produce what you perceive is in front of you. The front part of the eye is where light first enters. Light strikes the cornea and then the lens. As it passes through, light gets bent or refracted and this produces an image at the back of the eye. The job of eyeglasses is to adjust this light-bending power, either increasing or decreasing, to produce a sharp image where the natural structure of the eye is unable to do this. The bent light passes all the way through to the back of the eye where it hits the retina. The retina is the inner layer of the eye and is made up of three sub-layers (see **Figure 4.3A**). The deepest layer, farthest from the cornea/front of the eye, has light-sensitive cells. These are specialised neurones called photoreceptors that send signals when struck by light to another cell type they contact called bipolar cells. The bipolar cells connect to the cell in front called a ganglion cell, also a type of neurone. The ganglion cells possess a very long projection called an axon, which, together with the axons of neighbouring ganglion cells, are bundled together to form the optic nerve. This fibre bundle travels out of the back of the eye to carry the signal deep into the brain and towards the various regions that process and interpret visual information. Humans have two main classes of photoreceptor cells. The most abundant are called rods. The others are called cones. Light sensitivity comes from proteins made inside the photoreceptor cells, called opsins. These are concentrated in plate-like stacks at the end of the photoreceptor called the outer segment. Embedded within the opsin protein is a molecule derived from vitamin A with a kink-like structure that when struck by light changes shape. This change means that the opsin is now activated and contacts other proteins within the cell. The effect of this cascade of signals is to alter the electrical charge on the surface of the photoreceptor. In the case of rods, the cells become more negatively charged. When this happens, it interrupts the release of a neurotransmitter that communicates between the photoreceptor and the bipolar cell. That change prompts the ganglion cell to send nerve impulses down its axon and into the brain's visual system. Thus, photoreceptors convert incoming light into a signal that the brain can understand and thus you can 'see'. The signals from different photoreceptors are useful in different ways for vision. Under normal or daylight conditions, we use cone cell information. Cone pigments require stronger light to work. Humans have three different types, each with a different colour-sensitive pigment. This allows them to react to different wavelengths – colours – of light. By mixing and matching the signals coming from the three different cone cells, the brain can decode the colour of what we are seeing

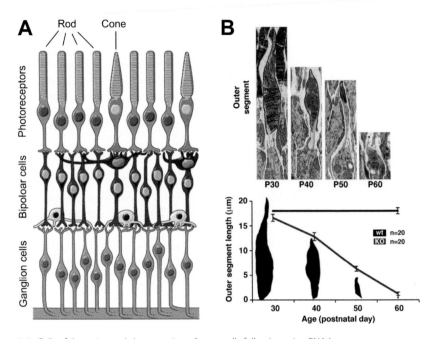

Figure 4.3 Cells of the retina and degeneration of cone cells following microRNA loss

Panel A shows the layers of the retina with the two types of photoreceptor cells, bipolar and ganglion cells (the axons of which form the optic nerve).

Panel B shows scanning electron microscopy images of cone photoreceptors in mice with a post-natal deletion (KO) of *Dgcr8*. The graph and the outlines of representative cones confirm the reduction in size over time compared to wild-type (wt) mice.

Source: Panel A image from Servier Medical Art. Servier Medical Art by Servier is licensed under a Creative Commons Attribution 3.0 Unported License (https://creativecommons.org/licenses/by/3.0/). Panel B reprinted with permission from Busskamp et al., *Neuron*, vol. 83, pp. 586–600 (2014).[123]

by comparing the signals from cones tuned to different wavelengths of light. This way, we cover the red-orange-yellow-green-blue-indigo-violet spectrum that we are able to see. Interestingly, most mammals, including mice, have only two types of cone cell, tuned to short (S) (blues) and medium (M) (greens) light wavelengths. Our third class, termed L cones, react to longer wavelengths and allow us to see the red end of the spectrum. Researchers suspect that these co-evolved as part of fruit-heavy diets in primate ancestors. Clever experiments published in *Science* by teams at the University of California and Johns Hopkins University in the USA demonstrated that if you insert the gene for the L cones into mice, this allows them to see the red end of the spectrum.[122]

Cones also give us sharp images. The ability to recognise small details and differences in what we are looking at with precision is a property called visual acuity. This is because right at the back of the eye, where light falls directly when we look straight at an image, is the fovea. Here, cone cells lie immediately in line with the bipolar and ganglion cells in a 1:1:1 ratio. So, if light strikes a cone, it sends a signal towards a single ganglion cell lying immediately in front of it. The rods are most useful when light levels are low. Rod photoreceptors are fantastically sensitive, able to react to a single photon of light, but they absorb light across a wider spectrum and there is only one 'flavour' of rod cell. So, information the brain receives from rod cells cannot be used to distinguish different wavelengths, but is great for low-light conditions. Rods are also poor at providing sharp images. Several rods are typically wired up to the same ganglion cell. The brain can't tell if the light struck a rod slightly to the left or to the right because they both send their signal to the same ganglion cell in the middle. The images generated are not as sharp as from cones. If you want to check this yourself, go into a dark room. Wait a few minutes to let your visual system adjust, switching to rod-only signals (the light is too weak to activate your cones), and then look around. You will notice two things. First, the image is a bit fuzzy and second, everything is shades of grey. That is your rod-only vision.

When researchers first began to study the effect of deleting *Dicer* in mouse embryos, they noticed that eye development was strongly impaired. Researchers then asked if microRNAs continued to be needed after formation of the eye. Taking this on board, and using the more specific approach of deleting *Dgcr8*, a team at the Friedrich Miescher Institute for Biomedical Research in Basel, Switzerland (where Filipowicz studied microRNA turnover) took on this challenge.[123] They also restricted the microRNA deletion to just cone cells. By the time the mice lacking *Dgcr8* had reached two months of age, most microRNAs were no longer detectable in cones, but were unaltered in the rods. This was accompanied by a major reduction in opsins inside the photoreceptor cells. In fact, the outer segment of the cone cell, the portion containing the opsins, degenerated in the mice lacking *Dgcr8* (see **Figure 4.3B**). Consistent with this, the cone cells of mice lacking microRNAs, while still present in the retina, no longer reacted to light. This could be partially rescued by introducing two of the most eye-enriched microRNAs, miR-182 and miR-183, into cone cells. These two microRNAs originate from the miR-183/96/182 cluster, a set of three microRNAs that originate from the same precursor, located in mice on chromosome 6.

The function of the miR-183/96/182 cluster has been tackled by a number of different teams using knockout approaches. In 2013, a joint team from universities in Chicago and Baltimore performed a knockout of the full cluster.[124] The mice survived and were generally healthy. The retinas of mice at five weeks of age looked normal. But recordings from the retina could already detect reduced functional properties, measured by a technique called an electroretinogram. As time went on, the structure of the retina changed, becoming thinner as cells were lost. The number and the size of contact points between photoreceptors and bipolar cells also reduced. By one year of age, the retina electroretinogram signal in mice lacking the microRNA cluster was almost undetectable. The retina deficit was worse for cone-related vision, suggesting that the rods were less reliant on these microRNAs. The retinas of mice lacking the cluster were also more easily damaged when exposed to very bright light. The team went on to find that more than 1,000 genes were being controlled by the miR-183/96/182 cluster. One of the genes encoded cone opsins, but there were many others, including increased levels of some transcripts that promote inflammation. The findings indicate that mice need microRNAs from the miR-183/96/182 cluster to maintain proper function and survival of cone cells.

The importance of the individual members of the cluster was further teased apart in a paper by a Chinese team from Wenzhou a few years later.[125] Rather than the full knockout of the miR-183/96/182 cluster, they inactivated only miR-183 and miR-96, leaving miR-182 alone. As with the complete knockout, the retinas of young mice were outwardly healthy. But, on closer inspection, subtle differences were found. This included a reduction in the size of the part of the cell containing the light-sensitive pigments. By the time the mice were a month old, electroretinogram responses were already abnormal and this persisted in older mice. Again, both rod and cone responses were diminished, but cones were more severely affected. And, as time went on, the retinas became thinner and signs of inflammation developed. The team also helped identify more of the targets of the cluster. One of the transcripts, called *Slc6a6*, encodes a transporter of the amino acid taurine. Taurine is required for photoreceptor function but, for reasons not fully understood, too much of it is toxic to photoreceptors. Indeed, when the team mimicked the effect of losing miR-183/96 by overloading photoreceptors with *Slc6a6*, the cells died. Of course, this is just one target. What about the hundreds of other genes that changed when miR-183/96 were deleted? Comparing the miR-183/96 findings to features in mice lacking only miR-182 indicates a more important role for miR-183 and miR-96. The study did not reveal whether combined or single actions of miR-183 and miR-96 were equally important.

Overall, these studies reveal the importance of this microRNA cluster in eye development and its necessity for ongoing retinal function in the adult eye. A final point of interest was that the mice lacking miR-183 and miR-96 had other sensory deficits that were not obviously related to the progressive blindness. The animals displayed unusual circling behaviour and an unsteady walk. The team found that the microRNA cluster was also expressed in other sensory organs and the researchers speculated that deficits in the vestibular system, which creates our sense of balance and orientation, may have been to blame.

What About Unique-to-Human MicroRNAs?

Most of what we have learnt about individual mammalian microRNAs we have learnt from mice. Less is known of the importance of more recently evolved microRNAs, including those unique to humans. We can 'humanise' mice to determine the importance of a microRNA unique to humans, but it is an imperfect solution. And there are hundreds of human-specific microRNAs. An easier approach is using human cells. We now have the ability to produce many different types of human cell. The technology of induced pluripotent stem cells (iPSCs) allows us to create a flexible cell source that, by feeding it with the right cocktail of chemicals or genes, can convert into any cell we want, heart cells, liver cells, brain cells and so on. So we can learn where these human-specific microRNAs are made in the body, use iPSCs to generate a model of that cell type, and then proceed to up- or down-regulate the microRNA and study how this affects function or predicted target genes. The technology to create organoids may take this further. Organoids are 3D cell clusters that, when grown properly, develop multiple cell types and the features of a tissue. These offer a closer step towards a model of an intact human that could be used to study the importance of a specific microRNA in human organ function. There are also additional options. Tissue is sometimes removed during biopsies for health surveillance, diagnosis or treatment. Keeping this tissue alive is another potential route to uncover what human-specific microRNAs do. We must also remember that finding a phenotype when knocking out a specific microRNA does not tell us which of the target genes is responsible. That is, which of the possibly hundreds of targets of that microRNA, now more abundant because of the loss of a layer of microRNA control, drives the observed abnormality. This requires a further experiment to mutate 3' UTR sites for that microRNA and find which one 'phenocopies' or matches the microRNA knockout. This is a challenging experiment. While a single site or a few sites could be mutated, perhaps picking those most conserved or where the biological pathway is most plausibly linked to the observed phenotype, complete assessment would require multiple and possibly hundreds of edits to 3' UTRs. We are approaching a time when this is technically possible. Genome editing tools such as CRISPR allow precise edits to sequences at scale. But it could be a fool's errand. The modest repressive effect of most microRNAs on their targets would require exquisitely sensitive assays to detect an effect of disrupting a single or a few microRNA targeting points on a given mRNA. We will see whether there is an appetite among researchers, and the people who fund the work, to engage in such efforts.

The First MicroRNAs to the Show

Let us now look at the earliest moments of life. When do the first microRNAs begin to fine-tune gene expression? Which microRNAs are specific to this period and what are some of the processes they control? **Figure 4.4** provides a simple outline of the early stages of human embryo development. I will focus on mammalian development and draw mainly from work on mice since the limited availability and the ethical restrictions on studies of human embryos mean that our understanding is less complete.

The broad requirement for microRNAs at very early stages of development had been demonstrated back in 2003 by Hannon's team. Deletion of *Dicer* in mice had resulted in the arrest of embryo development by the end of the first week, a third of the way through the normal 21-day gestational period of a mouse. Earlier that same year, Sharp's team at MIT had found sets of microRNAs that were specific to embryonic stem cells in mice.[30] These cells make up a structure called the inner cell mass of the blastocyst, from which the embryo develops. They are a very special type of cell, capable of dividing indefinitely. They are also a blank slate, able to become any cell type in the body given the right signals. The blastocyst stage of embryo development happens three to four days after fertilisation in mice and about five days after fertilisation in humans. The stage before the blastocyst is called the morula, when the early embryo is a ball of just 16 cells. Before that were eight, four and two cells, having undergone the first cell division after fertilisation of the egg by a sperm. A set of transcription factors are critical at this time, before cell differentiation takes place, including OCT4 and NANOG. Their activity is essential for maintaining cells in an undifferentiated state and allowing rapid cell division and exponential growth. From the morula stage, cell differentiation leads to three defined structures. Trophoblast cells form an outer wall and surround a cavity that contains the inner cell mass. In humans, blastocyst formation happens towards the end of the passage through the fallopian tube and about two days before implantation in the wall of the uterus. Within the blastocyst, several further rounds of cell division occur and there are about 200–300 cells by the time of implantation. The trophoblast will go on to combine with the endometrial wall of the uterus and form the placenta. The blastocyst's inner cell mass, also known as the embryoblast, comprises a ball of embryonic stem cells from which two key structures develop. One part is called the primitive endoderm and will develop into the amniotic sac in which the embryo grows during pregnancy. The second part is the epiblast, from which the three so-called germ cell layers form: endoderm, mesoderm and ectoderm. Together, these three layers generate the more than 200 major cell types in the human body. The first of these, the endoderm, will

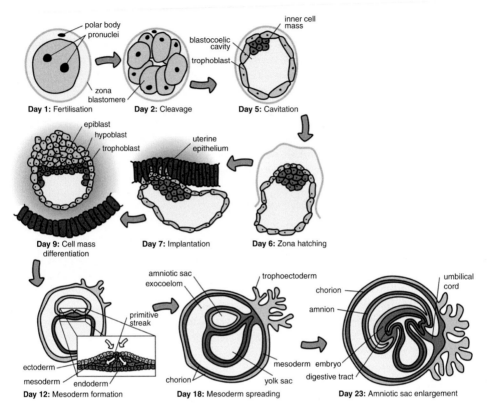

Figure 4.4 Stages of human embryonic development

This shows an illustrated sequence of some of the early stages of human embryonic development, beginning with fertilisation and up to the third week post-fertilisation.

Source: Adapted (some panels removed for simplicity) from original by Zephyris – SVG version of, CC BY-SA 3.0, https://commons.wikimedia.org/w/index.php?curid=10811330.

give rise to the epithelial cells of the body that line the walls of various organs, including a large part of the gut and lungs. The mesoderm gives rise to all three types of muscle (heart, skeletal and smooth), the notochord (a key organising structure and component of the future vertebrate column), tissue of the skin and bone, kidneys, gonads and red and white blood cells. The ectoderm gives rise to structures including the brain, the spinal cord and peripheral nerves as well as skin cells.

Embryonic stem cells possess pluripotency, the ability to form any cell type in the body, and self-renewal, the ability to divide indefinitely. The identification of microRNAs in embryonic stem cells therefore reflects active roles shaping two fundamental cellular processes with scientific and medical applications. Sharp's team searched for microRNAs in undifferentiated embryonic stem cells from mice, using the presence of the *Oct4* transcript, which is dramatically down-regulated upon differentiation, as one of the markers of undifferentiated stem cell-ness. At the time, no microRNAs had been obtained from early embryos. Extracting short RNAs from the embryonic stem cells, they were able to identify various microRNAs, some of which had never previously been described. This included a set of six microRNAs, numbered miR-290 to miR-295. All six microRNAs came from a common precursor, a microRNA cluster termed miR-290~295. Their expression was not detected in more differentiated cells or adult tissues. This indicated a role restricted to embryonic stem cells and the period of time before implantation of the embryo. Importantly, there were human versions of the embryonic stem cell cluster microRNAs. That was as far as the study went, so the targets of these were unknown. But that knowledge gap began to close quickly with follow-up studies. Later studies would show that miR-290~295 cluster microRNAs regulate a step in the cell cycle in embryonic stem cells. This is the cycle of duplicating DNA and then splitting the cell in two (mitosis). Embryonic stem cells have a shorter phase called G1, a growth phase when the cell readies itself for DNA replication (S phase) and prior to splitting to create two daughter cells. This is critical to the ability to rapidly generate new cells. The miR-290~295 microRNAs suppress inhibitors of the G1/S phase transition, thereby maintaining a fast cell division cycle. Among the identified targets were p21 (cyclin-dependent kinase 1a), a known inhibitor of the G1/S phase transition, as well as other regulators of this cell cycle phase. Thus, these microRNAs maintain the proliferative ability of embryonic stem cells via control of the molecular machinery of the cell cycle.

More recently, a team from the Swiss Federal Institute (ETH [Eidgenössische Technische Hochschule]) in Zurich took a systematic approach to identifying the targets of this microRNA cluster. They generated mouse embryonic stem cells lacking *Dicer*, *Drosha* and *Agos 1* and *2*, to completely remove microRNA production and function from the cells.[126] This resulted in de-repression of all transcripts controlled by microRNAs, including any regulated by the miR-290~295 cluster. The gene lists were refined further based on alignment predictions and AGO pull-downs, resulting in a set of 759 targets. This represented 7 per cent of all expressed genes, suggesting that microRNAs repress a relatively smaller percentage of targets at this early stage of organism development. The predicted point of interaction of the microRNAs on these mRNAs was overwhelmingly in the 3' UTRs and used 7-mer seeds. This demonstrated that the early embryonic period abides by the standard rules of engagement. Some of the mRNA targets displayed large numbers of sites for microRNAs, indicating cooperative actions of microRNAs. Half of all the mRNA targets that changed in the mutant embryonic stem cells were predicted to be regulated by one or more members of the miR-290~295 cluster, confirming a major role for this group of microRNAs. Complementary experiments deleting the miR-290~295 cluster from mouse embryonic stem cells resulted in increased levels of more than 1,000 transcripts. This list was then refined to a set of about 100 high-confidence direct targets of the six microRNAs in the cluster. Among these were a set of 14 transcription factors that control early pluripotency. One of these, TFAP4, was experimentally validated as a master regulator. When the researchers modelled the effect of microRNA control on TFAP4 expression, it changed the levels of nearly 500 genes, a sizeable portion of all the genes regulated by the cluster. Many of those genes have functions in differentiation and stem-ness. The ETH study also found that deleting the miR-290~295 cluster in mice resulted in failure of many embryos to develop beyond an early stage. The findings reveal that large-scale control of gene expression in embryonic stem cells is achieved by a small number of microRNAs via actions on a small number of transcription factors. The miR-

290~295 cluster effectively restrains the various programmes that are ramping up to move beyond the blastocyst stage, ready to forge ahead to generate endoderm and epiblast. The microRNAs from the miR-290~295 cluster are there to curb the enthusiasm of all this developmental machinery.

A second embryonic stem cell–specific cluster of microRNAs was identified in 2004.[127] This was a set of eight microRNAs, later named the miR-302/367 cluster, and was located on human chromosome 4, a different chromosome from the miR-290~295 cluster. This provided a more complete picture of how the transcriptional programmes in embryonic stem cells are coordinated. The miR-302/367 cluster is not restricted to mammals, and is present in some form in all vertebrates, probably evolving at the branch of the animal kingdom that led to tetrapods. It is therefore older in evolutionary terms than the miR-290~295 cluster. Various targets of these microRNAs have been identified. They include cell cycle control enzymes that regulate the G1-to-S phase transition, including p21. There are also targets of miR-302/367 that control DNA methylation, important for the soon-to-begin phases of shutting down certain genes as development proceeds. Thus, both clusters converge on some of the same targets and processes, strengthening repression and ensuring redundancy for what is a critical phase of embryo development.

Some of the mechanisms which ensure that the right amount of these embryonic stem cell cluster microRNAs is produced are also understood. Sequences around the miR-290~295 and the miR-302/367 cluster loci attract transcription factors active in embryonic stem cells, including OCT4 and NANOG. Thus, expression of the embryonic stem cell microRNAs is driven by key transcription factors that maintain the pluripotent state. Another transcription factor linked to switching on the miR-290~295 cluster is growth arrest and DNA damage 45, GADD45. Teams from Guangzhou, China, showed that GADD45 binds to the promoter region of the miR-290~295 cluster and creates a more open chromatin state, permitting access to the transcriptional machinery.[128] The transcription factor c-Myc has also been shown to promote expression of a member of this cluster (miR-294). But if the embryo is to transition to the next stage, with production of the three germ cell layers, then key factors maintaining embryonic stem cell states must be silenced. This includes OCT4, which has been active pre- and post-fertilisation of the maternal oocyte, guiding the gene expression programmes that maintain pluripotency and self-renewal. The Oct4 gene locus becomes closed down by epigenetic processes including methylation of the DNA. In 2008, Filipowicz's team demonstrated that a key function of the miR-290~295 cluster is to coordinate the switches that transition from pluripotency to differentiation.[129] They showed that in the absence of miR-290~295 microRNAs, a set of transcriptional repressors, which included retinoblastoma-like 2 (RBL2), block the machinery for DNA methylation, leaving Oct4 active. A key function of the cluster, therefore, is to suppress these transcriptional repressors, and facilitate epigenetic silencing of Oct4 in embryonic stem cells. Since OCT4 as well as the transcription factors SOX2 and NANOG promote expression of the embryonic stem cell microRNAs such as the miR-302/367 cluster, their levels follow a similar fate, declining in expression until they too become silent. The shut-down of the microRNA core support for embryonic stem cells is normally permanent in differentiated cells. However, studies show that these microRNAs can be reawakened in cancer where they can contribute to self-renewal once again that leads to uncontrolled proliferation and disease. Studies continue to explore the number, type and function of microRNAs during the earliest stages of embryo development. The clock has been pushed even further back, with researchers identifying microRNAs after first division, when the embryo is in the two-cell stage. MicroRNAs are present from the very beginning and their levels increase rapidly even before the blastocyst stage.

MicroRNAs, Hox Genes and Patterning the Developing Embryo

Perhaps fittingly for a book on the conductors of the molecular orchestra, we come now to Hox genes. These genes are conductors of embryo development, switching on early to direct the correct patterns of gene expression that produce the anterior–posterior (front–back) axis of the body and features such as limbs and vertebrae.[130] Humans have 39 Hox genes, on 4 different chromosomes, organised in sets running in sequence together, a formation known as colinearity. Their expression is highly organised with both spatial and temporal components. The Hox genes at the front or 3' end of the cluster are expressed earlier and in more anterior structures, whereas those members expressed at the tail or 5' end of the gene cluster are expressed later in development and at the posterior end. Hox genes switch on in a staggered fashion, with waves of expression working collectively in specifying features during development. All proteins encoded by Hox genes are transcription factors, capable of promoting or repressing expression of genes during development. This is important since a role of Hox genes is to ensure that a feature such as a rib is not only present where it should be but absent from locations where it should not be. The coordinate actions of Hox genes ensure such correct body plan patterning. Their encoded proteins all share a DNA binding region called a homeobox and most eukaryotes (animals, plants and fungi) have Hox genes. They are kept silent during the blastula phase, beginning to switch on during the gastrulation phase of embryo development. Their effects on the body plan are highly conserved, as demonstrated by classic experiments that showed a chicken version of a Hox gene could substitute for the deleted equivalent in the fly *D. melanogaster*.[131]

Expression of Hox genes is tightly controlled through promoters and enhancers and intensely regulated post-transcriptionally by microRNAs. In fact, microRNA genes are embedded among Hox gene clusters. It was Tuschl's group who, in a paper in 2003 identifying a further 31 microRNAs in mouse and human, first mapped a microRNA to a Hox gene locus, lying between *Hox4* and *Hox5*.[24] However, it was Bartel's team who first experimentally demonstrated that microRNAs regulated Hox gene transcript levels (**Figure 4.5**). In a 2004 study in *Science*, the team identified near-perfect complementarity between miR-196 and a sequence in the 3' UTR of *HOXB8*.[132] Expression of miR-196 appears towards the end of the first week post-fertilisation, indicating a role in gene expression during early embryogenesis. Consistent with the extensive homology between microRNA and target, miR-196's main mode of action was cleavage of the *HOXB8* mRNA. Several other Hox family transcripts were also found to be targets of miR-196, albeit with less complementarity, indicating that miR-196 was a master controller in early development via coordinated suppression of Hox levels. This is facilitated by the physical positioning of the gene for miR-196 in the genome, behind the Hox genes it targets. Owing to the sequential colinear expression, the Hox genes are activated first, followed by their microRNA repressor, to facilitate fine-tuning and switch-off. Additional processes regulated by Hox genes have also emerged as being under microRNA control. These include muscle development, a process repressed by HOXA11, the transcript for which is targeted

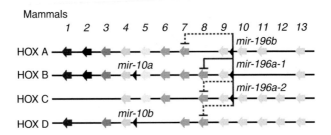

Figure 4.5 MicroRNAs embedded among Hox genes

The figure shows the genomic organisation of Hox clusters. The arrows indicate Hox genes representing 13 paralogous groups (genes related through duplication events). The black arrowheads indicate microRNA genes. The dotted lines indicate repression supported by predicted (bioinformatics) evidence only. The vertical dark-grey line indicates that microRNAs from any of the three loci could repress the targets.

Source: Reprinted with permission from Yekta et al., *Science*, vol. 304, pp. 594–6 (2004).[132]

by miR-181. This microRNA relieves the blocking effect of HOXA11 and promotes muscle cell differentiation. It later became clear that microRNAs could regulate expression of almost all members of the Hox gene family. As more microRNAs capable of regulating Hox gene expression emerged, a further feature was noted. The Hox-embedded microRNAs were skewed towards those Hox genes that expressed first, influencing the patterning of forward structures. Furthermore, the 3' Hox genes bore higher numbers of seed sites for microRNAs such as miR-196 than those expressed posteriorly. This imposes stronger regulation of those Hox gene transcripts. This has the effect of creating less restriction for the actions for posterior Hox genes, which creates posterior prevalence.[133] This is thought to be important for correct timing and patterning during vertebrate development, allowing later-expressed genes to exert their effects on a background of prior anterior Hox gene activity. In addition to providing a localised and tight regulatory environment for the genomic programmes that control major steps in development, the microRNAs embedded among Hox genes have been critical for vertebrate evolution and development.

MicroRNAs Make Gametes

Taking a step further back, there are important roles for microRNAs in the germline cells that give rise to gametes – sperm and egg cells.[134, 135] Development of germline cells and the gonads occurs very early during embryo development. The precursors of sperm and eggs are called primordial germ cells and originate from cells of the ectoderm and endoderm. This happens between five and six days post-fertilisation in the mouse and about two to three weeks post-implantation in humans. Specific signals ensure that key genes that drive differentiation, such as the Hox genes, do not switch on, while pluripotency factors, including OCT4, remain active. The primordial germ cells then migrate to where the gonads will eventually form, after which they differentiate to form germline stem cells and supporting tissue to produce gametes. A key role for microRNAs during this process in lower animals including *C. elegans* is the 'clearance' of maternal mRNAs from the primordial germ cells to ensure that they do not differentiate into somatic (i.e. non-reproductive) cells. MicroRNAs are also involved in regulating the cues that signal the migratory route of primordial germ cells. Classic studies in zebrafish showed that miR-430 performs several tasks that ensure the correct routing of these cells.[136] This includes clearing the directional cue protein stromal cell-derived factor 1α (SDF1α) during transit from previous domains. Another function of microRNAs is to support the maintenance of germline stem cells, where they regulate the process of cell division, for example regulating the G1/S phase checkpoint by repressing cell cycle inhibitors. This includes miR-7, which, along with other microRNAs, promotes germline stem cell divisions and maintains a pluripotent state, in part by repressing transcripts that would trigger differentiation. But differentiation is necessary to produce gametes. Here, other microRNAs have been found to be involved. MicroRNAs of the miR-17~92 cluster repress the E2F1 transcription factor, avoiding meiotic cells such as gametes being triggered to undergo programmed cell death. MicroRNA activity is also critical to the function of supporting 'nurse' cells within the testes. Loss of Dicer from these cells prevents production of sperm and leads to degeneration of the testes. Likewise, the cells that support the developing oocyte require microRNAs, with deletion of *Dicer* impairing development of the follicle cell mass that surrounds immature oocytes. Indeed, microRNAs perform key roles ensuring correct transcript levels of the various genes that regulate follicular development and oocyte maturation. Hormonal control of oogenesis and spermatogenesis is also regulated in a feedback loop by specific microRNAs. The microRNA machinery is not essential for gametogenesis in all species, however. For example, the germline cells in zebrafish can produce sperm and eggs without Dicer.

MicroRNAs That Ready the Next Generation

Can we step back further? Is there an earlier moment when microRNAs have an effect on organism development and future trajectories? Perhaps. Evidence has emerged that microRNAs are present inside the gametes, travelling as part of the molecular mix at the time of fertilisation. There was some initial scepticism about the biological importance of the transferred microRNAs owing to the low amounts involved. This view has changed and it is clear that gamete-borne microRNAs can have biological effects on the developing embryo. Remarkably, parental experiences affect the specific complement of these microRNAs and research suggests that this has the potential to convey effects on the offspring that alter embryo development enough to produce a measurable phenotype in the progeny. This is what is called parental or *intergenerational* effects. But *transgenerational* effects are also possible.[137] That is, environmental and other experiences in one or other parent are passed through to the second generation. Something a grandparent experiences shapes the grandchild's biology. The factors reported to convey the memory of ancestral environmental exposure include exposure to toxins, infection, altered diet and metabolism, and stress. The system appears to have evolved as a supplement to inherited genetic material to better prepare subsequent generations for conditions they will encounter, providing offspring with a survival advantage. But while such an ability has clear advantages for short life-cycle species such as *C. elegans*, where conditions met by the offspring may be very similar to those met by the parents, the value for long-lived species such as humans is less clear. Indeed, studies in mammals indicate that not all such inter- and transgenerational effects are beneficial. There are examples that are maladaptive and detrimental to the progeny. Gamete-delivered microRNAs are implicated in both inter- and transgenerational effects.

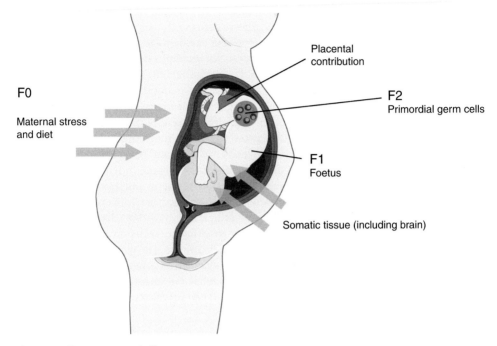

Figure 4.6 Transgenerational effects

Concept of maternally transmitted transgenerational effects. Maternal stress or diet perturbations (F0) can be transmitted via the placenta, resulting in timing-specific effects on the developing foetus (somatic tissues) that can lead to changes in long-term health outcomes in the first (F1) generation. In addition, primordial germ cells, which contribute genetic and epigenetic information to the second (F2) generation, are also present and undergo *in utero* programming during embryonic development.

Source: Adapted with permission from Dunn et al., *Hormones & Behavior*, vol. 59, pp. 290–5 (2011).[138] Main image from Servier Medical Art. Servier Medical Art by Servier is licensed under a Creative Commons Attribution 3.0 Unported License (https://creativecommons.org/licenses/by/3.0/).

Let us first briefly review the inter- and transgenerational concept (**Figure 4.6**). This refers to non-Mendelian inheritance of traits, separate from the paternal or maternal DNA, by which experiences in the parents pass on to subsequent generations. A variety of mechanisms have been discovered by which life-exposures get wired into the gametes, conferring effects on the next generation. These include molecules present within the gametes that produce effects on the growing embryo. The passage of such information occurs via epigenetic mechanisms, meaning that the exposure or 'experience information' is carried by something other than changes to the sequence of DNA. This includes chemical modifications of DNA bases such as methylation, the actions of proteins on chromatin, and certain non-coding RNAs. Intergenerational adaptive effects would seem the most plausible, providing information of more immediate value to the next generation but transgenerational effects nonetheless occur. One of the mechanisms proven for transgenerational effects is disruption of the normal patterns of silencing of repetitive elements such as transposons in the embryo. The 'memory' for these patterns of transposon silencing during embryogenesis is inherited and, if disrupted or changed by environmental factors in the parent, can take multiple generations to restore, at least in model organisms such as *C. elegans*. The strength of evidence and the mechanisms of true transgenerational effects in higher animals and humans are rather contentious, however.

There are some famous examples of transgenerational effects in humans. These include studies on the descendants of a population in northern Sweden who experienced famine in the late 19th and early 20th centuries. In such studies, the first-generation offspring are referred to as F1 and the second, the grandchildren, the F2 generation. Records showed that mortality from diabetes in the F2 generation, the grandchildren, tracked with exposure of the paternal grandparent to abundant nutrition during the pre-puberty life stage. The mortality risk for granddaughters was associated with the paternal grandmother's food supply. A more recent Swedish study, this time using a much larger population from Uppsala, replicated some of these findings, reporting that pre-puberty exposure of the grandfather predicts male, but not female, grandchild mortality, although this was not specific to diabetes as had been reported for the Överkalix cohort.[139] A Dutch study followed the health outcomes in the grandchildren of women who bore children during the Second World War when the Nazi-occupied Netherlands experienced extreme food shortages.[140] Effects on birth weights and other outcomes have been detected transmitted from maternal grandmother through to granddaughter as well as through the male line. For example, the adult offspring (F2) of prenatally exposed F1 fathers had higher weights and body mass indices than the offspring of prenatally unexposed F1 fathers. No such effect was found for the F2 offspring of prenatally exposed F1 mothers. Of course, epidemiological studies cannot control for certain factors, but the effects of under- and over-nutrition of parents on the progeny are reproducible in multiple model species with both inter- and transgenerational effects demonstrated under laboratory conditions. For example, many studies show that feeding male mice a high-fat diet increases obesity in the next generation and the one after that. Such effects are influenced by the age of the parent at the time of exposure to the experience and the sex of the progeny. In some cases, counter-intuitively, both low- and high-sugar diet exposure has been reported to produce similar effects on adiposity, the amount of fat/fatty tissue, in the next generation. Besides diet and nutrition, there are several other factors that can have transgenerational effects. These include cigarette smoking and drug use, stress and parental behaviours. The effects of stress are one of the most intensely studied and bring in the wider issue of inter- and transgenerational effects on brain development.[141] Studies in mice show that traumatic stress, modelled by unpredictable maternal separation combined with unpredictable maternal stress, transmits multiple effects onto the F1 and F2 offspring.[142] These include lower innate anxiety and fear-responses, which can be interpreted as increased risk-taking, as well as depressive-like behaviours. The F2 offspring in this model also display hypermetabolism and increased insulin sensitivity. There are also cross-over effects with dietary exposures affecting brain-related functions. The Dutch children of the adults from the hunger winter of 1944–5 were also at higher risk of psychosis, suggesting transmission of nutritional effects that can affect neurodevelopment.

The idea that factors besides the genome sequence are contained in gametes has been known for some time. This includes several proteins in sperm cells that are critical for fertilisation to occur. But these do not convey transgenerational effects. Researchers have been trying to identify what it is, besides DNA, in the gametes that conveys such exposure information. In the early 2000s, this list grew to include microRNA.[143] While not abundant, there are a variety of different microRNAs that have been identified in sperm, including sperm that are predicted to have fertilising capacity in humans. Oocytes also contain a diverse catalogue of microRNAs. These are not the same microRNAs as are expressed in the embryonic stem cells. They include a set that have been shown to be absent in the unfertilised egg, present in one-cell embryos after fertilisation, but absent again by the two-cell stage. This indicates that the microRNAs came from the sperm and the list includes miR-34b, -34c, -99a, -214, -451 and -449. Studies have confirmed that these, such as miR-34c, are bound to AGO2 in sperm and thus ready to function. Experiments proved that the transfer process can work by loading artificial microRNAs into sperm and confirming their later presence in the zygote. The transferred microRNA can have important effects during embryogenesis. For example, inhibiting miR-34c in the fertilised zygote at the one-cell stage occasionally prevented first division and the formation of the two-cell embryo, at least in mice.[144]

Several factors associated with intergenerational and transgenerational inheritance of traits can affect the composition of microRNA in gametes, including sperm.[137, 141] The microRNA contingent of the gametes appears to be able to convey core environmental exposures, in the broadest sense, to the next generation. Using the unpredictable maternal separation combined with unpredictable maternal stress paradigm, researchers found that the sperm of F1 mice display elevated levels of various microRNAs including miR-200b, miR-375, miR-466 and miR-672. MicroRNA levels were also altered in brain structures associated with stress responses in the F1 mice. The traumatic stress experience did not extend to affecting the microRNA composition of F2 sperm,[142] although altered brain microRNA levels were found in these animals, suggesting a partial transgenerational effect on microRNAs in response to stress. In another study, the injection of sperm RNAs from traumatic stress–exposed males into wild-type fertilised oocytes resulted in offspring with comparable metabolic and behavioural changes to the trauma-exposed mice. There are other examples of stress effects conveyed by microRNAs in sperm. Exposing mice to chronic variable stress, a mixture of physical restraint, light exposure and predator odours, either during puberty or as adults, results in a general increase in microRNA content in sperm as well as differences in sperm microRNA profiles between those animals exposed at the two different life-stages.[145] Some of the microRNAs overlap between studies, such as elevated levels of miR-375. Later functional studies modelled the altered patterns of microRNA in sperm by injecting fertilised zygotes at the one-cell stage with a set of nine microRNAs (miR-29c, miR-30a, miR-30c, miR-32, miR-193, miR-204, miR-375, miR-532 and miR-698).[146] The injected zygotes were then implanted into surrogate females. When the offspring were studied, they were found to display subdued stress responses compared to the offspring from oocytes with a normal microRNA contingent. A key brain region central to stress responses, the paraventricular nucleus, displayed altered levels, mainly down-regulation, of nearly 300 genes. The findings provide evidence that sperm RNA can mediate intergenerational effects and highlight how early-life exposure to traumatic experiences can have effects across generations.

There are also studies showing that parental health and environmental exposures affect sperm microRNAs, potentially conveying effects to future generations. When male mice are fed a high-fat diet that produces obesity but not diabetes, the F1 and F2 offspring, despite been maintained on a normal diet, develop obesity and insulin resistance.[147] The sperm of the founder males again has been found to contain higher levels of a set of microRNAs. Environmental contaminants including nicotine have also been demonstrated to alter the microRNA content of sperm, potentially providing a route of transmission of information that could affect the health of the next generation.

How do sperm microRNAs produce the transgenerational effects? There appear to be several mechanisms. The most direct is via suppressive effects on mRNA transcripts, altering patterns of early gene expression by modifying levels of key transcription factors in the embryo. This has been directly demonstrated, with injection of microRNAs linked to intergenerational stress-related changes resulting in down-regulation of transcripts in single-cell zygotes including *Sirt1*, a coordinator of transcriptional activity.[146] Another, non-mutually exclusive mechanism is via effects on DNA methylation. MicroRNAs may adjust epigenetic marks leading to differences in the accessibility of certain genes to transcription.[147] Taken together, this research reveals that parental experience and environmental factors can alter microRNAs in the gametes to produce effects on the developing embryo. These effects quite possibly result in lifelong changes to health, including metabolism and brain development. They may even be capable of passing on to the next generation. The multitaskers have branched out to fine-tune the next and future generations.

Using MicroRNAs to Create Stem Cell-ness

The ability to create any cell type using any starting cell material has transformed scientific research and offers unlimited potential in medical applications to restore damaged and diseased tissues and organs. For example, the possibility to restore mobility by replacing vital lost brain cells in Parkinson's disease. Some of the key advances came from Shinya Yamanaka, winner of the 2012 Nobel prize for physiology or medicine for his work to determine the combination of factors that could convert an adult cell back into a pluripotent state. That is, turn back the process of differentiation to a point when a cell can be coaxed into forming any other cell in the body. The 'Yamanaka factors', reported in *Cell* in 2006, were the transcription factors OCT4, SOX2, KLF4 and c-Myc.[148] If delivered into an adult cell, the cell returned to a primordial state from which, given the right growth factors and conditions, it could become any cell in the body, including neurones. Researchers around the world have benefited from these discoveries. For example, neuroscientists can create neurones of any type in a dish by taking a skin or blood cell from someone. If the person has a genetic disease, the neurones that harbour that mutation can be created and studied; potentially, then a drug can be found that corrects any abnormal physiology. It is a technology my own lab has benefited from, examples of which can be found in later chapters.

A stem-like state is also detected in certain forms of cancer, that is, cells that have acquired the ability to self-renew and differentiate. Analysis of the composition of cancer stem cells has found genes associated with the activity of OCT4, SOX2 and NANOG. However, the transcription factors themselves were not consistently found, suggesting another culprit. This led to testing whether one or more microRNAs from the two microRNA clusters associated with embryonic stem cells might be able to substitute for the Yamanaka factors. In 2008, teams from Los Angeles and researchers in Taiwan showed that over-expressing miR-302 in two cancer cell lines generated cells that bore embryonic stem cell–like molecular and cellular features.[149] These included expression of OCT4, SOX2 and NANOG, proteins that were hardly detectable in the parent line. The over-expression of miR-302s also removed some of the epigenetic marks that become applied as cells differentiate. Last, treatment of the microRNA-converted cells with specific growth factors could differentiate them into a broad range of cell types. This proved that certain microRNAs, when introduced, can create a pluripotent stem cell–like state. This held significant advantages over the approach being taken with the Yamanaka factors in terms of simplicity, efficiency and safety because it avoided the need to deliver four large transcription factor genes via a virus into a single target cell. The same approach worked with other microRNAs from the clusters. In 2009, researchers showed that transfecting members of the miR-290~295 cluster into differentiated (i.e. somatic) cells could substitute for the absence of one of the four Yamanaka factors (c-Myc), generating pluripotency.[150] Of those tested, miR-294 was the most effective member of the cluster and was sufficient on its own to de-differentiate cells. Using the microRNA did not produce identical effects to c-Myc, but the resulting cells could readily generate any of the three germ-cell-layer types. Again, it was evidence that microRNAs could substitute for the Yamanaka transcription factors in creating induced pluripotent stem cells.

Refinements of microRNA-based cell re-programming later emerged. If you are only interested in generating, say, neurones, from adult cells, experiments show that there is no need to go all the way back to an embryonic stem cell–like state. It is possible to directly convert adult cells into neurone-like cells using a microRNA-based approach. This borrowed an idea from Bartel and colleagues' 2005 study, which showed that HeLa cells could be transformed towards a neurone-like state by loading them with the brain-enriched miR-124.[35] Research showed that it was possible to treat fibroblasts, a cell type common to connective tissues, with a combination of miR-124 plus miR-9, and to generate cells with neurone-like physical and molecular properties, including components that neurones use to communicate.[151] Not all types of neurone have been able to be generated by this approach, however, suggesting that some additional factors are required for some subtypes. The mechanism by which miR-124 and miR-9 achieve this cellular conversion is not fully understood but includes repressing an inhibitor of neural development and transcription of non-neuronal genes. The direct re-programming also works for other cell types. For example, using different combinations of microRNAs including miR-1, researchers have been able to convert fibroblasts into muscle cells.[152, 153] The transition can be relatively fast, with markers of heart muscle or cardiomyocytes appearing within three to six days of exposure to the microRNAs. This includes electrical properties and contractile movements. Excitingly, this doesn't just work in cell culture. Delivery of the muscle cell programming microRNA combination was able to convert non-myocyte cells into myocytes in the injected hearts of mice, and this could restore some properties, including heart pump function, in a model of cardiac arrest.[154] Given the enormous health burden of heart and brain disease worldwide, approaches such as these to repair tissue could have a transformative effect as medicines of the future.

Brain Development

There is a pervasive use of microRNAs during the formation of the brain.[59, 135, 155] This was known from some of the earliest studies of microRNAs (see **Figure 4.7**). Brain development involves highly constrained and genetically organised gene expression programmes coordinated by the actions of transcription factors and the cohorts of genes they command.[156] Each step features shaping by the actions of microRNAs. MicroRNA expression is controlled in both space and time, generating exquisite waves of microRNA activity

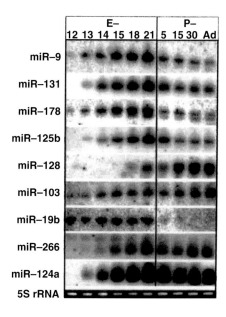

Figure 4.7 MicroRNAs switch on during brain development

Early evidence for the up-regulation of microRNAs during mammalian brain development. The RNA was extracted from embryonic (E) or post-natal (P) brain tissue from mice at different times (days – numbered). MicroRNAs were then detected by a radio(33P)-labelled oligonucleotide probe and exposed to film. Note that some of the nomenclature of these early-identified microRNAs was later updated.

Source: Reprinted with permission from Krichevsky et al., *RNA*, vol. 9, pp. 1274–81 (2003).[31]

that coordinate and sharpen the edges of the gene expression programmes that initially maintain high rates of cell birthing, then drive transitions that push cells to lose their ability to self-renew and begin the long journey of migration and acquisition of the hallmark features of neurones and support cells in the developed brain. There are examples of the same microRNA being switched on to guide expression of genes at one stage of development before disappearing, only to re-emerge later, brought back to target other genes in later maturation processes. There are more than 4,000 research papers on microRNAs in brain development. Thus, there is space for only a light review of key events and the microRNAs found to shape them. Moreover, while the main phases and processes are understood, the development of the brain is staggeringly complex and gaps and details remain to be fully worked out, especially for humans. For simpler animals such as *C. elegans*, we have reached the moment when we have mapped every gene in every brain cell, the place where the cell came from and to what it connects (although a complete connectome version with microRNAs is not yet available).

We can split brain development into five phases. Neurogenesis is the process of generating the vast numbers of cells that will become neurones (the term gliogenesis is used for the equivalent that generates the support cells of the brain). Migration is the process whereby cells are guided to the right parts of the brain to integrate into the networks and larger-scale structures of the brain. Differentiation is the process by which immature neurones lose their ability to divide and acquire their specialised features. Elimination is when excess cells are removed. Finally, myelination sees the insulating of the axons ('wires') that are the long projections from one neurone to another. Human brain development begins early, around the third week post-fertilisation. Neural progenitors derive from the epiblast and form owing to secreted molecular guidance cues received by migrating cells along the midline of the embryo. Further signals during gastrulation serve to set up the front–back organisation of the embryonic nervous system. The order of the migrating cells and further signals specify the regional identities of the neural progenitors and the major divisions of what will become the brain. The first major subdivision of the ectoderm forms the neural tube, the first defined structure, which forms along the midline from the neural progenitors. The hollow inside will eventually form the ventricles, the cavity system inside the brain through which cerebrospinal fluid circulates. Front segments of the tube grow rapidly, forming the early forebrain and midbrain, with further subdivisions forming the structures called the telencephalon and the diencephalon. These will eventually form the cerebrum, which is the largest part of the brain containing the cortex, and structures such as the hypothalamus, a key coordinator of homeostatic functions such as temperature control, respectively. Progenitors behind this region form the hindbrain and the spinal cord. The rudimentary structures and the main compartments of the nervous system are defined by the end of the embryonic period. By four weeks post-conception, what will become the two hemispheres of the brain can be distinguished. During the foetal stage of development, from the ninth week of gestation, the folds of the cortical surface appear (later becoming the sulci and the gyri). Progenitor cell divisions switch from symmetrical (split/divide equally) to asymmetric, with the production of one immature neurone as well as a further progenitor per division. The soon-to-be neurones are now post-mitotic and will not divide again. They leave the proliferative zone towards the developing brain structures, migrating with guidance scaffolding provided by a specialised cell called radial glia. A second major source of neurones develops called the medial ganglionic eminence, which floods the brain with what will later become inhibitory neurones. In fact, there is increasing awareness of multiple origins and migratory routes during human brain development. The clock is also being wound back on when cortical neurones first appear, with the 2006 discovery of so-called predecessor cells around one month post-fertilisation, when the entire human embryo is only a few millimetres in length.[157] The six-cell-layer structure of the cerebral cortex forms based on the order of arrival, with the earliest-migrating neurones forming the deepest layers. Major neurone production is completed mid-gestation, but brain growth increases significantly postnatally and brain maturation continues long after birth, beyond childhood into late adolescence and perhaps into adulthood. The process of differentiation completes with the neurones in place and involves formation of the extensions from neurones that will receive and send nerve impulses, honing in on recipient cells via the actions of secreted attractant and repulsive guidance molecules. Major regional connections, such as the thalamocortical pathway, that transmit sensorimotor information are established by the 26th gestational week in humans. Proliferation and migration of the supporting glial cells occurs later than for neurones, completing postnatally and into childhood. Myelination is also a largely postnatal process, performed by specialised cells called oligodendroglia. Hox gene activity is critical for nervous system development. The activity of the different Hox proteins demarcates boundaries that will become the various cranial nerves, lobes and substructures during brain development and helps direct the correct path of migrating neurones and subsequent differentiation. Hox gene expression remains active through to the postnatal stage and their expression can be detected in the adult brain. Key postnatal roles include ensuring appropriate connectivity through maturation and elimination of contact points between brain cells.

Neurogenesis As discussed previously, the human brain is distinct in a number of ways from the brain of other primates and lower mammals, most obviously in the density of neurones and the surface topology, with a massively increased surface area created by the folding of the cortex. Setting the number of cells in the brain is a combination of factors, each of which is controlled by microRNAs, including the number of progenitors, the number of cell divisions they can undergo and the duration of the cell cycle. The unique cell generative capacity in the human brain has been linked to a greatly expanded germinal zone called the outer subventricular zone. This is a cell-birthing factory for the brain. Evolutionary genetics have traced the genes responsible for this expansion and identified sets of microRNAs that co-evolved with those genes. Humans also have a protracted period of activity of neural stem cells. This is made possible by the actions of microRNAs, which target cell cycle genes and other processes to extend the period of proliferation. This includes members of the miR-17~92 cluster of microRNAs, which target transcription and other regulatory factors, including phosphatase and tensin homolog (PTEN) and T box brain protein 2 (TBR2), that direct progenitors towards differentiation. Thus, the actions of this cohort of microRNAs keep proliferating cells from entering the next phase before sufficient cells have been generated. Other microRNAs that have been identified as promoting proliferation of neural progenitors from human embryonic stem cells include miR-9. Indeed, mice lacking miR-9 display severely reduced brain growth. A second early role for miR-9 is in preventing migration of early-stage neural precursors. These early anti-migratory effects of miR-9 are owing to suppression of stathmin, a motility-promoting protein. Let-7 family microRNAs are important in ending the cycles of cell division, many of which (e.g. let-7a, b, d or g) down-regulate the pluripotent factors OCT4, SOX2 and NANOG in embryonic stem cells. Thus, a set of microRNAs helps to ensure that the right number of rounds of cell division occur before moving on to chaperone cells during the next stage.

Migration Several microRNAs have been identified that exert important effects on where cells end up and the correct layering of neurones within the brain. These include some of the most abundant microRNAs in the adult brain such as miR-9 and miR-128. Studies show that altering the levels of miR-9 or miR-128 during development changes the positions of certain neurones in the cortex. That is, the neurones end up in the wrong layer. Several recently evolved human microRNAs have been identified as being switched on during early phases of human brain development and thus influencing the structure of key brain regions, including the frontal lobe of the brain.

Differentiation Differentiation is one of the best-studied processes, with microRNAs helping to turn a relatively uncommitted cell down a path towards specialisation and holding it there. The ability of microRNAs to promote differentiation of brain cells is via complementary actions on cell cycle factors, RBPs and transcription factors. Five microRNAs dominate the differentiation process: miR-9, miR-124, miR-125, miR-128 and let-7. Levels of miR-124 ramp up in differentiating and mature neurones. Among the targets are transcripts that code for proteins that are important for neural progenitors. Thus, a key function of miR-124 is to suppress progenitor gene expression, thereby facilitating differentiation into mature neurones. Also, miR-124 suppresses neurone-restrictive silencer factor (NRSF), a repressor of neuronal genes. By blocking NRSF, miR-124 enables widespread switch-on of neuronal genes. This is enhanced by miR-124 targeting an RNA splicing factor, polypyrimidine tract binding protein 1 (PTBP1), which switches cells to generate transcripts that code for proteins present in mature neurones. Also targeting NRSF is miR-9. Conversely, in neural progenitors, NRSF is actively expressed and prevents expression of miR-9 and miR-124. Unusually, the passenger strand of miR-9 (miR-9*) is also used in brain development.

Notably, miR-9* and miR-124 display almost identical patterns of expression during brain development. The actions of miR-124 and miR-9* also serve to limit the number of cell divisions. Later functions of miR-9 and miR-124, which begin upon neurones reaching their final destination, include promoting the outgrowth of structures that neurones use to receive signals. A 2009 study in *Nature* showed that this is achieved by coordinated targeting by these two microRNAs leading to down-regulation of a protein complex called BAF53a that remodels chromatin.[158] Again, and unusually, it is the mi-9* strand that is active. The actions of the microRNAs via targeting seeds in the 3' UTR of *BAF53a* down-regulate the protein product and allow the expression of a physiological opponent complex called BAF53b to start. It is the actions of BAF53b on gene expression that drive formation of the specialised structures on neurones for receiving signals called dendrites.

If microRNA activity is suppressed during specific phases of brain development, it prevents the formation of the support cells in the brain, glia. Among the list of tasks performed by let-7 during brain development is coordinating the differentiation of the progenitors of glial cells into what will eventually become astrocytes, the most abundant class of glia in the brain. Steering neural progenitors towards becoming glia requires the simultaneous activation of genes that define these cells while suppressing neural programmes. A key driver of astrocyte differentiation is signalling by Janus kinases (JAKs) and signal transducer and activator of transcription proteins (STATs). There is also a specific member of the SOX family, SOX9, that promotes differentiation into astrocytes. The dual task driving glial features as well as inhibiting neural features is shared with the miR-125 family of microRNAs. Experiments show that this microRNA suppresses inhibitors of astrocyte differentiation, that is, it blocks the molecular barriers to astrogliogenesis.

Elimination An important event during brain development is removal of excess and under- or mis-connected cells. Approximately half of the neurones within a brain region are eliminated during brain development. This occurs through the process of programmed cell death, a gene-directed cell suicide programme. Such cell death is important for correctly balancing cell numbers and types within brain networks and mainly occurs prenatally. There is also massive pruning and elimination of early contact points between maturing brain cells, which mainly occurs postnatally. A number of microRNAs have been identified as important to these processes, including miR-34a, elevated levels of which target anti-apoptotic transcripts and promote apoptosis, a form of programmed cell death.

Myelination Myelin is produced by specialist glia cells called oligodendrocytes. The processes of these cells are rich in this protein and wrap around and around the axons, which are the long projections from neurones that convey messages. This serves as a type of electrical insulation and strongly increases the speed of nerve impulses. The process of myelination of axons continues over many years postnatally and is a major contributor to the increasing weight of the brain. Thus, ensuring the correct numbers of cells are in place and directing them to come out of earlier progenitor states and on through development to oligodendrocytes is critical for brain function. There are several phases of oligodendrocyte differentiation and myelination and each involves microRNAs. Broadly speaking, the process sees the gradual decline and removal of transcripts that maintain self-renewal ability and neuronal gene expression, while genes that provide the key attributes of oligodendrocytes ramp up. Thus, as with other aspects of brain development, the process requires complex coordination of shifting gene expression patterns and actions of microRNAs to shape these into the mature cell type and away from immature and uncommitted forms. The most critical microRNAs in the early phase of directing neural precursors towards an oligodendrocyte lineage and, later, in the conversion of oligodendrocyte precursor cells towards oligodendrocytes are miR-219 and miR-338. The two have different targets at different stages. Early on, their actions are directed towards transcription factors that maintain a proliferative state, being replaced later by targets linked to neurogenesis and transcripts enriched in non-oligodendrocyte cell types. The abundance of miR-219 and miR-338 increases along the path towards cells becoming oligodendrocytes and inhibition of their function blocks maturation to oligodendrocytes. Members of the miR-17~92 family are also important in the survival and proliferation of these cells, as evidenced by the reduced numbers of oligodendrocytes in mice with a targeted deletion of the cluster. Another microRNA, miR-138, was shown to block the SOX4 transcription factor and promote the final differentiation to mature oligodendrocytes and conversion to their active myelinating form. Expression of miR-219 and miR-338 remains high in mature oligodendrocytes, indicating roles in maintaining cell identity after differentiation.

Finishing the Job

The part of the human brain that develops latest is the prefrontal cortex. This region controls executive functions such as planning, switching between tasks, and working memory. There are important differences in the prefrontal cortex of humans compared to our close primate cousins, in size but also in the complexity of organisation and the sophistication of the wiring. A range of human brain diseases and developmental disorders arise because of differences and abnormalities in how this part of the brain develops and the environmental factors that influence function. Accordingly, identification of the development and maturation of this critical structure that makes us so 'human' is important to resolve. A major boost to this effort came from teams at the Allen Brain Institute, in Seattle in the USA. The institute was founded in 2003 by Microsoft co-founder Paul G. Allen and has been a major source of reference data for the neuroscience community. The institute works to generate detailed molecular and cellular maps of the mouse brain and the human brain. The treasure trove of data includes atlases of the mouse brain and the human brain, detailed down to the level of single cells, enabling researchers to navigate and study any part of the brain at key stages of development. The genes expressed in each cell in each region have been determined, meaning that for any gene you can find out where it is made and how much of it there is. Among these resources, made freely available to the research community, are microRNA datasets. Collections of carefully preserved, donated human brain samples have been processed and subjected to small RNA sequencing. Thus, we now have extensive coverage of the microRNA landscape spanning the early postnatal period to the adult in humans. This allows researchers to follow which of the various families and individual microRNAs switch on during different phases of human brain development and how this differs between regions at different ages. The first comprehensive analysis of the Allen Institute's microRNA data appeared in 2013, led by teams in the USA and the UK, reporting findings from 82 brain samples.[159] The expression of more than 900 microRNAs was analysed. The greatest changes in microRNA expression occurred during the transition from infancy to early childhood and the largest differences in microRNA expression occurred in the dorsolateral prefrontal cortex. In addition to being the region with the greatest changes in microRNA expression during development, the microRNA contingent of the dorsolateral prefrontal cortex also showed large sex differences. Forty microRNAs showed sex-based differences in levels in this brain region, most of which happened in samples around the time of puberty, and most of the differences were higher levels of microRNAs in female brains. The seemingly greater microRNA activity in the female compared to the male brain in this brain region may shape disease risk or severity, since dysfunction of the dorsolateral prefrontal cortex is linked to psychiatric diseases, such as schizophrenia, in which sex differences have been reported. The targets of these microRNAs are not fully resolved, but prediction-based approaches found many to be transcription factors. Together, the findings support microRNAs having broad and multifaceted effects shaping the neural networks and sex-based differences in this important brain region during development. What is missing, however, is any cellular resolution. At the time, there was no way to link differences in microRNA levels to specific cell types. We are edging towards sequencing and other 'omics technology that should provide that. In 2018, a team at the University of California at Santa Barbara led by Kenneth Kosik reported in *Nature Neuroscience* a catalogue of all genes expressed in individual brain cells at different stages of human brain development.[61] Remarkable enough on its own, the study featured a method of sampling small RNAs that made it possible to measure the microRNAs expressed in many of these different cell types. This created a microRNA-target atlas of the developing human brain at single-cell resolution. This has revealed which microRNAs are acting in what cells at distinct phases of human brain development. The mapping was of active, AGO2-loaded microRNAs and was performed to coincide with key moments such as peak neurogenesis (gestational week 15). More than 900 microRNAs were found to be AGO2-loaded during different phases of human brain development. Many of the microRNAs that showed differences in levels between stages of human brain development were those most recently evolved. A total of 3,693 transcripts were being targeted at early stages of development, about a thousand more than at later times when gliogenesis was more prominent. This indicates a slowing of the level of microRNA activity. Many of the targets were transcription factors, chromatin modifiers and signalling pathway components, consistent with how microRNAs are able to exert effects across a wide expanse of the gene expression landscape. Looking further into their specific identities, many targeted transcripts were known to be markers of well-defined cell types. This is consistent with microRNAs driving and maintaining cell identities during and after brain development. When the team performed the combined analysis of microRNAs and mRNAs in the same ~300 individual cells, they learnt that almost all microRNAs detected were enriched in specific cell types. Neurones taken from the upper layer of the brain contained different microRNAs from lower-layer neurones, which also differed from progenitors present in still-maturing regions that were not fully differentiated. For example, miR-124 was enriched in the mature neurones, whereas it was hardly detectable in the progenitor cells in an intermediate stage of differentiation. The study hit on a basic feature of how microRNAs were acting during human brain development. They work to repress genes not normally expressed in a cell type or are made to regulate the levels of genes expressed in that same cell type. The study also reinforced earlier insights about target switching during brain development. Several microRNAs, including miR-9, targeted different transcripts at different stages of human brain development. Thus, many microRNAs change their roles along the course of development.

Reflections

Building an organism, even a simple one like *C. elegans*, requires coordination of gene expression on a grand scale, with thousands of genes switching on and off at precise moments as cells divide, move and acquire their specialist features. The instruction programmes for this are ancient, but continue to evolve. It is not only the number and the diversity of genes but how and when they are used and for how long that has been instrumental in the development of more complex organisms, including ourselves. MicroRNAs begin to shape these programmes at the earliest moments of life. As microRNAs go through their own on/off moments, they sculpt the gene expression landscape, acting on transcription factors and the signals that trigger the bursts of growth, renewal, the signs of distinct features and the final resting place of cells. Nowhere is this more spectacular than the brain. We still have much to learn. We have tracked only a small percentage of the microRNAs and their targets in complex brains during development. Completing this mapping exercise will take time. We may one day know what every microRNA is doing in every cell during human development. This would not only represent a heroic scientific achievement but also have applications in medicine, allowing, perhaps, new ways to prevent or correct the disorders of development that devastate the lives of those affected and their families. The symphony that is organism development is perhaps the greatest of all conducting tasks, with the most at stake. Some of the microRNAs that are pivotal to brain development never reappear. Others pick on new targets. Some help to keep the status quo, making sure that cell features are robust. Others, as we will see in Chapter 5, find themselves busier than ever.

MicroRNAs Shape the Machinery of Our Minds

Neuroscience is by far the most exciting branch of science because the brain is the most fascinating object in the universe.

Stanley Prusiner, discoverer of prions (Nobel prize, 1997)

We have seen that one of the most important and extensive uses of microRNA occurs as animals develop and grow. MicroRNAs steer the complex gene programmes that ensure the right number of cells are generated in our tissues, organs and systems. They make sure that cells end up where they should be and what they should be. There is perhaps no organ where getting this right, the wiring, is more complex and important than the brain. The human brain contains an estimated 86 billion neurones. These form elegant communication networks that collectively generate the capabilities we are familiar with: control of breathing, heart rate, sleep, thought, planning, sensing, movement, emotion, memory and so on. For this to all work, billions of cells have to make connections, both local and long-distance, to one another. An estimated 100 trillion contacts. We have seen how microRNAs shape the developing brain, controlling the gene programmes that help fill the brain with cells and turn these into the various cell lineages that possess the necessary physiological properties. For some microRNAs, this was their crowning achievement. The genes they once regulated now switched permanently off, there is no need for them either. Having finished shape development and differentiation, the settled brain also stops making some of its microRNA controllers. For other microRNAs, their work is only just beginning.

The human brain expresses around 16,000 different genes, about 76 per cent of all the protein-coding genes in your genome.[160] As you might expect, it is heavily stocked and continues to produce a remarkable diversity of microRNAs, more than 1,600 different microRNAs by some estimates.[159] Some of the microRNAs needed during development find new targets in the adult brain. Repurposed; nature being efficient once again. Other microRNAs switch on for the first time, peaking after the brain has gone through development. Settling down to keep neurones behaving themselves. What are they doing? The adult brain struggles with two somewhat opposing demands. On the one hand, it must be extremely resilient, capable of executing and re-executing myriad functions with precision. On the other hand, it must be adaptable, capable of reshaping its circuits to learn.[161] MicroRNAs help the adult brain serve these apparently contradictory goals, ensuring that neurones send, receive and react to the signals that comprise their day-to-day functions with complete fidelity. They enforce stable gene programmes for the circuits that underpin who you are, your personality and attributes, your intellect. When we look across at other animal species, we see similar dependence on microRNAs for mature brain function. We know that the human brain's expansion benefited from and may have been driven by microRNA expansion, but we are not alone. Other animals have created more brainpower by enhancing their microRNA repertoire. In this chapter we look at some of the processes that microRNAs regulate in the adult brain, the functions that microRNAs perform once brain development is complete and the circuits and structures are all in place. While the macro-level structure of the brain and its circuits becomes 'fixed' beyond a certain period of development, other aspects of our brains remain malleable. One of the best-understood actions of microRNAs underpins how neurones can adjust the strength of their connections with one another, the process of synaptic plasticity.

Basic Neurophysiology and Cell-to-Cell Communication

Before we get to how microRNAs shape communication in the adult brain, a short review of the basics. The mammalian brain has two hemispheres: each is organised into a series of lobes that each display some degree of specialisation. For example, the occipital lobe, which is found at the back of the brain, receives information from the optic nerve and performs key steps in the early processing of visual information. The temporal lobes, on the left and right sides of the brain, serve roles in memory, emotions and processing sensory information. If we keep going down in scale, through an imaginary microscope, we will eventually reach a scale of circuits made up of different combinations of neurones and glia (**Figure 5.1A**). Four out of five neurones in the human cortex are excitatory. When an excitatory neurone's signal reaches its target it causes the receiving neurone to become activated and more likely to 'fire' a signal. Mixed among these, the remaining 20 per cent or so are inhibitory neurones. When inhibitory neurones fire, they can block or reduce the firing of the next neurone. It is the balance of these activities that is necessary for brain networks to function, to correctly receive and code information. It is important to briefly cover how this occurs because, as we will see shortly, microRNAs directly influence the amounts of proteins that are critical to sending and receiving signals between brain cells. The signal that the brain uses to send information is called an action potential or 'spike'. Of the various major cell types in the brain, only neurones can generate action potentials. Their ability to do this is based on their electrochemistry, an ability to control the position and movement of charged ions and, by adjusting their location, send the charge from one end of the neurone to the other. How is this done? At rest, the inside of a neurone is negatively charged with respect to the outside. The charge difference or *membrane potential* is set up by a series of pumps and channels in the outside of the nerve membrane. The first step in generating this is to separate two main ions across the neurone's outer (plasma) membrane. Potassium (K) is concentrated inside the cell and sodium (Na) is pumped out of the cell to concentrate it on the other side of the membrane. Each ion carries an equal positive charge: K+, Na+. The pump that does the separating, called the sodium-potassium ATPase, sends three sodium ions out of the cell for every two potassium in. This creates a small electrical difference and a negative charge on the inside. A second process, the leak of potassium ions from the inside to the outside, carries away more positive charge, increasing the negative charge inside the neurone. This leak is allowed only for potassium. The membrane does not allow the sodium ions to creep back in; sodium ions can move in, but only when special gates for them open. Combined with one or two other features of the chemistry of these cells that we will skip, the inside of a neurone at rest is about 70 millivolts negative (−70mV) relative to the outside (**Figure 5.1B**).

An action potential, the nerve impulse, comprises a brief reversal of the membrane potential: from negative to positive and back again, in combination with the transmission of

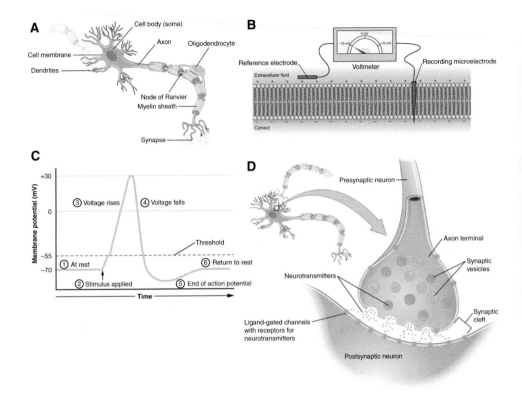

Figure 5.1 Neuronal structure, function and synaptic transmission

Panel A shows the basic parts of a typical neurone.

Panel B shows neurones at rest carrying a negative charge inside, generated by the unequal separation and movement of ions such as potassium.

Panel C shows the sequence of events during an action potential. It is the opening of voltage-gated sodium channels that generates the rising phase of the signal.

Panel D shows the synapse, the point where synaptic transmission occurs.

Source: Images from openstax.org.

this signal from one end of the neurone, close to the main cell body where the nucleus is located, down the axon to the end of the neurone. During the action potential, for the briefest of moments, channels for sodium open. Sodium ions flood into the neurone, taking positive charge with them and briefly the inside membrane goes from negative to positive. Then the channels shut off, no more sodium can enter and channels for potassium open. Potassium ions move out. This takes positive charge out, restoring the membrane's potential to negative and the neurone goes back to resting. This sodium open/sodium close/potassium open process takes about a millisecond, so neurones can fire hundreds of action potentials per second (**Figure 5.1C**).

When an action potential reaches the end of the neurone's axon, it causes the release of a small amount of substance, stored at the nerve terminal, called a neurotransmitter. The neurotransmitter crosses a tiny gap before arriving onto the next neurone where it binds to protein receptors on the surface. The region where one neurone communicates to another and the gap in between is the synapse. The process of signal transfer is called *synaptic transmission* (**Figure 5.1D**). What happens next depends on the type of receptor that the neurotransmitter has bound. At many synapses, the binding of a neurotransmitter to the receptor causes the immediate opening of channels that allow sodium into the cell. This will make the inside of the neurone more positive and push the next neurone towards a tipping point, about −50mV, when it will send a new action potential. That is what happens at an *excitatory* synapse. The neurotransmitter sent across at the largest number of excitatory synapses in the brain is called glutamate. However, the opposite effect can also be achieved. Some neurotransmitters open channels that cause the membrane potential to remain in a negatively charged state and thus less likely to send an action potential. These are *inhibitory synapses* and the neurotransmitter has the effect of reducing the likelihood that the neurone can send on an action potential. The most common neurotransmitter at these synapses is called GABA (gamma-amino butyric acid). There are several other neurotransmitters. Some of these are household names, such as dopamine and serotonin. They can all produce either excitatory or inhibitory effects, depending on the receptors they encounter. Brain function involves this mixture of excitatory and inhibitory signals. Without inhibitory neurones, information would be noisy, the message garbled. And we could get mass firing of all neurones, creating an electrical storm. We know this because drugs that block the activity of inhibitory neurones trigger seizures, the hallmarks of the brain disease epilepsy (more about that in Chapter 6).

The Wider Cell Community in the Brain

Information is coded by the frequency of action potentials being sent around networks in the brain. Modern neuroscience techniques allow us to record and visualise in real time the firing of brain cells and to analyse the distinct gene activity in different cell types. This has revealed that we have dozens of subtypes of neurones. Each has a distinct structure, neurotransmitter, pattern of firing behaviour and connection partners, performing specific roles in brain networks. Interspersed among the neurones are glia cells. Two of the three major classes of glia, astrocytes and oligodendrocytes, we met in Chapter 4. The other, microglia, are related to immune cells. As the brain develops, they invade and help shape the wiring of the brain before settling down to sit and monitor the local environment around synapses. If the brain is ever damaged, they react quickly, transforming into an amoeboid shape and moving to sites of damage to help clear up debris. We will not touch further on the functions of microRNA in glia in this chapter since the literature on neuronal microRNAs is extensive enough. So, at the risk of upsetting the glia researchers, this chapter will by and large focus on neuronal microRNAs.

Not All Synapses Are Created Equal

Coming off the main body of a neurone is a series of branches called *dendrites* that look rather like the roots of a tree. Dendrites serve as the information-collecting sites. Axons from other neurones form synapses all over these branches. If you look under a microscope, the branches of excitatory neurones are covered by small protuberances. Imagine acorns or leaves on a tree branch. These are the dendritic *spines* and most excitatory inputs arrive onto them. The released neurotransmitter binds to receptors on the top of the spine. If the receptor reacts and opens a pore that allows sodium ions to flood in, we get a change in membrane potential to a less negative potential. The amount of that change is, however, rather small. That is, a single input from a single spine is not sufficient to trigger a new

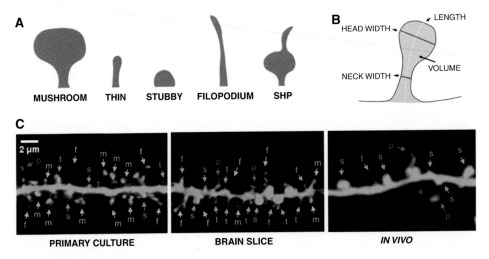

Figure 5.2 Dendritic spines

This shows the morphological diversity of dendritic spines.

Panel A shows the main spine shapes: mushroom (m), thin (t), stubby (s), filopodium (f), spine-head protrusions (SHP; p).

Panel B shows how the types are defined (morphometric parameters).

Panel C shows microscopic images of dendritic spines obtained from *in vitro* (primary culture), *ex vivo* (brain slice) and *in vivo* (cranial window) imaging. Scale bar: 2 μm.

Source: Reprinted with permission from Bączyńska et al., *International Journal of Molecular Sciences*, vol. 22, pp. 4053–74 (2021).[162]

action potential. And the farther the event occurs from the neurone's cell body, the weaker the effect. In order for a new action potential to occur in the receiving neurone, signals must summate, add together either in space or in time. For example, two or more synaptic inputs from the same axon arrive straight after one another, or action potentials at two or more sites on the branch arrive at the same time.

There are other factors besides summation which influence whether or not a synaptic event produces a meaningful response in the receiving neurone. Dendritic spines each vary in their shape and size. This affects the strength of the signal that can pass through. A good spine for synaptic communication is one that has the shape of a mushroom (see **Figure 5.2**). Stronger depolarisations can be measured at larger spines. Thin or undeveloped spines, by contrast, are incapable of transmitting signals. Thus, the shape and the number of dendritic spines are important elements of how neurones communicate. Repeated and persistent firing of a neurone at certain frequencies can trigger growth of spines in the post-synaptic neurone. This results in synaptic strengthening and is a cellular basis for how we learn, sometimes simplified as 'neurones wire together if they fire together'.

Proteins of Plasticity

As the collection points for incoming signals, dendritic spines are fundamental to brain function. Consequently, anything that affects their properties is important. This includes, of course, the proteins of the dendritic spine, which serve one of three main tasks. There are proteins that provide structural support. This includes a protein called actin, which works somewhat like the scaffolding around a building under construction, only the scaffolding is on the inside. Actin can form various shapes by extending into chains or clumping together into balls. This in turn changes the shape of the spine. If the long chains collapse into a ball, the spine itself shrinks and folds in. The second type of protein we find are those involved in initial receipt and transmission of the incoming signal. These proteins include the receptors on the surface of the spine which bind the incoming neurotransmitter. The third class are the proteins that transmit that signal farther down the line.

The proteins at synapses come from two sources. Some are transported there from the cell body, but many are produced locally by translating mRNAs. One of the leaders of this field of research is Erin Schuman at the Max Planck Institute for Brain Research in Frankfurt, Germany.[163, 164] Estimates from her team's work suggest that as many as 4,000 mRNA transcripts can be detected at dendrites.[165] This amounts to as much as a third of the total present in the cell body compartment. Interestingly, the type of transcript and the abundance vary along the length of the dendrite. That is, some of the transcripts are different in the dendrites closest to the cell body compared to dendrites farther away. This presumably reflects adjustments in molecular composition to optimise the different segments' ability to receive and transmit signals. In general, rates of translation of these mRNAs vary according to their abundance. Higher amounts of mRNA give rise to higher amounts of the translated protein. But there are exceptions, where rates of translation are lower than would be expected based on mRNA abundance. Where there is a disconnect in the translation rates of an mRNA, it is often for those transcripts that harbour long 3' UTRs. Thus, neurones store an enormous wealth of transcripts, not just proteins, close to their synapses. About a tenth of the transcripts are specifically enriched in this compartment, indicating that neurones actively transport and concentrate them in dendrites. Together, the trafficked proteins and the ones made locally will determine what effect an incoming signal has at that synapse.

Why keep a large repertoire of mRNAs close to synapses? Why not just shuttle all the proteins needed from the cell body? The answer is that being able to locally produce the proteins needed provides finer control and the ability to rapidly respond to ongoing and incoming signals, turning these into physical changes to the structure of the synapse. Dendrites from excitatory and inhibitory neurones have quite similar mRNAs, suggesting that the raw materials for making these adjustments are shared. In contrast, the mRNA landscape of the soma, the main body of the neurone, differs more between excitatory and inhibitory neurones. Thus, among different neurones there is a variety of gradients and distributions of RNAs which serve common functions as well as creating their unique physiological properties. As we understand more about how learning and memory works, it has become clear that physical changes to synapses are critical. Gene expression within the nucleus is also involved, and synergism, a dialogue between the compartments, is thought to be required. As learning occurs, synapses undergo changes in their size and chemical composition. This directly changes the electrical properties of neuronal circuits in the brain. That is, incoming information, for example a sensory experience, produces particular patterns of neuronal activity that bring about changes in the circuit involved. Some of these changes are long-lasting, while others are not. If these changes are retained, it is thought to be the basis for memories. There are a number of key proteins involved in synaptic memory formation, including calmodulin-dependent kinase II (CaMKII), a calcium-responsive enzyme that works primarily by adding a phosphate group to other proteins, bringing about a change in their activity. By some estimates, about 1 in every 100 proteins in your brain is a molecule of CaMKII. Memories formed as a result of synaptic changes require new CaMKII synthesis.

Research on the mechanisms that regulate synaptic plasticity converged with interests in microRNA in the early 2000s. It was known that the 3' UTR was necessary for some mRNAs to be synaptically localised and functional. Experiments in mice had shown that spatial and other forms of memory were all impaired when the 3' UTR of *CaMKII* was mutated. The discovery of microRNAs now connected some of the dots. The 3' UTR sequences were important for the mRNAs being translated at synapses during memory formation because they held binding sites for microRNAs. As we will see shortly, microRNAs are critical to adjusting how much of the various proteins there are at the synapse. By doing this, they are contributing to tuning the signal strength that can be received at a particular site on a neurone. Thus, microRNAs are part of the brain's plasticity machinery. Several microRNAs are present at dendrites where they locally regulate how much of each synaptic protein is present. This includes miR-134, miR-138 and miR-181a. In turn, the production of active microRNAs is closely regulated and responds to shifting patterns of communication at synapses. By regulating protein levels at synapses, microRNAs are fundamental to the control of overall brain function. Neurones respond to the amount of information they receive by physically changing the contact points on their dendrites. If signals are sent at certain frequencies, the strength of synaptic connections can either increase or decrease. The changes in strength relate to physical changes to the structure of the dendrite and the receptor machinery expressed there. This is backed up by extensive research showing failings in brain function upon disruption of some of the microRNAs that work at the synapse. Examples are found later in this chapter and in Chapter 6.

MicroRNA Enrichment in the Brain

Before we look at how specific microRNAs regulate communication in the brain, we return to the early days of microRNA discovery. Experiments led by Tuschl in 2002 had searched through the soup of RNA from tissues of mice looking for microRNA sequences.[20] When it came to the brain, they separated out three parts of the brain that each served different functions: the cortex, the cerebellum and the midbrain, the last of which contains fibre tracts and structures important for sensorimotor processing and communication. Tuschl's team found that miR-124 represented nearly half the microRNA molecules they counted in all three brain regions. They also found several others unique to the brain. These included miR-128 and miR-134. The team also noted that each of these brain-enriched microRNA in the mouse was also present and identical in humans. The brain had a special selection of microRNAs not produced anywhere else in the body, and humans and mice shared a number in common.

Within a couple of years, dozens more brain-enriched microRNAs had been identified, many expressed only once brain development was complete. Attention turned to synapses. As it was already known that the protein composition at synapses could rapidly change and that the 3'UTR of mRNAs were important, this pointed squarely to a role for microRNAs. Indeed, if proteins are locally made at synapses, then you need to have a system for buffering and fine-tuning the amount of those proteins. Distributing microRNAs to synapses also solved one of the big challenges for microRNAs in general, namely, how to play important roles in regulating gene expression when their abundance is low relative to target mRNAs.

Co-locating the microRNA at a structure of major functional importance and concentrating it there solves this problem. If sequestered in a restricted space where their actions are important, microRNAs could produce strong effects. Effectively, this is what has been discovered for many neuronal microRNAs: that they are enriched at sites of importance for neuronal function.

Within a few years it was clear that the brain was the most microRNA-rich organ in the body. It expressed the greatest diversity of microRNAs and the most microRNAs by abundance. This fitted with the observation that the brain also expresses the greatest diversity of protein-coding genes. Let us put some numbers on this. Studies that have measured sets of neuronal microRNAs in the brain and compared these computationally to genes expressed at the same site which contain binding sites in their 3' UTRs for those microRNAs reveal the average number of targets of a neuronal microRNA in the hippocampus (at least in the rat brain) to be around 500. It has also been estimated that three-quarters of the microRNAs expressed in the brain are present to some extent within synapses. Thus, thousands of brain transcripts are regulated by microRNAs. At an individual microRNA level, the degree of synaptic enrichment greatly varies. Some microRNAs appear to be concentrated at synapses, whereas others show higher levels in the main cell body region. This reflects the range of processes being controlled by the microRNAs. MicroRNAs that perform roles in synaptic function tend to be enriched at synapses, whereas microRNAs with housekeeping jobs or involved in earlier developmental roles tend to be less enriched there. The system of synaptically located microRNAs to control the structure and function of synapses appears to have been recognised early in evolution as a solution to fine-tuning neuronal networks and building-in responsive circuits that adapt to the information they receive. Indeed, *C. elegans* uses microRNAs to adjust the structure of its synapses. So, this system, or versions of it, was already in place hundreds of millions of years ago.

MicroRNA Machines at the Synapse

Simply locating a microRNA molecule by a synapse is not enough for it to do its job; we need other components such as AGOs. Soon after microRNAs were first identified at synapses, researchers began to look for co-located biogenesis components, asking is the machinery for microRNA function also present at synapses? Once antibodies were generated that recognised Dicer and other biogenesis components, it was possible to stain brain tissue sections to see where these proteins were located. This showed abundant staining of neurones for these proteins in the adult brain. A synaptic location was quickly suspected because, in addition to staining of Dicer around the outside of the nucleus, there was a telltale pattern of punctate staining (think of beads on a string) that extended outwards from the cell body consistent with presence at what looked like spines on dendrites. Wherever you looked in the brain and found neurones, you also found staining for Dicer. Glia cells made less Dicer than neurones, hinting that neurones relied much more on microRNAs to regulate gene expression than the brain's support cells.

In early studies to confirm that microRNA biogenesis components were present at synapses, researchers took pieces of brain tissue, homogenised them to create an emulsion and then spun this using a powerful centrifuge. Different compartments of the cell separate as layers or sediments, with the heavier parts of the cell at the bottom, lighter on top. Using low speeds of centrifugation, you get the nucleus. At the very highest speeds, 100,000 times the force of gravity, you can collect a pure fraction of the watery cytosol, lacking all other heavier components of the cell. In between, when the spin speed is just right, you can get clumps of synapses. The purity of the different fractions is checked by testing for the presence of known proteins and the absence of contaminants. A team at the University of Illinois in Chicago in the USA found Dicer and AGOs in the purified synaptic fraction of the adult mouse brain.[166] They also found that the synaptic fraction was rich in precursors of microRNAs,[167] suggesting that inactive microRNAs were shuttled down to the synapse ready for maturing later. We will return to that shortly.

Resolving the synaptic location made use of ever greater magnification methods, to try to see microRNA components within or below a dendritic spine. Synapses are very small structures: if you really want to be sure that a protein is there, you cannot use light-based microscopy because the wavelengths are too long and the images will not resolve; electron microscopy is needed (Note: this situation is changing as new techniques, including super-resolution microscopy, are achieving ever greater magnification power and sharper images. But this did not exist at the time of these early experiments on the synaptic location of microRNA components). By firing electrons at a tissue section treated with a chemical fixative, we can image at much greater magnification. At this scale, synapses and their substructures are large enough to see. If we apply an antibody to the protein of interest, for example a gold bead attached to Dicer, then we can see where it lies. And synaptic location was exactly what was found. Both Dicer and AGO proteins can be seen within dendrites, close to where excitatory transmission occurs.

Signposting the Synapse: How MicroRNAs Know Where to Go

How do the transcripts that are to be locally regulated, as well as the microRNAs themselves, know to go to the synapse? Do they just float down? Some do appear to do this. There is a general gradient of transcripts between the cell body and the dendrites. But neurones also have efficient and precise transport processes for moving RNAs around.[168, 169] This is particularly critical for neurones where axons and dendrites can extend great distances. It is no coincidence that failures of cell transport systems are implicated in several neurodegenerative diseases. A set of rules has been uncovered that direct mRNAs to synapses. First, a localisation sequence is needed, which is usually in the 3' UTR of the mRNA. These are recognised by RBPs. Upon recognition, these assemble into a complex ready for transport along a protein scaffolding system comprising microtubule proteins and a 'motor' protein. Upon reaching their destination, they disembark like passengers from a train and go to a waiting zone. Typically, they become anchored below the synapse, probably to structural proteins such as actin. They are then ready for activity-dependent translation and/or microRNA regulation. But why not just send the already translated protein? Because by only sending the mRNA, the synapse retains the ability to decide whether and when the protein is made. It is a secure layer of control that is required for proper synaptic function. This system also serves as an economy of sorts because mRNAs can generate several rounds of translation and thus more copies of a protein.

It appears that microRNAs destined for synapses are also recognised and transported in a similar way. This hasn't been worked out for all, but we have some examples. Gerhard Schratt's team, now at the Swiss Federal Institute of Technology (ETH) in Zurich, identified both the sequence within a dendritically localised microRNA and the protein that takes miR-134 to the synapse.[170] They discovered that the loop sequence of the precursor molecule of miR-134 (i.e. pre-miR-134) had a sequence of nucleotides, ACUUU, that ensured that it was delivered to the synapse. Grafting the ACUUU sequence onto a microRNA that was normally not located at synapses resulted in it being synaptically located. Changing the loop sequence of pre-miR-134 stopped miR-134 accumulation at synapses. Using the loop, they fished for proteins that could bind it and found a single protein called DHX36. A closely related protein called DHX9 binds many other microRNAs. Without DHX36, miR-134 did not accumulate at synapses. Once at synapses, pre-miR-134 appears to be released from its chaperone before it can function. So, synaptic microRNAs have a trafficking system that delivers them to where they need to be.

Connecting the Amount of a MicroRNA to Synaptic Activity

Locating microRNAs within synapses helps solve the problem of how to locally regulate protein levels and this is an important step in how synapses can be plastic. It gives autonomy to the spines. Individual spines have the resources they need to adjust the proteins that enable synaptic communication based on the inputs they receive; in other words, they make local decisions based on incoming information. As we will see shortly, this can happen in near real time. That is, within seconds of an incoming synaptic event, microRNA levels change in order to make adjustments to the local protein repertoire. In some cases, the response is to grow the spine, reinforcing its ability to receive and transmit onwards a strong signal. MicroRNAs can also contribute to shrinking the spine, reducing the strength of signal that passes through. But simply co-locating the microRNAs, the biogenesis machinery and the mRNA targets is not sufficient. We need a system that responds proportionately, a way to link the *strength* of the incoming signal to switch the microRNA on and off. If we want to make sure that the incoming signal is converted into changes in synapse strength, we need ways to regulate the amount of the active, AGO-loaded microRNA that is at the synapse and able to do its job. We need a way to couple synaptic activity to the production and loading of microRNAs. And this system needs to be able to provide control over microRNA production in both space, at the synapse, and time (ready when we need it).

We can imagine ways in which coupling of synaptic signals to microRNA responses could work. A neurone might use a signal sent from the synapse back to the nucleus where the main machinery of transcription is present. Transcription of microRNAs would then ramp up and new microRNAs would be sent out to the synapse. There is evidence that this is how expression of some activity-regulated microRNAs is controlled. Nearly 20 years ago, studies recognised that some of the brain-expressed and activity-regulated microRNA genes had sequences in their DNA that allowed known activity-responsive transcription factors to bind. In particular among these were recognition elements for a transcriptional controller called CREB. The CREB protein can respond to changes in neuronal activity because it is regulated by a small molecule called cyclic AMP (cAMP), which is related to ATP and which is generated when neurones are active. Once cAMP binds to CREB, the complex attaches to various sites in the genome and switches genes on and off. Having a microRNA under the control of CREB is a handy way to couple it to neuronal activity. A team from the Vollum Institute in Portland, Oregon, USA, just across the river from where my colleagues were studying the same microRNA in stroke models, were the first to show that CREB linked levels of miR-132 to neuronal activity.[171] They showed that CREB bound to a DNA regulatory sequence close to the *Mir132* gene and would respond to signals from outside the cell, including from the brain-derived neurotrophic factor (BDNF), a nerve growth factor. Exposure of neurones to BDNF resulted in a strong increase in levels of miR-132. Studies since have identified transcriptional mechanisms that link neuronal activity to changes in expression of other microRNAs.

The second way to couple the amount of a microRNA to synaptic activity is to have systems for sensing changes in synaptic activity located on the microRNA biogenesis machinery itself. As we have seen, key components of the microRNA biogenesis system are present at synapses. Could their activity be linked so they respond to synapse activity by changing the local production of microRNAs? Such a system could respond to signals that come through the receptor proteins on the surface of the dendritic spine and lead to increased or decreased activity of enzymes such as Dicer or AGOs. Evidence has accumulated that this second system also operates. The microRNA biogenesis components at the synapse can sense and respond to changes in neuronal activity. In particular, intracellular calcium levels have emerged as the key link. This again meshed with a lot of what was already known about how synaptic strengthening worked. One of the receptors for the neurotransmitter glutamate is the NMDA receptor, named after N-methyl-D-aspartate, an amino acid derivative that selectively activates this receptor but not other glutamate receptors. When NMDA receptors open, they allow a short pulse of calcium to enter the cell. This activates a pathway that leads to changes in gene activity. Blocking NMDA receptors interferes with many learning and memory processes. It was about to be discovered that microRNA activity also responds to these local, NMDA receptor–mediated calcium signals.

Coupling Synaptic Activity to MicroRNA Production

A key breakthrough that helped us understand how microRNA activity is coupled to neuronal activity came from the team of Schuman.[172] At the time the study was published, in *Science* in 2017, it was clear that microRNA levels at the synapse varied in response to neuronal activity and that components of the biogenesis machinery also responded to neuronal activity. But no one had yet seen this occurring at the level of individual synapses. This required a way to image microRNA activation events at synapses. The team developed a molecular sensor that could achieve this task. It was based on the precursor form of miR-181a, one of the most abundant microRNAs in the brain and one known to be located at synapses. Within the sensor was a fluorophore, a type of coloured dye. This was placed within the sequence in a way that meant it was blocked by the loop region of the pre-miR-181a. Cleavage of the precursor meant that the loop 'quencher' region was removed and the production of a mature microRNA was accompanied by a flash of light, detected by an ultra-sensitive camera attached to a microscope hovering over the synapse. There was now a way to monitor, in real time, the Dicer-mediated processing of microRNAs at synapses in response to changes in neuronal activity. After introducing the probe into neurones, they showed that depolarising neurones triggered the cleavage of the precursor to release the mature form of miR-181a. Using their high-magnification imaging, they applied puffs of glutamate close to the synapses and recorded the local production of mature miR-181a at single synapses (see **Figure 5.3**). This occurred in the shaft region or the head of the dendrite, indicating that this was highly localised and, within a dendrite, there is further specification of precisely where the processing of precursor microRNAs occurs. They found a short delay of one to five seconds between stimulation of the synapse and the processing of the microRNA and

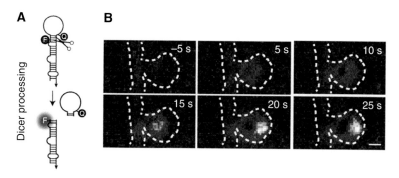

Figure 5.3 MicroRNA maturation at a single synapse

Here we are visualising the maturation of microRNAs at single synapses.

Panel A shows a schematic of the probe used to track microRNA maturation at single synapses. The design is a pre-miR-181a sequence containing a fluorophore (F) and a quencher (Q) near the base of the loop. If Dicer cleaves the pre-microRNA, it releases the quencher and the 'active' microRNA can now be detected.

Panel B shows time-lapse images of probe fluorescence in a dendritic spine during local glutamate uncaging, which was used to trigger activation of the spine. Scale bar, 2 μm.

Source: Reproduced with permission from Sambandan et al., *Science*, vol. 355, pp. 634–7 (2017).[172]

after a few seconds the signal was gone. This tells us that activity-dependent microRNA processing is rapid and short-lasting. Other experiments demonstrated that calcium was required for the activity-dependent production of mature miR-181a in response to glutamate release via NMDA receptors.

So, a mechanism exists by which microRNA levels are linked to synaptic activity. Using the same experimental system, the team could ask another question. How closely does synaptic activity link to microRNA-mediated suppression of targets? Using the sensor, they next counted the number of protein molecules of one of miR-181a's known targets, CaMKII. They found that in the location around where they recorded production of new miR-181a there was a reduction in the amount of its target protein. They proved that this was truly a microRNA-mediated event by showing that the effect was lost when *CaMKII*'s 3' UTR site for miR-181a was removed. This remarkable series of experiments established three fundamental principles of microRNA control over mature brain function. First, microRNA activity is directly linked to synaptic activity. Second, it is calcium entry into the synapse which couples these, via stimulation of Dicer in the dendrite. Finally, locally generated mature microRNAs act on their targets at synapses to reduce protein production. We now had a better understanding of the mechanism by which microRNA function is coupled to synaptic activity.

Some questions still need to be answered about the coupling process. We know that different frequencies of synaptic input can produce different effects on synaptic strength. Certain firing rates result in spine expansion and increased synaptic strength. But at another frequency we get what is called long-term depression (LTD), namely, a reduction in synaptic strength. What happens to microRNA production in these different settings? There is presumably a way for the system to be frequency-dependent. Does the same calcium-dependent mechanism of Dicer-related activity work in both situations? Does Dicer switch between processing from some microRNAs to others? How is that decided? Both Dicer and

AGOs can undergo extensive post-translational modifications affecting their activity.[38] Which of these shape the different possible outcomes of a given synaptic input? Last, we should not think of these two microRNA activity systems – the one that signals to alter transcription in the nucleus and the one that controls at local synapses – as mutually exclusive, as one or the other. We need both systems to work. This is because while we have a system for locally coupling synaptic activity to maturation of microRNAs, we will eventually run out of microRNA precursors at the synapse. We must replenish the pool of synaptically localised microRNA precursors and that requires the engagement of nucleus-based transcription.

Further Tuning of MicroRNA Control at Synapses

Other components of the RISC have been found that help tune microRNA activity to synaptic activity. One of these is a protein named MOV10.[173] (The 'MOV' stands for Moloney Leukemia Virus – a retrovirus that causes cancer in mice). It physically binds to the RISC, jamming itself against the protein complex, and is an additional part of the system controlling microRNA function. In a manner similar to Dicer, the function of MOV10 is regulated and tuned to synaptic activity. Increased neuronal activity, or the activation of NMDA receptors by glutamate, activates an enzyme complex which digests the MOV10 protein. This results in rapid lowering of MOV10 levels and any mRNAs that are being suppressed by microRNAs at the synapse are released and translated. Indeed, reducing MOV10 levels in neurones was found to result in dozens of synaptic mRNAs becoming translated. These were involved in spine structure and function – glutamate receptors and downstream signalling components such as CaMKII. The increase in protein levels was often in the range of ~20 per cent, consistent with the amount of suppression we know that microRNAs typically cause. This happens relatively quickly. Measurement of the kinetics of the response showed that higher protein levels of microRNA targets could be detected just over 10 minutes from when neurones were stimulated. Another lesson from this study was the finding that not all synaptic mRNAs began to undergo translation once this microRNA brake was released. This means that while certain mRNAs at synapses are under resting microRNA control, others are not. Why the preferential treatment? Presumably this comes down to sequences within the microRNA, mRNA and RISC activity. Of course, such experiments are really gathering RNAs from a variety of synapses, all with varying amounts of active stimulation. Experiments in the future should help to clarify the rules.

These and other experiments reveal an expansive set of microRNA mechanisms at work at the synapse. Synaptic activity can stimulate an increase in microRNA production as well as relieve microRNA repression. Some microRNAs are sitting pre-loaded and actively suppressing translation, whereas others become engaged once synaptic events occur. The microRNA findings also reconciled some of the earlier puzzles of the relationship between protein production and synaptic plasticity, specifically the seemingly contradictory evidence that both protein degradation and synthesis were required for synaptic plasticity. The experiments on MOV10 provided a neat explanation. You need to release the microRNA brake to synthesise new proteins for synaptic plasticity and for that to happen you need MOV10 to be degraded. How this is all integrated appears to depend on the strength and the timing of the incoming signals, the particular type of neurone and even the position of a synapse along a dendrite.

MicroRNAs That Control Synapse Structure and Function

By the mid-2000s, researchers had moved beyond documenting the presence of microRNAs at the synapse and begun to establish what they were doing there. This would lay the groundwork for our understanding of how microRNAs control synaptic strength. Among the early work was a study led by a Harvard University team that included Schratt. At the time, several microRNAs were known to be brain-specific. The team made a new observation, that the highest amount of one of these, miR-134, coincided with peak synapse development.[174] They also found that making neurones fire repeated action potentials caused an increase in the level of the precursor, pre-miR-134. This suggested that the microRNA might be involved in adapting synapses to incoming signals. Importantly, when they labelled neurones from the hippocampus, a key part of the brain involved in learning and memory, they found that the microRNA was localised to dendrites. Synapse-rich preparations of rodent brain samples made using centrifugation also showed enrichment of the microRNA. Experiments since, using a technique called atomic force microscopy, which allows nanoscale imaging, show miR-134 to be present at the base or within the shaft of dendritic spines.[175]

To understand what miR-134 was doing at synapses, the Harvard team looked at the relationship between the amount of miR-134 and the structure of the spines. Lower amounts of miR-134 were associated with larger, mature and active spine heads, whereas higher numbers of miR-134 molecules were found at immature spine heads. This suggested that the presence of miR-134 could be a molecular marker of inactive or irrelevant spines. To prove that miR-134 was involved in the switch between spine types, they began altering the amount of miR-134 in neurones. They did this using a chemically modified sequence of nucleotides that was complementary (i.e. antisense) to miR-134. This is called an antimir (or 'antagomir' if complementary to the complete mature microRNA).[176] When they exposed neurones to the miR-134 inhibitor, they found that the size of the dendritic spines changed. Specifically, blocking miR-134 made the spine heads grow slightly larger. Conversely, introducing more miR-134 into neurones led to reductions in spine volume. It appeared that miR-134 functioned as a negative regulator of spine morphology.

How was miR-134 altering spines? Schratt and colleagues searched for potential targets enriched in neurones, and found LIM kinase 1 – LIMK1 for short – a protein previously known to cause spines to grow when activated. A binding site for miR-134 was present in the 3' UTR of *Limk1* and when this was mutated, changes to miR-134 levels no longer had effects on spines. This meant that miR-134's effects were being mediated through its actions on *Limk1*. Since the team already knew that levels of miR-134 were sensitive to synaptic activity, the model proposed was that as neuronal activity increased, levels of miR-134 also increase, resulting in a fail-safe to oppose overgrowth of spines. They had discovered the first microRNA feedback loop for controlling synaptic strength.

Later experiments by the same team showed a second effect of miR-134 on dendritic branches. When levels of miR-134 were increased, it produced a reduction in the complexity of dendritic branches in neurones.[177] This could also serve to reduce the extent to which an individual neurone is connected to its neighbours, both close by and long distance. A sort of de-networking effect. Another synaptically-enriched microRNA, miR-138, seems to perform a similar function to miR-134, reducing spine size. Within synapses, miR-138 has been found to target the transcript for an enzyme called acyl-protein-thioesterase 1 (APT1 – encoded by *LYPLA1* in humans). The enzyme removes a fatty acid molecule from proteins that control actin in the spine. This promotes spine growth. Like miR-134, the level of miR-138 is tuned to synaptic activity.[178] In models of synaptic strengthening, levels of miR-138 decline, whereas simulating conditions of synaptic depression increases miR-138 levels. So miR-138 negatively regulates spine size, playing a role in adjusting down synaptic strength, albeit via targeting different transcripts. At least in cell culture. What about in an intact brain? Mice in which miR-138 is inactivated display changes in behaviour and cognition consistent with some of these findings.[179] When placed in a maze, mice lacking miR-138 move and explore normally, but they have problems in tasks that test short-term memory. But not long-term memory. Curiously, the dendrites on neurones of miR-138-deficient mice were found to be normal, in contrast to what was seen when miR-138 was blocked in cultured neurones. This is a discrepancy from the observations in isolated cells which underscores the importance of investigating microRNA functions using both *in vitro* and *in vivo* ('within the living') methods. An equivalent experiment of knocking out just miR-134 is still awaited. So far, the cluster of microRNAs in which *Mir134* resides has been deleted and mice studied, but the interpretation of the results is complicated by the cross-effects of deleting several microRNA genes.[180]

The Net Effects of Spine Changes on Excitability

Let us look in more detail at the chain of events by which miR-134 produces the change in spines. We know that LIMK1 is important for maintaining the protein scaffolding inside the dendrite. When active, LIMK1 adds a phosphate group to a protein called cofilin. This inactivates cofilin and has the effect of expanding the spine head because cofilin normally works to depolymerise actin; it switches it from a fibre-like shape to a globular form. Effectively, cofilin collapses the spine head, so blocking cofilin retains the spine size and shape. By reducing levels of LIMK1 protein, miR-134 would cause a small shrinkage of the spine head. What effect is that likely to have? As explained earlier, the dendritic spine head is the primary site of glutamatergic input and the synaptic currents and the strength they convey are proportional to the volume of the spine head. Studies show that glutamate produces larger currents when released onto large-volume spines. Larger currents through a spine make it more likely, overall, for an action potential to occur in the recipient neurone. A circuit or feedback loop therefore links increased synaptic activity to a microRNA that blocks a spine-growth protein. By regulating levels of LIMK1, miR-134 can avoid overgrowth of spine heads and the accompanying increased signal strength at that synapse. It acts as a sort of circuit-breaker. But what if the system also functions in inhibitory neurones? An increase in synaptic input onto inhibitory neurones that increases miR-134 levels would reduce spine volume. If we reduce the excitatory drive onto an inhibitory neurone, we could end up reducing the brain's ability to dampen excitability. We'd be removing a layer by which excitability is kept in check. So, it is important that we know not only if a microRNA and its target is present in the same synaptic structure but also the cell type, be it inhibitory or excitatory.[181] In the original studies by Schratt's team, they used cultures of rat brain neurones. These would be mainly excitatory neurones because of the way standard cell culturing conditions favour the normal ratios of cell types.

Similar questions arise if we think about microRNAs that might affect the number of spines. Several of these have been identified. A reduction in spine number could reduce the number of potential inputs and reduce network excitability. An increase in spine number should increase the potential input sites and so favour greater excitability. However, there are experiments which show that spines can also function as a filter on excessive excitability. A reduction in spines could indicate a less-connected neurone, perhaps one that has fewer inhibitory inputs and is thus more excitable, and does not take account of a potential change to the balance of excitatory and inhibitory input. And changes to spines are not always accompanied by changes to synaptic strength. Studies have shown that fully blocking synaptic transmission produces only modest changes to dendritic spine dynamics. Finally, the actin depolymerising agent latrunculin A, which reduces spine volume, actually causes seizures when directly applied to the rodent brain.[182] Thus, it is not simple to predict how a microRNA that targets the number or volume of spines may affect overall excitability.

One approach to getting a clearer sense of the function of miR-134 is to modify its activity in an intact brain. This is possible using antimirs to inactivate microRNAs. These work *in vivo* as well as *in vitro*. Researchers in my lab, having followed the miR-134 discoveries by Schratt, decided to look at what happened to spines when you inject antimirs targeting miR-134 into the mouse brain. Working with Javier DeFelipe at the Cajal Institute in Madrid, we shared brain slices from mice which they took and then individually filled neurones with a fluorescent tracer chemical.[183, 184] This diffused around the cell and then the entire neurone could be imaged under a microscope. The method was laborious and technically difficult and only a few cells could be labelled per brain section. That meant decisions had to be made on which cells to inject. We picked pyramidal neurones in the hippocampus because they are large excitatory neurones with elaborate dendritic trees covered in spines. What did we see? Treating mice with the miR-134 inhibitor caused an increase in the volume of spines in the neurones, matching what had been reported in cell culture. But we observed a second effect, a slight reduction in the number of dendritic spines. Changes to spine number were not found by Schratt's team when they manipulated miR-134 in rat hippocampal neurones. But that had been in a Petri dish–type experiment. We had been imaging neurones after blocking miR-134 in the intact mouse brain. After all, LIMK1 was not known to regulate spine number and a previous study found normal numbers of spines in *Limk1*-deficient mice. This indicated a new effect of blocking miR-134 *in vivo*. Perhaps in an intact brain a slightly different set of targets was under the control of miR-134? Or perhaps what we were seeing was an 'off-target' effect, something unrelated to blocking miR-134. What would be the net effect of these two changes? A reduction in spines on excitatory neurones might reduce excitability, but larger spine volume would be expected to transmit larger post-synaptic currents. To try to understand, we performed further experiments. First, we used a miniature version of an electroencephalogram (EEG) to record electrical activity on the surface of the brain. The EEG records weak signals from brain tissue that arise as signals are transmitted around the brain. The EEG recordings from the mice treated with the miR-134 inhibitor looked normal. But EEG recordings tell us only about things happening close to the surface of the brain and give very poor spatial resolution. That is, you can't be very certain which neurones you are detecting the activity of using an EEG. We decided to move deeper and joined forces with Stephanie Schorge at University College London (UCL), part of a collaboration that had started through a large European project called EpimiRNA that I was coordinating. The UCL team included Gareth Morris, who was an expert in electrophysiology. He was able to record the activity of neurones using miniature electrodes placed directly on the surface of thin slices of the brain structure called the hippocampus. He could also gather information about how networks of neurones behaved by placing the recording electrode outside the cell, within the spaces occupied by dendrites. Now we could ask questions about how neurones behaved when we manipulated miR-134 with much greater precision. Were neurones firing differently when we manipulated the microRNA? Did they produce stronger or weaker action potentials? Did they synchronise more or less? Gareth found that most of the properties of individual neurones were normal across several tests.[185] He made recordings of what are called miniature excitatory post-synaptic currents. These are the weak but nevertheless detectable pulses of current that occur as pockets of excitatory neurotransmitters reach their target receptors and cause brief openings of an ion channel that let sodium or calcium into a cell. The recordings looked normal. He measured action potentials by directly injecting current into a neurone, bypassing the need for neurotransmitters to bring the cell up to a threshold for firing. Again, things were normal. So, he decided to push the network a bit harder, to in effect stress-test the whole hippocampus by giving it a 'seizure'. There are several ways this can be done. You can electrically stimulate the tissue at a high frequency. You can wash in a drug that blocks inhibition, for example a drug that blocks GABA or mimics an excitatory neurotransmitter. An electrical storm can also be triggered by changing the amount of potassium in the bathing solution around the neurones. This is because the membrane potential depends in large part on the differences in potassium concentration between the outside (low) and the inside (high) of neurones. Adding more potassium to the solution bathing the tissue changes this ratio and the membrane potential shifts in a positive direction, which can cause neurones to fire more action potentials. When Gareth washed the potassium solution onto brain slices, he could see typical high-firing 'epileptiform' activity. When he ran this experiment in the presence of the miR-134 inhibitor, he found that this was greatly reduced. Blocking the microRNA prevented neurones from synchronising and firing at very high frequency. It had blocked the electrical storm. What changes in the various machines of synaptic transmission were being changed by inhibiting this microRNA? Was it the changes in the dendrites? Reshaping some of the synapses or their number? The experiment was not designed to get that answer, but it had helped move a step forwards in our understanding of this particular microRNA. There were also implications for miR-134 inhibition as a possible drug to stop seizures. We will return to this in detail in Chapter 6.

Other Spine-Tingling MicroRNAs

A whole trove of microRNAs has been found to control dendritic spine function. We've now met some of these – miR-134, miR-138 and miR-181a. Another is miR-132, which we met in the context of how neurones link synaptic activity to transcription of new microRNAs. The effects of miR-132 on synapse structure are roughly the opposite to miR-134 and miR-138. When miR-132 levels are increased in neurones, it causes dendrites to extend and branch more. This has the ability to adjust communication in the brain by making more connections between neurones. The changes to structure occur because miR-132 targets a transcript that encodes a protein called p250GAP (in humans, the *ARHGAP32* gene).[186] This protein promotes disassembly of the scaffolding inside dendrites. If you deplete p250GAP from neurones then dendrites grow larger and more complex. A rise in levels of miR-132, which occurs when you stimulate neurones, as we saw earlier, puts a block on p250GAP, leading to dendrite growth. This is all calcium-dependent, and it goes away if you block NMDA receptors at the same time as the stimulation is given. So, here is another microRNA-controlled circuit that regulates the structure of dendrites in response to activity. This set of microRNAs therefore act somewhat like physiological opponents, working as a team at synapses. As synaptic inputs arrive, an increase in miR-134 and miR-138 acts to dampen signal strength, while an increase in miR-132 promotes outgrowth and expansion of the dendritic receptive field. The balance between these affects whether or not a synapse is adjusted. We don't fully understand who wins this battle at the level of individual synapses because it is difficult to measure all the various components at once while recording synaptic strength changes. The outcome at the individual synapse probably comes down to its composition and balance of microRNA and target transcript levels, the recent history of inputs, specific calcium changes and probably other factors we are yet to discover.

Many of the findings described so far used antimirs to tease out what the microRNA is doing, but antimirs are not perfect tools. Only a fraction of the antimir introduced to a system probably makes it inside cells to engage their microRNA targets, so total inhibition cannot be guaranteed. Genetic evidence, meaning manipulating the DNA for the microRNA, is important to corroborate important discoveries. The same team at the Vollum Institute who linked CREB to miR-132 generated a mouse in which the *Mir132* gene could be deleted, using the floxing technique.[187] This meant that the timing and even the cell type in which miR-132 is deleted could be controlled by treating mice with the Cre enzyme. The team delivered the Cre enzyme packaged inside a virus into the hippocampus of mice, deleting miR-132 from various neurones. When they studied the structure of the miR-132-deficient neurones, they found fewer, shorter dendrites with dramatically reduced complexity. Where dendrites were properly formed, they had fewer spines. This fully backed up the earlier studies that used antisense inhibitors (vindicating antimirs as a tool for microRNA research in the brain). But do the effects of manipulating miR-132 translate into something we can recognise as a change in brainpower? Notably, an earlier experiment found that levels of miR-132 increase in the brains of mice as they learn to navigate a maze, an effect mediated through CREB. Using a reverse of the Vollum Institute approach, a mouse was generated in which miR-132 levels could be increased in CaMKII-expressing excitatory neurones.[188] When the cognitive ability of mice mildly over-expressing miR-132 was studied, the results were remarkable. They learnt to navigate a maze more quickly and made fewer mistakes in repeat trials. This tracked with an increase in spines. The team had made smarter mice by elevating levels of miR-132. But the benefits of extra miR-132 were dose-sensitive. When they increased levels too much, the opposite effect was observed. The mice performed worse than normal in a maze. So, too much of a good thing . . . Perhaps excess spines and complexity reach a point where they negatively affect network activity. The brain becomes too 'connected'. This has been seen in some neurodevelopmental disorders. For example, there are extra spines on the neurones of children with fragile X, which is associated with severe problems with learning. Interestingly, increased levels of miR-132 are a feature of models of the brain disease epilepsy in which excessive networking of neurones may be an underlying mechanism and cognitive problems are also common among patients.

A Wrinkle to the MicroRNA-Synapse Control Story

This section has focussed on how microRNAs contribute to matching input and output during communication across synapses, in particular at dendritic spines, the most common site of excitatory neurotransmission (see **Figure 5.4**). But not all synaptic transmission occurs at spines on dendrites. I speculated earlier that the net outcome from changing spines

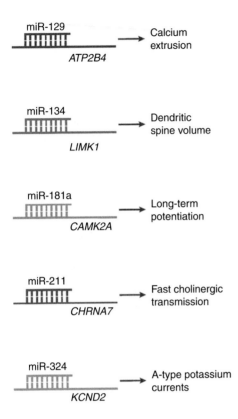

miR-129 → Calcium extrusion
ATP2B4

miR-134 → Dendritic spine volume
LIMK1

miR-181a → Long-term potentiation
CAMK2A

miR-211 → Fast cholinergic transmission
CHRNA7

miR-324 → A-type potassium currents
KCND2

Figure 5.4 Synapse-localised microRNAs and their targets

Examples of microRNAs and their targets that act locally at the synapse to regulate communication.

Source: Brennan & Henshall, *Nature Reviews Neurology*, vol. 16, pp. 506–19 (2020).[10]

would depend on whether the cell making them was excitatory or inhibitory. The situation is more complicated, however. The inputs and connections of the two main classes of neurones are actually quite different. The terminals of most inhibitory neurones converge closer to the receiving neurone's main cell body, the soma, including around the point where the axon branches off this part, called the axon initial segment. This creates a strong influence on the firing properties of the receiving neurone, placing inhibitory input close to the physical site where the action potential will manifest. If the incoming inhibitory transmission does not arrive onto dendritic spines, the coupling of microRNA activity to the structure of dendrites does not apply. That is not to say that there are no inhibitory synapses at other points; there are, and some do fall on dendrites. But some of the microRNA control mechanisms will have limited significance for inhibition in the brain.

What about the input to inhibitory neurones themselves? Most mature inhibitory GABA-releasing neurones are not encrusted with the dendritic spines seen on excitatory neurones. An exception is the medium spiny neurones of a brain structure called the striatum. The synaptic input for most GABA-releasing interneurones arrives directly onto the shaft of their dendrites. While inhibitory neurones express the receptors for glutamate, and thus can be activated by excitatory neurones, they generally lack a substantial NMDA receptor complement. Despite these differences, Schuman's and other studies that labelled newly synthesised proteins confirm that there is very active translation, with protein synthesis in the dendrites of inhibitory neurones. And there are thousands of mRNA transcripts present in the dendrites of inhibitory neurones. Some of these are the same as those in the dendrites of excitatory neurones, but others are not. For example, GABA-releasing neurones do not have in their dendrites the transcript for CaMKII, a key protein in activity-dependent changes to excitatory synapses. Last, the synaptic dynamics of a given inhibitory neurone acting on different target excitatory neurones are the same. This suggests a degree of non-plasticity in this form of inter-neurone communication and it contrasts sharply with excitatory neurones which display varied synaptic strength on different targets, presumably owing to prior activity-dependent plasticity. The point is that much of what we know about microRNA function at synapses has come from studying dendritic spines on excitatory neurones. This means that a large and important class of synapses has been understudied. Many of the expressed transcripts in inhibitory neurones display 3' UTRs rich with microRNA binding sites. Studies show that inhibitory neurones express a large contingent of microRNAs, but, given the afore-mentioned differences in synaptic communication, it is possible that microRNAs in inhibitory neurones have other roles than those their cousins perform in excitatory neurones. Notably, the Vollum Institute team showed that miR-134, one of the most studied of the microRNAs that control dendritic structure, is active in inhibitory neurones.[189] If spines are less important for inhibitory neurones, then the attention of miR-134 will be switched to other, non-spine targets. Researchers working to resolve these issues are beginning to focus more on the functions of microRNAs in inhibitory neurones. In studies by Schratt's team, the most pronounced increase in transcripts after genetic deletion of *Mir138* occurred in inhibitory neurones.[179] This suggests that miR-138 is important in defining inhibitory neurone features by suppressing a pool of transcripts. As mentioned, mice lacking miR-138 display short-term memory deficits. Experiments showed that these can be replicated by blocking miR-138 exclusively in inhibitory neurones in the hippocampus of mice. That is, the memory faults in mice lacking miR-138 are owing to a change in inhibitory neurone function. Recordings from excitatory neurones, which are critical to these memory events, detected enhanced incoming inhibitory signals in mice lacking miR-138 in their GABA-producing neurones. This implied that faults in memory were owing to over-inhibition in the hippocampus. Thus, correct amounts of inhibitory signalling depend on the actions of this microRNA, with an excess of inhibition blocking new memory formation. Notably, many of the genes controlled by miR-138 in inhibitory neurones have been linked to schizophrenia. The links between microRNAs and this psychiatric condition are discussed later in this chapter.

MicroRNAs and Making Us Smarter

The studies on miR-132, miR-134 and miR-138 show that microRNAs at synapses exert powerful influence on structure and function. The ability to change synaptic strength could have several applications. As we'll see later, adjusting levels of these microRNAs could represent new ways to treat brain diseases in which there is too much excitability. If higher amounts of miR-134 reduce the size or block the growth of synapses, this could affect plasticity and potentially reduce the ability to learn. Could blocking miR-134 do the opposite, that is, improve our ability to learn? Make you *smarter*?

We have thought about this question. In reality, specific synapses change on specific neurones in response to very specific types of incoming information that vary in strength and timing. So, probably, blocking miR-134 in a general way could not make us smarter. There is also the issue that while inhibiting miR-134 in the brain increases spine volumes, it also slightly decreases spine numbers, at least in mice. The latter effect may get in the way of seeing any benefits of the former. Simply growing spines in a general way would be unlikely to create conditions that make us smarter. But the results with miR-132 were impressive and so we tried an experiment. We ran a series of tests on mice and rats given a miR-134 inhibitor.[183-185] In one test we simply observed the animals doing their everyday activities, such as grooming, rearing and exploring. Everything looked normal. We then put the rodents into small rooms with objects both familiar and novel and looked at whether they showed any more interest in one over the other. Rodents are naturally curious and will tend to go over to a new object, or one that has been moved, and check it out. If you calculate the ratio of time between the old and the new object/position then you have a very crude measure of memory or cognition. But the rodents given the miR-134 inhibitor showed no more or less interest than the controls. So, a broad-acting inhibitor of miR-134 doesn't seem to make a rodent smarter; it doesn't make it dumber, either. It remains possible, of course, that if we could target the synapses in a way that was more selective, we might be able to do better. Something for the future perhaps . . .

A Fault in the Spines

We weren't the first or only people thinking about miR-134 and brainpower. A team at MIT found a link between miR-134 and learning in a study reported in *Nature* in 2010.[190] This actually began as a study of a gene called *SIRT1*, a member of the sirtuin family. These are truly ancient genes. A homologue is found in yeast, an organism we last shared a common ancestor with about a billion years ago. The gene encodes a protein that seems to sculpt the genome, shaping and adjusting it to switch genes on or off. The MIT team came across miR-134 when they were studying mice in which a segment of the *Sirt1* gene responsible for catalytic activity had been selectively inactivated in neurones. What they found was that mice without functional SIRT1 had learning impairments. The actual test measured whether the mice could associate a stimulus with a context. In one experiment, mice heard a sound followed by getting a small electric shock from the cage floor. A normal mouse quickly learns that if the sound happens, they're going to get a shock and they freeze as soon as they hear the sound. A natural fear response. The SIRT1-mutant mice didn't freeze. They hadn't learnt to associate the sound with a soon-to-happen foot-shock. The team checked all sorts of other reasons why the mice might not freeze, for example they couldn't hear properly, and ruled them out. The cognitive problems were pervasive. For example, when introduced to a new object in their cage, a mouse will normally spend time exploring it. The SIRT1-mutant mice spent no more time with the new object than the old. And the mice were poor at learning about where things were in space. A classic test of learning is to have a rodent swim around in a tank of opaque liquid. In one place there is a submerged platform. Animals will eventually find the platform, after swimming around in a random way. Next time they're placed in the pool they swim straight for the submerged platform. When the mice missing SIRT1 were put in a swim test, they failed to remember the location of the underwater platform. Each test they would swim around as if it was their first time.

The team suspected that this could all be owing to faulty spines. When they looked, they found that there were fewer spines than normal in the neurones in the SIRT1-mutant mice. To prove that this had consequences, they tested synaptic strength and plasticity. One way this can be done is to deliver a train of electrical impulses into the hippocampus. After a short delay, you find that the response of future stimulations is larger. Routine electrical responses in the mutant mice were normal, but when they gave a prolonged train of electrical impulses to mimic a strong experience, the expected increase in synaptic strength failed to materialise. They started to look for clues as to what was wrong as a result of the loss of SIRT1. They found a fault in the BDNF signalling system which links increased synaptic activity to the growth of spines during learning. This was traced in turn to lower levels of CREB in the SIRT1-mutant mice. But levels of the mRNA transcript for *Creb* were normal. This tipped them off that a post-transcriptional process was altered. One or more microRNAs were suspected and miR-134 turned out to be the culprit. They checked the levels of miR-134 in the brains of the SIRT1-mutant mice and found that they were abnormally high. They found that the *Creb* transcript had a binding site for miR-134. Things were coming together. Through a set of further experiments, they proved that miR-134 could down-regulate CREB whereas blocking miR-134 increased levels of CREB. This helped explain the memory problems in the SIRT1-mutant mice. We know that CREB is critical for long-term memory formation, from a discovery that can be traced to classic experiments in the 1990s by later Nobel prize–winning neuroscientist Eric Kandel in experiments on learning in a model organism (a gastropod called *Aplysia*). We share a similar, albeit more complex, molecular learning pathway as *Aplysia* (as do mice). So, too much miR-134 and you end up with lower levels of CREB, which means you can't learn. But why was miR-134 elevated in the SIRT1-mutant mice? It turned out that SIRT1 controls a repressor protein called yin yang 1 (YY1) that blocks miR-134. The removal of SIRT1 interrupted this brake and led to higher levels of miR-134 in neurones, knocking on to interference with the CREB pathway. Importantly, they showed that just increasing miR-134 alone created similar learning and memory problems in normal mice that were seen in the SIRT1 mutant mice. Blocking miR-134 in the SIRT1-mutant mice returned their learning and memory to normal. Interestingly, they never mentioned the behaviour of normal mice given the miR-134 inhibitor. So, we are left to wonder if miR-134 inhibition, at least some targeted version of it, could do some good in conditions where learning and memory are impaired. Could miR-134 inhibition help with any of the various brain diseases in which learning and memory are affected?

Dendritic spines and post-synaptic structures are not the only places microRNAs are found at synapses. Studies have also detected microRNAs within the part of a neurone that is presynaptic. That is, the axon terminal. Just like dendrites, there is local control of translation in axons.[169, 191] This is perhaps best studied in the growth cones of neurones, the tips of growing axons seeking to connect to a neurone. This local control of protein synthesis is critical for determining how neurones respond to local environmental cues that guide their axon to its target(s). The first microRNA demonstrated to act at growing axons' tips was miR-9, which targeted a transcript encoding a microtubule structural protein in response to signalling from BDNF. The precursor of miR-181a is transported to growth cones of axons and locally matured in response to a signal from a member of the semaphorin guidance molecules. This contributes to correct and appropriate linking of the axon to post-synaptic structures. Once synaptic connections are formed, microRNAs continue to be present within axon terminals where they tune synaptic transmission by adjusting the proteins involved in the machinery of neurotransmitter release.

Sea-ing the Evidence That MicroRNAs Make Us Smarter

Before we move away from the topic of the contributions that microRNAs make to cognition, we touch on a surprising insight from studies on the octopus. Despite being an invertebrate and belonging to a branch of the animal kingdom that includes molluscs such as slugs and snails, the octopus is known to be intelligent, clever and capable of solving puzzles and even tool use. Octopuses possess an estimated half a billion neurones, close to the number possessed by your average pet dog. But many of the octopus relatives have far simpler nervous systems. So, octopuses and other members of the coleoid family, which includes squid, offer a window into the evolution of complex nervous systems. If we can unpick some of the mechanisms that distinguish them from similar-sized but less-brainy counterpart cephalopods such as the *Nautilus*, we may find clues as to what helps build a smarter brain. A study in 2015 found that coleoids showed high rates of RNA editing.[192] This is a post-transcriptional mechanism unrelated to microRNAs that introduces base modifications to RNAs. It serves to create more diversity than is encoded in the genome. Research on the octopus showed that this editing happened most for transcripts with nervous-system functions. The octopus was expanding the pool of proteins that could be generated from the same basic gene instructions. If post-transcriptional changes to RNA are different in octopuses compared to other cephalopods, then what other post-transcriptional mechanisms might also differ? What about microRNA? Indeed.

Drawing inspiration from the RNA editing finding, a study in 2022 led by a team at the Berlin Institute for Medical Systems Biology searched RNA transcripts from octopuses for more clues to their unusual intelligence.[193] When mRNA transcripts were sequenced from the tissues of octopuses, they were found to be similar to other invertebrates with one exception. Octopus transcripts had much longer 3' UTRs, a classic 'tell' that they may be under the influence of microRNAs. Small RNAs were then pored over and microRNAs identified. A total of 164 microRNA genes were identified in the common octopus *O. vulgaris* (probably an underestimation, given gaps in sequencing and what is known about the genome). A remarkable 43 microRNA families were found in the coleoids that were not present in *Nautilus*. So, there was a large expansion of the microRNA repertoire during octopus evolution. And these 'new' microRNA families were being made in the nervous system. In fact, four out of five of the microRNAs unique to octopuses were present just in the nervous system. Many were expressed during brain development. Identification of the targets of these microRNAs is underway, but more than 10,000 microRNA response elements – conserved seed sites for binding – were identified among the 3' UTRs of octopus protein-coding transcripts. Predictions can be made that they have contributed to new cell types and wiring patterns that underpin complex neural networks. Again, all this points to microRNAs being linked to the development of complex brains and the emergence of higher intelligence in animals. **Figure 5.5** summarises the study and its findings.

Cell Type–Specific MicroRNAs: The Right Place at the Right Time

As we have already seen in earlier chapters of this book, for example Chapter 4, the co-location of microRNA and target in the same cell is of enormous significance. The molecular components for a given process may all be potentially under microRNA control. But the microRNA must be expressed in the same cell. A lot of research is performed using what is called bulk analysis. A piece of tissue or a mix of cells in culture is used as the starting material, then RNA is extracted from this mix. The cells from which the RNA originated

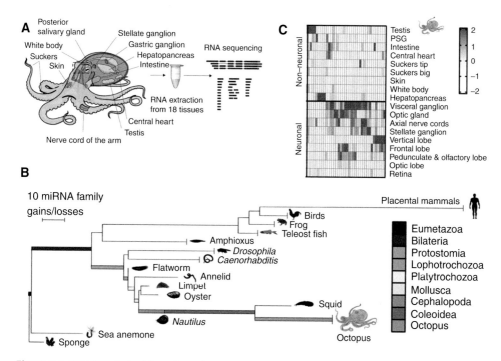

Figure 5.5 MicroRNAs helped the octopus become smarter

Analysis of the transcriptome of *O. vulgaris* revealed 35 novel microRNA families restricted to this species as well as long 3' UTRs in nervous-system expressed genes.

Panel A is a schematic of the tissue sampled for RNA sequencing.

Panel B shows a phylogeny of animal groups with the branch lengths reflecting gains of microRNA families (minus the losses). The vertical lines at the end of branches represent shared complement of microRNAs. Note the dramatic expansion of microRNAs in *O. vulgaris*.

Panel C shows the novel *O. vulgaris* microRNAs (columns) across tissues (rows), highlighting the gain in neural tissues.

Source: Reprinted with permission from Zolotarov et al., *Science Advances*, vol. 8, eadd9938 (2022).[193] Distributed under a Creative Commons Attribution License 4.0 (CC BY).

cannot be traced back. Thus, we might 'know' that a microRNA is expressed in the brain, but whether it is actually expressed in the cells in which we are studying a process of interest cannot be known for certain without somehow imaging the microRNA and the target. There are various ways to do this, but they are slow, technically challenging and do not often lend themselves to quantitation. This last limitation is important because, as we learnt earlier, stoichiometry is critical when it comes to how strong an influence a microRNA may have on a given protein or pathway. If there is a similar number of microRNA molecules to the target mRNA, it is likely that the suppression may be strong. But if there is a mismatch, with a small amount of the microRNA and a large amount of the target mRNA, the suppression will be weak or non-existent. But it is not sufficient to know that the microRNA and the target(s) are co-expressed in the same cell. Both microRNAs and their targets can be trafficked to different locations in the cell. So, a microRNA with a target recognition site for a synaptic protein that is present only in the soma of the cell would effectively be unable to regulate that target. It would be as if the microRNA were not even there.

To bring this together, knowing that a microRNA and a target are both present in brain tissue does not prove that one regulates the other. We need to be sure that they are present in the same cell and, further, within the same part of the same cell. This is all a moving target because the abundance of both changes with ageing and neural activity. Finally, we'd like some certainty regarding the abundance of each in order to have some confidence that the regulation occurring would be biologically meaningful. We can achieve some of these aims using in situ hybridisation, a technique that uses a chemical label or probe which attaches to the target RNA in the original place. That is, it allows anatomical localisation of a specific RNA. If a brain is sectioned into very thin slices, then these can be mounted onto microscope slides and stained for the molecules of interest. The cell types can usually be visualised or identified by other staining methods. The result is usually a spot of colour wherever your target is. By using a microscope, you can magnify this to the point where microstructures such as dendrites are visible and see if your microRNA is where you think it should be. By using two different coloured labels, it is possible to check if the target is also within a short-enough distance to be targeted by the microRNA. That is, if you label the microRNA red and the target green, then see yellow under the microscope, there's a good chance that the two are in close proximity. This doesn't easily solve the issue of the number of each molecule. Most methods at best give an idea of the relative amount of one versus another. Precise counts of individual molecules are challenging. Huge effort has gone into adapting techniques to improve sensitivity, which is important for low abundance molecules like the microRNAs that are present at synapses, and to improve signal-to-noise and quantitation. We are getting ever closer to methods that give actual copy numbers of each microRNA and target mRNA inside a cell.

Identifying all the protein-coding transcripts in all the different cell types in a tissue all at once is now possible. The technique is called single cell sequencing and it has transformed the fields of neuroscience and biomedical research. It is possible to measure the levels of every gene in any cell type. There are even ways this can be done on intact tissue sections. That means you can measure the levels of the expressed genes in cells within a structure. But this technology has not fully reached the microRNA world. There has been work to measure the microRNA composition of individual cells, but it is not fully developed and there are challenges. But when that technology becomes available, it will make it possible to sequence microRNAs and find out which are made in what cell type and how abundant they are relative to their transcripts. This could help resolve long-standing questions such as does the increase in microRNA diversity really account for the additional diversity of the human brain? Do patterns of microRNA expression change sharply and drive cell types to undergo additional rounds of specialisation? At what point, and in what combination of microRNAs, is the cell's final state fixed? What about looking at cell type–specific microRNA content in a disease context or after a treatment. How do microRNA levels change in different cell types as a brain disease develops? How is this altered by an effective treatment?

From the trickle of studies on this topic to date, sequencing microRNAs in specific cell types, we can expect major breakthroughs soon. Indeed, in Chapter 4 we saw the insights possible from single cell sequencing of microRNAs in the developing human brain.[61] That study confirmed that the mRNAs present in the AGO2 complex in the developing human brain were many of those that define individual cell types. For each of the 312 brain cells analysed, most microRNAs were enriched in one particular cell type. MicroRNAs that controlled proliferation were present in immature and still dividing cells, whereas those such as miR-124 with a role in fixing neuronal identity were present in mature neurones.

Brain cells use microRNAs to repress transcripts not needed or wanted in that cell type. And the study showed temporal switching and efficiency, calling up specific microRNAs to repress transcripts at one time, then using the same microRNAs later to control other transcripts. In closing the main part of this chapter, we have seen how microRNAs fine-tune synapses. They are themselves fine-tuned by the very signals they respond to, being adjusted by locally arranged biogenesis machinery. Their reactions are fast, their target pool extensive. Their actions enhance the capability of neurones to receive signals or remove contact points, and everything in between, including simply holding spines steady. How many synapses are subject to microRNA-controlled plasticity, and understanding the distribution of microRNAs and targets and the rules which couple signals to plastic changes, requires more work. But we have a solid foundation for understanding how microRNAs shape the identities and excitability of neurones, creating exceptionally rich brain circuits and bestowing an enduring ability to react, to learn, to remember.

Macro-level Brain Functions Controlled by MicroRNAs

Let us now zoom further out from synapses and look at how some higher-order brain functions are affected by individual microRNAs. We have seen some hints that microRNA can affect memory. But what about personality? How you react to situations? How you process visual, auditory, emotional stimuli? These questions are important since many common brain diseases and the broader area of mental health feature problems with these macro-scale brain functions. Researchers have been exploring this through a combination of comparative studies on human brain samples donated after death from healthy controls and people who lived with diseases such as schizophrenia. These are then twinned with mouse and other model species studies, where microRNA levels can be adjusted to match the human condition. These experiments have been run in both directions, sometimes starting with a finding in the human brain and moving to a model and sometimes the reverse.

The amygdala is an ancient part of the brain, found in all vertebrates and located deep within the temporal lobe. It is extremely complex, comprising multiple groups of neurones arranged as 'nuclei' that work together to perform specific actions. A recent study found that the human amygdala, based on distinct transcriptional features, contains 45 different cell types.[194] It is highly connected to other parts of what is called the limbic system, sometimes nicknamed the 'lizard brain'. This includes the hippocampus. Among its best-understood functions are roles in the coordination of responses to fear and stress, anxiety and emotion. This has been learnt through studies of people with damage to the amygdala, through electrical stimulation and through brain scans that track increased activity in parts of the brain during specific tasks. Parts of the amygdala connect directly to regions involved in stress responses such as the hypothalamus and brain stem, and are part of the circuits that coordinate the flight, fright and fight response. There is strong evidence that elevated and chronic stress contributes to various mental and neuropsychiatric disorders.

The functions of several microRNAs have been linked to the amygdala and how we perceive, process and react to stress and anxiety. Indeed, the extent of neuronal cell diversity in the amygdala alone implies a target-rich environment for microRNAs. This idea has been led by the team of Alon Chen, working originally at the Weizmann Institute in Rehovot, Israel. They studied changes to both protein-coding transcripts and microRNAs when mice were exposed to stress. Levels of multiple microRNAs increased in the amygdala and a remarkable 85 mRNAs associated with responses to stress were predicted targets of 1 microRNA family: miR-34s.[195] They set about trying to understand what microRNAs might be doing within this part of the brain. To prove that microRNAs were important to the amygdala in a general way, they took the blanket approach of knocking out the amygdala's ability to make new microRNAs. They did this by taking floxed *Dicer* mice and injecting the amygdala on both sides of the brain with a virus expressing Cre. This depleted Dicer just in this part of the brain, leaving microRNA production unscathed elsewhere. After a two-week wait, and an assumed decline in mature microRNA levels in the amygdala, they tested the mice. Mice are naturally inquisitive, but their evolved tendencies direct them to avoid situations where they might be spotted and eaten. Mice dislike open and bright spaces. When the mice lacking microRNAs in their amygdala were placed in test areas and given the choice of being in open or bright spaces, they avoided them in favour of being close to walls and dark areas. This is normal, but the level of avoidance in these mice was well above normal. They were hyper-anxious. Getting back to miR-34, the team were able to show that elevating the amygdala levels of one of the family members restored levels of anxiety to normal in the mice. The mice were still cautious, but would spend longer exploring the open, bright spaces. Delivery of the microRNA had an *anxiolytic* effect. The loss of Dicer from the amygdala did not cause any gross changes to structure and no neurodegeneration, at least at that time point. The mechanism was narrowed down to an effect on one of the key components in the stress response. A seed site for the miR-34 family member was found in the transcript for the receptor for corticotropin-releasing factor (CRF). This receptor is activated by CRF, which itself is released from the hypothalamus as part of the stress response. Thus, the microRNA was modifying the ability of the amygdala to sense the fear-provoking effects of the stress response.

Later studies by the same group identified a microRNA linked to the mechanisms underlying chronic stress.[196] To model chronic stress in mice, they repeatedly exposed animals to a more dominant animal. This had both a physical component, where direct contact was allowed between the animals, and a sensory phase, where they could see and smell the aggressor mouse but were physically separated. The short physical encounters result in anxiety which, over time, consolidates into chronic stress and depression-like symptoms. Levels of one microRNA in particular, miR-15a, were elevated in the animals chronically stressed by social defeat. When they modelled this change in normal mice, they found no initial effect. Elevated miR-15a did not change mouse behaviours in test mazes. Similarly, reducing levels of miR-15a had no obvious effects in the maze tests. But an effect was seen after exposing mice with lower levels of miR-15a to chronic social defeat. The animals were hyper-anxious (**Figure 5.6**). This suggests that miR-15a is somehow involved with recovery from chronic stress. Although this work in mice lacks the myriad complexities that underlie chronic stress in humans, levels of miR-15a were found to be elevated in blood samples from children exposed to childhood trauma.

This tells us that a functioning microRNA system is required for an appropriate amygdala-driven fear and stress response. It is part of our coping mechanism. By attenuating stress-related gene activation, microRNAs in the amygdala place limits on this complex, multi–brain region–coordinated response to visual and sensory stimuli directing motor and behavioural changes in the animal. Without microRNA control, the neurones within the amygdala are prone to eliciting exaggerated signals and triggering behaviours above what are natural and appropriate. Since the functions of the amygdala are highly conserved, this suggests that disruption to microRNA control may be a cause of affective and psychiatric

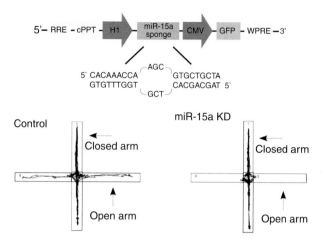

Figure 5.6 miR-15a protects against chronic stress

The schematic (top) shows the viral vector design including the segment containing a 'sponge' sequence that when expressed in cells knocks down (KD) miR-15a. The elements either side (H1, CMV, GFP, etc.) contribute to expressing or visualising the vector. The lower panels are traces of mouse movement in the elevated plus maze, a test for anxiety. The maze has two barrier walls and two open arms. After being exposed to chronic social defeat and then tested in the maze, the miR-15a knock-down mouse no longer enters the open arms of the maze.

Source: Reprinted with permission from Volk et al., *Cell Reports*, vol. 17, pp. 1882–91 (2016).[196]

conditions in humans, including post-traumatic stress disorder. If this is the case, it could open up new diagnostic and therapeutic strategies for disorders associated with excess and chronic fear and anxiety.

Disturbing Thoughts of MicroRNAs

There have been significant efforts to discover microRNA imbalances that may underlie mental health problems and the severe psychiatric disorder schizophrenia. Schizophrenia and other forms of psychosis are devastating to the lives of those affected and their families. Progress is needed as these are among the highest-burden brain diseases, often emerging in adolescence. While many people recover, schizophrenia for many sufferers will come and go throughout a person's lifetime. Two main types of symptom characterise schizophrenia. One set is called 'positive' and comprises changes in behaviour, including delusions such as paranoia and the feeling of being persecuted, and hallucinations such as hearing voices. Current treatments combine mental health support with medications called anti-psychotics. These comprise drugs that modify how dopamine and other neurotransmitters work in the brain and are moderately effective in controlling the positive symptoms. The 'negative' symptoms are much harder to treat. These include becoming socially withdrawn, unresponsive, emotionless and uninterested in the world. The causes remain poorly understood. There does not appear to be a gene 'for' schizophrenia. But genetics play a role. We know this from twin studies and other genome sequencing efforts. Environmental factors are also important, including events and exposures *in utero* and later-life psychological stress.

Notably, schizophrenia is one of the most common symptoms in people with DiGeorge syndrome, in which one of the missing genes is the microprocessor component *DGCR8*.

Mouse models of the syndrome feature impaired microRNA biogenesis and the animals display some psychosis-like behaviours. More broad evidence that microRNA dysregulation contributes to the risk of the disease has come from genetic association studies where DNA is sequenced to find variants and mutations. Large consortia have pooled together the genomes of tens of thousands of patients and compared these with controls. What they have found at higher frequency than the general population are sequence gaps and changes in the code for microRNA biogenesis genes and 3' UTRs of transcripts involved in neuronal function. Most often, the variants found are predicted to impair the normal production and function of microRNAs, but complete loss of a biogenesis gene is rare. Most people with schizophrenia do not have faults in the genes of the microRNA pathway.

A number of specific microRNAs have been linked to schizophrenia through these genetic studies.[197] One of the first was miR-137. Sequence variations in the precursor, but not the mature sequence, were found to be more common in patients than controls. Experiments suggested that the effect of the variant was to impair maturation, leading to lower levels of miR-137. Carriers of two copies of the variant develop earlier and worse symptoms and tend to have detectable changes on brain scans, including shrinkage. Notably, some of the targets of miR-137 are themselves genes implicated as risk factors in schizophrenia. This link has been backed up by studies in mice engineered to produce half the normal amount of miR-137 in the nervous system.[198] Mice with a partial loss of miR-137 have multiple differences in the structure and function of the brain. Dendrites are longer and covered in more spines than normal. Tests of synaptic plasticity show impairments and the mice are poor learners in maze tests. In tests that specifically measure neuropsychiatric symptoms, the miR-137-mutant mice exhibited elevated anxiety, reduced sociability, excessive self-grooming when in contact with unfamiliar mice and a general increase in repetitive behaviours.

But herein lies the rub. Despite them sharing similar psychiatric-like behaviours, many of the features in the miR-137-mutant mice are very different from animals lacking *Dgcr8*.[199] The DGCR8-mutant mice display fewer spines and lower dendritic complexity. Assuming that these discrepancies are not of some experimental design or technical factor, it becomes hard to reconcile the synaptic differences having anything to do with the altered behaviours, unless *any* change in spines and dendrites from the norm, too few or too many, can produce the same phenotype. This could be explained if a sort of goldilocks zone exists for spine density and dendritic complexity, above or below which we get impaired states of synaptic connectivity.

Another approach has been to start by measuring levels of various microRNAs in brain structures most strongly associated with the disordered function and symptoms of schizophrenia. This includes the prefrontal cortex, a large area at the front of the brain that is involved in executive functions such as coordinating problem-solving, reasoning and control over thoughts and actions. Notably, one of the microRNAs found to be lower in patient brain samples, miR-1202, is primate-specific and brain-enriched.[200] Targets of this microRNA include transcripts that support neuronal communication. We will need human and animal models to explore whether or not this is causally involved or has functional importance. Other microRNAs continue to be identified with links to neuropsychiatric disease. These include miR-499 and miR-1908, which were recently linked to bipolar disorder, a neuropsychiatric condition marked by episodes of extreme mood swings. Levels of miR-499 are elevated in bipolar patients and following isolation stress in young rats, and directly treating neurones with dexamethasone to chemically mimic a stress response triggers an increase in levels of miR-499. This microRNA is also enriched in synapses where a key target is a calcium channel–encoding gene called *CACNB2*, for which variants are known to predispose to bipolar disorder.[201] The neurones in which levels of miR-499 were elevated displayed altered structure, including reduced complexity of their dendrites. And calcium responses were subdued in the neurones with elevated miR-499. Bringing this together, elevated miR-499 may impair calcium entry during normal signalling and disconnect neurones from their proper circuits and contact points. Interestingly, there is a negative correlation between levels of miR-499 and the volume of a key temporal lobe structure, the left Wernicke's area. This is involved in language development and social cognition; the processing, storage and application of information. Brain scans show that people with the highest level of miR-499 have the smallest volume of that structure. Although correlative only, this finding suggests a link between high levels of this microRNA and the structural underpinnings of a complex brain disorder. Here, therefore, is another microRNA-controlled circuit that, by altering neuronal microstructure, can cascade towards brain-wide dysfunction that may contribute to neuropsychiatric disease.

These and other studies suggest that deficits and disordered microRNA function contribute to the molecular patterns that drive altered brain structure and function. There is a considerable way to go, however. Studies are needed to better understand what drives changes in microRNA levels and what those changes drive. Systematic efforts to map normal and neuropsychiatric-related microRNA expression are needed with high cellular and temporal resolution. This should be performed at different life stages, to assess the pre- and post-natal effects of known precipitants of psychosis. And we need better models. For example, the negative symptoms of schizophrenia are difficult to reproduce in mouse models. There are other conditions where microRNA dysfunction may also play a part, such as personality, sexual identity and eating disorders. Work to explore these is urgently needed.

Motor Control

A final example of where microRNAs serve critical roles in large-scale processes controlled by the brain relates to movement and the coordination of our voluntary muscles. Voluntary (skeletal) muscles are those we can consciously control and are one of three main types of muscle in the human body, the other two being smooth muscle, which we find in large blood vessels and certain hollow organs in the body, and cardiac or heart muscle. The control of voluntary movement is highly complex, featuring initiating, integrating sensory information, directing and then grading the firing of the motor nerves – motoneurones – which exist in different brain regions and the spinal cord, termed upper and lower motoneurones, respectively. The neurones that ultimately trigger voluntary muscle contraction extend beyond the central nervous system, which is the brain and spinal cord, and run out to the muscles in the periphery. Motoneurones have some distinct physiological properties that integrate the contractile forces generated within their target muscle cells. You can guess the consequences of damage or disease within our motor control system – paralysis. This can be owing to trauma, such as spinal cord injury and stroke, or one of several progressive neurodegenerative diseases. Probably the best known of these is motor neuron disease or amyotrophic lateral sclerosis (ALS), which is sometimes known as Lou Gehrig's disease in the USA and known worldwide because of affecting Stephen Hawking, among many others. There are also several severe childhood diseases of the neuromuscular system. One of these is spinomuscular atrophy (SMA). This usually has a single gene cause, a mutation in the survival motor neuron gene (*SMN*). The effect is often apparent when the carriers are still babies, striking within months of birth. The severity ranges but can be life-threatening owing to progressive weakening of muscles, including those used for breathing.

A failure of the microRNA system has been found to cause certain neuromuscular diseases. A link between microRNA and diseases of the neuromuscular system was already on the horizon when, during the mid-2000s, a series of discoveries was made on genes that caused ALS. Mutations were found in a subset of ALS patients within genes that coded for RNA binding proteins and those proteins were known to inhabit parts of the cell where microRNAs were active. This led a team from the Weizmann Institute to test what happened when you block microRNAs from functioning just in motoneurones.[202] Mice with impaired microRNA production, achieved by knocking Dicer out of the cells using the Cre system, developed motor control problems within a few weeks. They became slower and lost grip strength. Analysis of the muscles and motoneurones revealed active degeneration of both cell types and breakdown of the nerve-muscle junctions. Without certain microRNAs, levels of key proteins became disrupted, including the neurofilaments required for the survival and function of the motoneurones. Interestingly, although this study targeted Dicer, the levels of many microRNAs were found to be normal at the time that symptoms were appearing. This suggested that only certain microRNAs are required for proper motoneurone function and it prompted a search for the key microRNAs. Several were later identified, in models of SMA and ALS. The most important was miR-218. This was found to be the most enriched microRNA in developing motoneurones of the spinal cord. When the *Mir218* gene was knocked out in mice, the motoneurones failed to make connections with their muscle cell targets.[203] Over time, the motoneurones became hyperexcitable and began to degenerate. So, loss of this single microRNA was able to recapitulate multiple features of neuromuscular diseases such as ALS. Later studies showed miR-218 to be a master regulator of genes in motoneurones, repressing more than 300 different transcripts.[204] Those genes controlled neurotransmission and transport systems, including potassium channels, and all bore miR-218 binding seeds. In normal motoneurones, the level of these transcripts is significantly lower than neighbouring non-motoneurone cells, meaning that miR-218 establishes a unique pattern of gene expression in this neurone subtype. Such pervasive gene suppression is uncommon, but not unique. The abundant miR-124 switches off hundreds of transcripts expressed during early neuronal development to steer neurones to a mature phenotype. These findings raise further questions. How does the gene set targeted by miR-218 convey the special properties of motoneurones? What is it about higher levels of those genes that is so toxic to motoneurones? Does miR-218 do a similar job in humans?

We do not yet have the answers to the first of these questions, but we have for the last. Like the mice, human spinal cords and human motoneurones in cell culture express high levels of miR-218, while levels of miR-218 are lower in spinal cord samples from people who died of ALS. Not only that, but levels of miR-218 were the most reduced of all microRNAs in the patient samples. And the same genes over-expressed in the mice deficient in miR-218 were up-regulated in the spinal cords of the ALS patients. Importantly, genetic association studies found rare cases of variations in the precursor of the two versions of miR-218 present in the genomes of ALS patients.[204] This was proven to impair biogenesis of miR-218, leading to lower levels of the mature form, suggesting that this may increase risk or directly cause the disease. As with the studies in neuropsychiatry, these findings tell us important functions of this microRNA in establishing normal physiological features of specific neurone types. And that without them, in fact with just half the normal level, there emerges profound disruption to neuronal function that extends to impact major systems controlled by the brain, leading to devastating disease. We will see examples in Chapter 7 of how findings such as these are being used to develop new therapies.

Summary and Reflections

Throughout this chapter we have seen examples of how the microRNA system is active in the adult brain, adjusting to changes in patterns of neuronal behaviour and feeding this back, as well as underpinning the mechanics of communication, how we learn and remember. Much of our understanding has come from studying individual neurones and the microRNAs enriched at synapses. Here, they form a rapid response system that adjusts the protein composition of the synapse, changing the shape of contact points and the receptor and signalling mechanics, and increasing or decreasing the strength of signals that can pass through. But there is also a large pool of microRNAs in brain cells working to tune many other processes. We don't have all those details. Some processes lend themselves more easily to experimentation and not all the people able to perform those studies have yet shifted their attention to microRNAs. When and if they do, I expect we will see many additional processes central to neuronal function having a microRNA story. Scaling up, we have seen examples of microRNAs that, by influencing cell physiology, can extend to affect patterns of complex animal behaviour, in a molecular version of the 'butterfly effect'. And we have seen the stark impacts that faults in the microRNA system can have on the brain and the body functions under its control.

Our understanding of microRNAs and their targets in the functioning brain remains patchy. Full of gaps but moving towards a more complete picture. We are close to being able to determine what every microRNA in the brain is targeting in specific cell types. This will generate a more granular understanding of the roles of each microRNA. Research on microRNA contributions to brain disease is currently rather unbalanced. Tipped as you might expect to the most scientifically famous and those diseases where the burden is greatest. So let us finish by asking another question. Is there an(y) aspect of brain function that is not reliant on microRNAs? A disease where no dysregulation is detectable? Perhaps processes regulated by 'older' parts of the brain? Control of the autonomic nervous system such as respiration, heart rate, thermoregulation? Not so far. A glance at the literature finds microRNA links to these topics, albeit fewer than those for, say, psychosis. So probably the reach of microRNAs in the brain is pervasive. We know, however, that not all genes, including many expressed in the brain, possess sequence elements that render them subjects of microRNA control. For example, many of the non-cell-specific and maintenance genes lack elements in their transcripts that would render them under microRNA control. And there are diseases that can be caused by defects in those systems. However, the cascading events of any neuronal or glial cell dysfunction will change local, network and regional patterns of signalling so would ultimately hit the processes that are under microRNA control. Will we find a brain process outside of microRNA control? I'm not sure, but I look forward to knowing the answer.

Centre of the Electrical Storm
MicroRNAs and Epilepsy

6

When Lia was about three months old, her older sister Yer slammed the front door of the Lees' apartment. A few moments later, Lia's eyes rolled up, her arms jerked over her head, and she fainted. The Lees had little doubt what had happened. Despite the careful installation of Lia's soul during the *hu plig* ceremony, the noise of the door had been so profoundly frightening that her soul fled her body and became lost. They recognised the resulting symptoms as *quag dab peg*, which means 'the spirit catches you and you fall down'.

From The Spirit Catches You and You Fall Down: A Hmong Child, Her American Doctors and the Collision of Two Cultures, *by Anne Fadiman (Farrar, Straus & Giroux, 1997, p. 20)*

The Calm Before the Storm

The above quote comes from a book written about the experience of a family with a child who has epilepsy, and the clash of cultures between their traditional beliefs as an indigenous people from South East Asia and the world of modern (Western) medicine. There are an estimated 60 million people living around the world with epilepsy. In some respects, epilepsy is one of the 'oldest' brain diseases. There is a detailed description of epilepsy in one of the collection of Babylonian tablets at the British Museum, which dates to the middle of the first millennium BCE. Translated, it gives clinical observations of what we would recognise as the main seizure types and some of the different epilepsy syndromes. There are written accounts of people with epilepsy, thoughts on the causes and suggestions of treatments that date back centuries. In the past, epilepsy was called the 'sacred disease' on account of it being thought to be owing to divine or malign intervention. Hippocrates attempted to dismiss the idea of it being brought on by divine interference, reasoning that it was a disease like any other. There is a long and tragic history of the mistreatment of people with epilepsy; they were often blamed and tortured for being possessed by devils. To this day, it remains one of the most stigmatised diseases and surveys of attitudes towards epilepsy continue to find high levels of misunderstanding of what it is and what causes it. I have spent most of my career investigating the molecular differences found in brain tissue samples from people who underwent neurosurgery to relieve treatment-resistant epilepsy. What my studies over the past decade have shown, along with research by many others, are extensive changes to the microRNA system in the parts of the brain from which seizures arise or to which they spread. We have found changes to the microRNA biogenesis machinery and levels of dozens of microRNAs. This drives adjustments to genes and pathways that are responsible for the control of brain excitability. Some of these represent beneficial adaptations, an effort by cells and networks to keep stable. But other changes are maladaptive, contributing to the problem and driving and sustaining epilepsy, as well as compromising the effectiveness of medicines. This chapter will delve into this brain disease and the discoveries made about microRNAs. The applications of this knowledge include potential future medicines and diagnostic tests.

So, what is epilepsy and what causes it? It is a brain disease whose primary symptom is the recurrence of seizures.[205–208] Seizures are brief disturbances of brain function in which groups of neurones or entire brain regions undergo highly synchronous, high-frequency neuronal discharges. The synchrony becomes an electrical storm that temporarily disrupts the function of any brain region in which it arises or which it passes through. What is experienced or observed from the outside depends on where the seizure is occurring. Seizures in a part of the brain that processes sensory information may cause unusual tastes and smells, or visual or auditory disturbances. If a seizure spreads to the motor cortex, the part of the brain that connects to the neurones that contact your skeletal muscles, it will trigger sequential stiffening and contractions of the muscles of the limbs and trunk. If you have ever witnessed a seizure, this is probably the type of seizure that occurred. You may have witnessed other seizures without knowing it. Many types of seizure do not give rise to such physical changes and would be unremarkable to the untrained eye. Petit mal epilepsy, now called absence epilepsy, is an example of this type of epilepsy. Seizures in this form of epilepsy are very brief and cause only temporary disruption of awareness.

We do not fully understand what causes a seizure. At a very simple level, it is because a tipping point is breached between excitation and inhibition in the brain. There is either too much excitatory drive or too little inhibitory drive or a mix of the two. This idea comes from several sources of evidence: from studying brain samples from people who have epilepsy, the genes found to be linked to the disease, electrical recordings and imaging of the brain during a seizure, and our understanding of the mechanisms of action of various drugs that prevent, and neurotoxins that promote, seizures. Let's start with the last of these. If we give an animal such as a mouse a drug that repeatedly activates glutamate receptors to boost excitatory neurone activity, a seizure will develop within a few minutes. If we block inhibitory neurone activity in the brain with other drugs, a seizure will also develop within a few minutes. Some of the genes in which errors have been found in people with epilepsy encode components of the GABA inhibitory neurotransmission system. Dravet syndrome is an example of a 'genetic' epilepsy caused by errors in the DNA sequence that encodes a sodium channel that is required for inhibitory neurones to fire at high frequencies. There are also genetic causes of epilepsy that are owing to errors in genes that work during brain development to coordinate genes switching on and off. Mutations in these can give rise to wiring errors that misplace inhibitory neurones in circuits. Other forms of epilepsy appear to have a less important genetic component or none at all. Epilepsy can arise, for example, owing to injuries to the brain and infections and is more common in old age and in Alzheimer's disease.[209] In fact, epilepsy can arise at any time of life.

Temporal lobe epilepsy (TLE) is the most common form of treatment-resistant epilepsy in adults. We met this structure in Chapter 5. The temporal lobe is responsible for a number of brain functions including processing sensory information; aspects of spatial navigation, so we know where we are in the world and can remember how to get back home; and the creation, storage and retrieval of certain types of memory, in particular episodic memories such as remembering your first day at school, and emotional memories. Deep within this

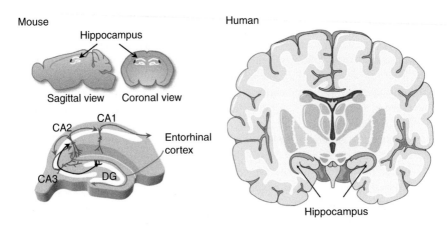

Figure 6.1 The hippocampus

This shows the location of the hippocampus in the mouse and human brain (in cross-section). The image at the bottom left is a schematic of the circuit connections between the sub-domains called the dentate gyrus (DG), CA1, CA2 and CA3; CA stands for cornu ammonis.

Source: Mouse brain schematics reprinted with permission from Chevaleyre & Piskorowski, *Trends in Molecular Medicine*, vol. 22, pp. 645–55 (2016).[210] Human brain schematic from Servier Medical Art. Servier Medical Art by Servier is licensed under a Creative Commons Attribution 3.0 Unported License (https://creativecommons.org/licenses/by/3.0/).

lobe is the hippocampus. **Figure 6.1** shows where this structure lies within the mouse and the human brain and the basic neural circuitry through which information flows.

The hippocampus is one of the most studied brain structures. Neuroscientists are very fond of the hippocampus. It has an elegant organisation comprising a three-part circuit through which information flows. Input to the structure comes mainly from a part of the temporal lobe called the entorhinal cortex via a bundle of axons called the perforant pathway. These synapse onto the first part of the hippocampus called the dentate gyrus. This is almost entirely composed of cells called dentate granule neurones. The axons of these neurones form synapses and activate large pyramidal neurones within a subpart of the hippocampus called the CA3 subfield. The CA3 neurones then target another set of pyramidal neurones in a region called the CA1. Finally, the axons of those neurones take signals out of the hippocampus and on to other connected regions of the brain. Interspersed with this circuit are inhibitory neurones that function to integrate signals and regulate firing of the excitatory, or principal, neurones. The hippocampus is also densely packed with all the major types of supporting glia cells.

What was noticeable to the first pathologists who studied the brains of people with TLE was that the hippocampus was shrunken and hard.[211] The shrinking reflected the loss of many neurones and the hardening reflected a scar formed by glial cells. Later, neurosurgeons began removing the hippocampus from patients with treatment-resistant epilepsy and found that this was highly effective at reducing or stopping seizures.[212] This proved that the damaged hippocampus was either the source of the seizures or an important part of the circuit. Neurone loss or the accompanying scarring process was suspected to cause this form of epilepsy. Both excitatory and inhibitory neurones have been found to be missing in resection specimens, which may tip the circuit towards seizures either because there are fewer inhibitory neurones or because there is a loss of excitatory neurones that activate the inhibitory neurones. This idea has been extensively supported using animal models of epilepsy. Electrical or chemical stimulation of the hippocampus of adult rats or mice causes neurone loss and, within a few days, epileptic (i.e. spontaneous) seizures. A recent study used an elegant technique to selectively delete just a single subtype of inhibitory neurone that releases a neurotransmitter called substance P in the hippocampus of mice. This caused epilepsy in all the animals within a few days.[213] Interestingly, when the brains of the mice were studied months later, many neurones besides the substance P inhibitory neurones were also missing. This proved two fundamental points. An insult to the brain that causes even subtle loss of inhibitory tone in the hippocampus is sufficient to cause TLE. Second, repeated epileptic seizures can cause further damage to the hippocampus that, over time, develops into the same pattern we see in patients with lifelong TLE. The rapid development of epilepsy in some models appears incongruous with most clinical observations, however. Our own studies have found that epilepsy in mice can emerge within two or three days from an inciting event, but many people have a first seizure out of the blue and quite separate in time from any conceivable brain insult. This suggests that the time frame for epileptogenesis (literally, the 'birth' of epilepsy) might be different in humans, perhaps because of species differences in cell types, cell density or other factors. Or, an initial insult seeds the epileptogenesis process deep within the brain and the time taken before the first clinical – that is, visible – seizure emerges reflects sub-clinical events that, over time, recruit more brain until a breakthrough seizure happens. The birth of TLE may occur a long time before it shows itself to the outside world. The debate over whether neurone loss is the most important cause of TLE is not settled. Added to which, surgical resection specimens from patients with long-standing TLE are occasionally obtained which lack any obvious neurone loss. In fact, the most consistent finding in the hippocampus of TLE patients is actually extra or expanded glial cells ('gliosis').[214] And neurone loss and gliosis are not the only pathologies found in resected TLE samples. Several other changes are also notable in most resection specimens. These include neuroinflammation, changes to the dendrites and axons, changes to the vascular supply, including leaky blood vessels, and changes to the extracellular environment, a matrix of proteins and other molecules that create structure for tissue. Experiments in rodents have shown that triggering any one of these processes is sufficient to create a TLE-like syndrome. It is this complex set of pathophysiological processes that makes microRNA-based treatments a good fit for treating TLE (see **Figure 6.2**).

The Beginning and the End

Despite the enduring changes in the brain, be it pathology or a gene defect, seizures are usually rare and brief events in people with epilepsy. Most of the time, the brain circuits are stable. So, what happens during transitions from 'no seizure' to 'seizure'? When seizures do occur, they are usually brief, so what makes a seizure stop? For some time it was thought that seizures began because inhibitory restraint on the brain network was temporarily lost. Several mechanisms for this onset moment are known and they are not mutually exclusive.[215, 216] There is broad agreement that it involves temporary changes to the inner chemistry of neurones that affect their ability to fire action potentials. For example, inhibitory neurones mainly use the neurotransmitter GABA. When released, GABA binds to an excitatory neurone and opens a gate for the movement of the chloride ion. This ion is

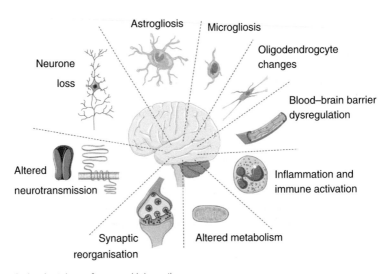

Figure 6.2 Pathophysiology of temporal lobe epilepsy

Examples of the various cellular alterations implicated in triggering seizures in TLE.

Source: Figure generated using images from Servier Medical Art. Servier Medical Art by Servier is licensed under a Creative Commons Attribution 3.0 Unported License (https://creativecommons.org/licenses/by/3.0/).

more concentrated outside the cell and carries a negative charge. Chloride entry makes the inside of the neurone more negative. Since action potential firing requires a change to a more positive membrane potential, entry of chloride effectively halts the firing of a neurone. But if these gates remain open too long then chloride will build up inside cells. This reduces the natural gradient that favours further chloride entry. At some point we reach a balance and chloride will no longer enter the neurone; it may even reverse and start to leave the neurone. If this happens, we have lost inhibitory tone, and excessive firing and synchronisation of surrounding excitatory (principal) neurones can occur. Another mechanism, described in Chapter 5, is via disruption of the potassium gradient. If potassium accumulates outside the cell, this reduces or depolarises the cell and neurones can lose the ability to reset their membrane potential between firing action potentials. This is a state called depolarisation block and if this happens to an inhibitory neurone then it will impair inhibitory control of the network. Experiments show that resetting inhibitory neurones back to their more negatively charged state allows them to restart firing and restore inhibitory balance. A mixture of these and other mechanisms underlies the neuronal synchronisation that signals the network shifting into a seizure. However, it is incorrect to think that seizures occur because inhibition fails. Human and animal studies in 2018 revealed that, counter-intuitively, GABA-releasing inhibitory neurone firing rates sharply increase immediately prior to seizure onset and may be the trigger for the subsequent synchronisation of excitatory (principal) neurones.[217, 218]

A seizure, whether it starts in one part of the brain and remains localised, or spreads, or begins on both sides of the brain at once, usually stops after one or two minutes. Why? One of the mechanisms is the build-up of adenosine outside neurones. This is a break-down product of ATP, the ATP having been co-released with many neurotransmitters. Receptors for adenosine are present at the terminals of excitatory neurones; when activated, they prevent further neurotransmitter release. We know that this helps to terminate seizures because blocking the formation of adenosine or the receptors it binds to causes seizures to continue for longer.[219] A second important seizure shut-down mechanism comes from the actions of protons (hydrogen ions/H+). This happens through the build-up of lactic acid and carbon dioxide (which forms a weak acid when dissolved in water) that accompanies metabolic activity during intense neuronal activity. The mechanism of this seizure-terminating effect is via acid-sensing ion channels. The binding of protons to the surface of these receptors causes them to open and allows sodium and calcium ions into the cell. The entry of calcium triggers neurotransmitter release. Because these specialised channels are present on inhibitory neurones, the build-up of acid activates inhibition in the brain. Experiments show that blocking these channels in animals results in seizures that fail to terminate.[220] Interestingly, acidosis brought on by inhaling carbon dioxide was known to inhibit seizures in people nearly a century ago; if some people with epilepsy hyperventilate and thus blow off too much carbon dioxide, making themselves slightly alkaline, this can bring on a seizure.

Treating Epilepsy

We can prevent seizures in people with epilepsy using drugs called anti-seizure medicines (ASMs). There are more than 30 available. But it was not always so. An account of the treatment of a person with nocturnal epilepsy called Janet Duncan, admitted to Glasgow Royal Infirmary in the 19th century, captures the awful reality of treatment efforts before the modern era of ASMs.[221] It reveals how poorly understood the disease was among health professionals, and how far we have come. Reported in History of a case of epilepsy, *Edinburgh Medical and Surgical Journal*, vol. 77, pp. 10–23, in January 1852, part of the description is as follows: 'on the 11th of September she had a number of severe attacks. Dr Alison saw her and bled her; ordered tartar emetic ointment to be rubbed on the head; gave her tartar emetic internally, and also pills, containing extract of colocynth, hyoscyamus, and croton oil.' Among the multitude of medicines and procedures given to the woman during admission was bleeding by leeches, croton oil to blister the skin on the head (that was tried several times), indigo powder, turpentine, a warm foot bath, wine (at one point a glass was ordered to be taken every hour), enemas (in general a lot of attention to bowel movements – both natural and medically induced) and tartrate of antimony – probably as an emetic (this was both given to her as a drink and rubbed on her head). She later died. If I had to guess, from human (iatrogenic) causes rather than the epilepsy.

The organised and systematic discovery of ASMs began in the twentieth century. One of the earliest drugs for epilepsy and one still in use today is phenobarbital. We have had this for 100 years. It boosts the amount of chloride that GABA causes to flow into neurones. There are other drugs that reduce sodium entry through channels, required during the first phase of an action potential, so effectively they work to temper the frequency of action potentials. Another drug, levetiracetam, modifies the mechanism by which neurotransmitters are released. Some ASMs work through a combination of actions. But there are problems with ASMs. First, not all patients get relief from their seizures. In fact, only about two out of three people with epilepsy achieve seizure control. Disappointingly, and despite the addition of further ASMs over the years, you are statistically as likely to be seizure-free today, in 2023, as you were in 1983.[222] Second, ASMs must be taken every day and often several times a day. Regular dosing is needed because our bodies rapidly break down and expel ASMs. Third, ASMs cause serious side effects for many people. Because they mainly work by dampening down brain excitability, patients often experience tiredness and a type of brain fog. There are other side effects, including liver and kidney toxicity. Some ASMs can trigger changes to mental state, including psychosis-like reactions. There are also rare immune reactions. One of these is called Stevens–Johnson syndrome, a skin reaction in certain individuals given the drug carbamazepine that can be life-threatening. Fortunately, a variant in a gene was discovered that predisposes people of Chinese ethnicity and different variants that predispose people of European ancestry. Warnings of these are now included on the medicine box and gene testing can be offered ahead of prescribing.

The other big problem is that ASMs do not cure epilepsy. They merely mask the symptoms – seizures. If you stop taking the medicine the seizures will return, regardless of how many years you have been taking the drug; ASMs do not seem to correct the underlying circuit faults. If we are to cure epilepsy, we need something that actually 'corrects' the brain network. This brings us to microRNAs. Could they offer a way to treat or prevent epilepsy? Could blocking microRNAs, and by doing so altering the functions of gene networks, be a way to treat a disease of brain networks? Which epilepsies would this work for?

Why MicroRNAs Make Sense in Temporal Lobe Epilepsy

Whether or not the inciting event is neurone loss or something else, most brain tissue from people with treatment-resistant TLE displays complex, multi-factor pathology. Replacing neurones is not easy, although researchers are exploring this, and while neurone loss might have been the sole inciting factor, the brain has usually changed extensively since and it may require changes to many processes to bring it back towards a stable network state. And layered on top of the enduring hyperexcitability is the problem of drug-resistance. Research shows that this is owing to a combination of changes in the movement of substances between the blood and the brain, as well as transporters and glial function, although the exact cause remains unknown. Disease modification will require the ability to adjust several processes and this is where microRNA come in. If a microRNA controls a series of pathways that are causing hyperexcitability and the pathophysiological processes that become altered in TLE, then there is a chance that targeting those – restoring levels if they are deficient or blocking them if they are in excess – could be a new therapeutic approach. **Figure 6.3** outlines this idea of microRNAs as being the right fit for a network disorder such as TLE. This concept can be exploited therapeutically, correcting multiple pathways by targeting the microRNAs that shape them; the approach is termed 'network therapeutics'.

Epilepsy and MicroRNAs

My laboratory started working on microRNAs in 2008. This was initiated by a brilliant neuroscientist with a flair for molecular biology, Eva Jimenez-Mateos. We were assisted by a team in the adjacent lab who had just discovered a link between microRNAs and the childhood cancer called neuroblastoma.[223] They generously shared some of their 'kit' and know-how, including a way to screen for microRNAs in tissue samples. Unknown to us at the time, a couple of other labs had also had the same idea. Three papers appeared within the space of a few months at the end of 2009 and in early 2010. The first of these, by a team at the University of California at Davis, found changes to microRNA levels in brain and blood samples from rats that were subject to different types of brain injury.[224] One of the insults

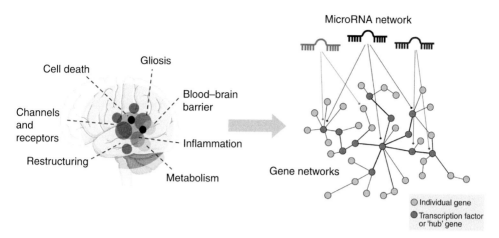

Figure 6.3 MicroRNAs control gene networks in temporal lobe epilepsy

The schematic on the left shows the temporal lobe and a selection of seizure-generating processes. These are in turn underpinned by altered gene expression networks (right). MicroRNAs regulate multiple targets within these gene networks, acting alone or in combinations on individual transcripts or more strongly via targeting gene control nodes. Darker lines between genes indicate stronger regulatory effects.

Source: Brain image from Servier Medical Art. Servier Medical Art by Servier is licensed under a Creative Commons Attribution 3.0 Unported License (https://creativecommons.org/licenses/by/3.0/).

was a prolonged seizure, triggered by an injection of a chemical called kainic acid. This is one of the most potent neurotoxins known. It was isolated from a red alga by a Japanese team in 1953. Tiny amounts are sufficient to kill neurones. The reason it is so toxic is that it activates one of the major types of receptor for excitatory neurotransmission in the brain. The receptor, known for a long time as the 'KA receptor' but now appropriately assigned another gene name, normally opens in response to glutamate. This causes a pulse of sodium ions to enter the neurone. Kainic acid mimics this, but, unlike glutamate, it is not broken down or removed quickly as a natural neurotransmitter would be, and it lingers, causing repeated activation of the neurone. Sodium overload begins and this then triggers osmotic swelling (water drawn in by salt); cascading secondary processes further damage the cell and within hours the cell is irreversibly damaged or dead. In addition to this direct toxicity, the kainic acid triggers waves of excitation that pass through the brain. This can create a permanently hyperexcitable state. The Davis team took samples from a group of rats that had been injected with kainic acid and measured the levels of microRNAs in the hippocampus. This revealed changes, both increases and decreases, in the levels of several. The two other studies published around the same time focussed on single microRNAs. One of the teams looked at miR-132, finding that it was strongly up-regulated by seizures in rodents.[225] The other study, led by wife-and-husband team Eleonora Aronica and Jan Gorter based at the University of Amsterdam, looked at miR-146a, which immunologists had recently found to coordinate inflammatory responses.[226] They found higher levels of miR-146a in the hippocampus from patients with TLE and showed that the same increase occurred in the same brain region when epilepsy was triggered in rats. In contrast to the very early and rapid rise in miR-132 that followed seizures, levels of miR-146a increased more gradually. The Dutch group took the important step of looking at what cell type was making miR-146a. It turned out to be astrocytes. In addition to hoovering up released neurotransmitter and generally contributing to the optimal environment surrounding synapses, astrocytes can mount powerful inflammatory responses after tissue injury. It appeared that miR-146a was a regulator of the inflammatory response in epilepsy, although, without manipulating the microRNA, it remained unknown whether this promoted or opposed neuroinflammation.

At the time these studies came out, we were sitting on our own data on microRNAs. We had used a microRNA screening kit to measure 380 different microRNAs in the hippocampus of mice given kainic acid, finding increases and decreases in the levels of 23 different microRNAs. We also had some of our own human data. For several years, we had been working with neurologist Norman Delanty at Beaumont Hospital in Dublin, a major centre in Ireland for the treatment of complex, drug-resistant epilepsy. The hospital specialises in the surgical treatment of epilepsy, procedures that were performed by neurosurgeon Donncha O'Brien. With the agreement of chief pathologist Michael Farrell, we worked to build up a collection of brain tissue samples donated after surgery by TLE patients. Then, using small pieces surplus to pathology's needs, we extracted RNA and measured levels of microRNAs, comparing these to levels found in autopsy samples donated to a brain bank. The levels in the human samples matched many of the changes we had found in the mice. We were about to publish this when the three other studies appeared. This put the brakes on our plans. We wouldn't be the first to publish on microRNAs and epilepsy, so the impact of reporting what we had found would be diminished. We decided to be patient and to add something more. Something no one else had tried: test whether altering one of the microRNAs would affect epilepsy. The ability to do this, to target a microRNA in a seizure model, was possible using antimirs. The main approach, at least for up-regulated microRNAs, was to inject an antimir into the brain of a lab mouse, engaging and blocking the targeted microRNA from working. We weren't chemists so we used a company that could synthesise a microRNA inhibitor for us. We just had to tell it which one we were interested in and it sent us a batch of the antimir. We actually picked antimirs to two microRNAs, but it was the results of testing the antimir to miR-134 that would change the direction and indeed shape the future focus of my lab for the next decade.

Blocking miR-134 Prevents Seizures

We met miR-134 in Chapter 5. There were several reasons to go after this microRNA. The link to neuronal microstructure was attractive because spines are conduits of excitatory neurotransmission and changes to dendritic structure were present in resected brain tissue from TLE patients. Our first job was to figure out how much of the antimir we would need to use. No one had inhibited this specific microRNA in the brain so we ran some pilot tests, eventually finding that injection of 0.12 nanomoles was sufficient to inhibit the microRNA (there are 6×10^{23} molecules in a mole, so this is about 10 billion times less). Having got the dose right, we checked how long the antimir effects lasted before wearing off. We found that the microRNA inhibitor had effects lasting at least one month. This prolonged duration of action was very exciting since it might allow us to generate long-lasting effects on the epileptic brain. We then designed two experiments. First, we would test what happened when we lowered the amount of miR-134 in the brain before giving kainic acid to mice. This would tell us if the microRNA controlled the excitability in the normal brain. The second experiment was the more exciting and ambitious. What if we inhibited miR-134 after we had initiated the epileptogenic process? Could we prevent epilepsy developing? Or at least reduce its severity? In both experiments, inhibiting miR-134 was protective. Mice in which we had lowered brain levels of miR-134 experienced less-severe seizures when later exposed to kainic acid.[183] We also found that signs of toxicity from the kainic acid and the seizures they caused, including neurodegeneration, were reduced. The results of the second experiment were the biggest surprise. Normally, mice begin to display brief epileptic seizures within a few days of kainic acid treatment. They continue to have these seizures regularly afterwards. The mice given the miR-134 inhibitor showed hardly any epileptic seizures and none at all during the first few days of monitoring. We kept watching and recording brain activity using our miniature EEGs, wondering if the effect would wear off. It didn't. Mice were still experiencing only rare seizures weeks and up to two months later. What we had found, it seemed, was something that could strongly suppress the development of epilepsy. But we had not fully prevented epilepsy. Perhaps we could, with some further adjustments to doses and timing of injections. To put this into context, ASMs have no such effect in preclinical models and nor do they prevent the development of epilepsy following brain injury in humans. The finding would set us on course to try to turn this into a medicine, a story we will pick up in Chapter 7.

Making Sense of the Mechanism

Over the course of the next few years, we tried to understand how the antimir might be producing these effects. We have identified three potential actions. The first, revealed by the first experiment, is an acute anti-seizure effect. This occurred when we injected the antimir, waited a day for it to take effect and then triggered seizures, which we found to be less severe than would be expected. While this was exciting, a drug that has to be given *beforehand* has limitations. That said, this is rather the way that epilepsy is treated currently. Patients take ASMs that lower the excitability of the brain, but they take them each day, even though an actual seizure might occur only rarely. So, although this finding did not rule out some clinical use, it was not what we were most interested in. What we most wanted to find, indeed where the majority of the focus is these days in the field of new treatments for epilepsy, is something that would modify the disease, actually change the underlying biological processes that are responsible for the disease. For example, switching certain genes off that were on, or vice versa, thus altering the connections between cells or other aspects of neuronal networks, could reduce their ability to synchronise and generate seizures. The results of our second experiment suggested that we might have an anti-epileptogenic or disease-modifying effect. The injection of the antimir resulted in far fewer seizures and this lasted for weeks. We think this is permanent because we tried to detect the presence of the antimir at the end of the experiments, weeks after the injection, and we couldn't find it. This suggested that over a period of a few days or maybe weeks, but not longer, the antimir had changed the circuitry at some level and disrupted the network that was triggering seizures.

We found one more benefit of the antimir. Epileptic mice that received the miR-134 inhibitor had more surviving neurones in their hippocampus. The molecule seemed to be *neuroprotective*. Was this a direct or an indirect effect of the antimir? If the antimir reduced the severity or duration of seizures, it might spare neurones from dying, but that would be an indirect effect. We suspected that the neuroprotection in the first experiment, where we gave the antimir before the kainic acid, was mostly because we had reduced the severity of the seizures. Less seizures = less damage. But in the second experiment we had given the inhibitor after the kainic acid and we still saw neuroprotection in the brains. This made it much more likely that the inhibitor was directly neuroprotective. We decided to perform a further experiment to settle the issue. We turned to neuronal cultures and set up three plates of cells. The first neurones were exposed to kainic acid alone. As expected, a check on the cells six hours later showed that half of the neurones were dying. The second plate of cells was treated with the antimir. These antimir-treated neurones all survived. The third plate contained cells given the antimir accompanied by double-stranded RNAs designed to lower levels of *Limk1* by RNAi. If the antimir was protecting the neurones by preventing miR-134's action on *Limk1*, effectively de-repressing LIMK1, then down-regulating *Limk1* should cause the neuroprotection to disappear. This is what we found. Virtually all the neurones that had been depleted of *Limk1* alongside treatment with the antimir in the plate died. This experiment told us that the neuroprotective effect of the antimir depended on LIMK1. Presumably, blocking miR-134's effects on *Limk1* caused the neurones to receive a less-severe toxic shock when the kainic acid was applied.

Work to understand the mechanism of protection is continuing. As with any microRNA research, the process of establishing which targets are important is complicated by the expanse of targets. I doubt that all the effects of the antimir are explained by rescuing any single target. The actions of microRNAs are context-dependent. We know that knockout of some microRNAs produces limited effects under control conditions, but upon stress or introduction of a pathology/disease context, strong phenotypes emerge. An antimir effect on a microRNA and its targets may change or be more complex as target levels and the site of action fluctuate in disease. And we must think too of the relationship between spines and epilepsy itself. Increased excitatory synaptic activity causes expansion of spines, but excessive stimulation (e.g. prolonged seizures) causes swelling and loss of spines. Severe dendritic alterations and spine loss have been reported in resected brain tissue from patients with TLE as well as genetically caused epilepsies. However, studies have also found rather normal dendritic morphology in brain samples from TLE patients despite a history of seizures, indicating that seizures alone may not always cause spine loss. Before moving on, there are two final experiments that clarify some of the mechanism of action of the antimir targeting miR-134 in the setting of epilepsy. We performed a mouse version of the cell culture experiment. That is, we lowered levels of *Limk1* at the same time as giving the antimir-134, but this time in mice that had been given kainic acid and were destined to develop epilepsy. The mice, given an antisense inhibitor of *Limk1* at the same time as the antimir, developed a higher number of spontaneous seizures.[227] That suggested that the seizure-reducing effects of blocking miR-134 in mice depend on the antimir restoring or protecting the amount of LIMK1. However, measuring levels of transcripts in the hippocampus of mice after they were given the antimir revealed changes to levels of 39 protein-coding genes in the mice given the antimir targeting miR-134 (see **Figure 6.4**). Among the different genes were elevated transcripts encoding potassium channel–related proteins, a transporter for sodium and a multi-drug transporter. Many other gene changes occurred at lower levels or less consistently. These could all be part of the anti-seizure mechanism(s). This captures the challenge of assigning a single mechanism to the observed effect of inhibiting this or any other microRNA. Efforts continue to understand how altering miR-134 protects against seizures. The answer could help with discovering future therapies.

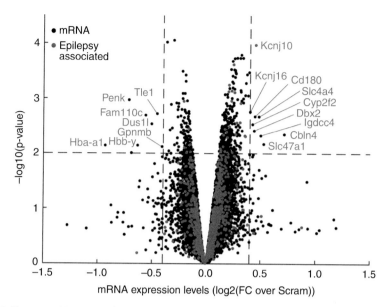

Figure 6.4 Changes to hippocampal gene expression after inhibition of miR-134

This 'volcano' plot shows gene expression changes in the hippocampus of kainic acid–treated mice 24 hours after inhibition of miR-134. Each dot is a unique gene transcript, with up-regulated transcripts right of centre, down-regulated to the left. The most important are specifically identified, based on statistical significance and fold change. Those genes previously associated with epilepsy are marked in lighter grey.

Source: From Reschke et al., *Molecular Therapy*, vol. 29, pp. 2041–52 (2021).[227]

Disappearing Dicer

We have also measured levels of miR-134 in human brain samples. The mature sequence of miR-134 is identical between mice, rats and humans and its functions in the brain may be similar since the seed sites for several experimentally confirmed targets are also conserved (*Limk1* might be an outlier here; the 3' UTR in the human transcript, *LIMK1*, does not possess a canonical miR-134 seed). Tissue samples from both the hippocampus and the overlying cortex of patients operated on for treatment-resistant TLE show elevated levels of miR-134. The up-regulation of the microRNA is therefore a conserved feature of TLE. This gives me confidence that if we are to develop a drug targeting this microRNA – see Chapter 7 – we have a good chance of it working.

During our studies we have found many other microRNA changes in human TLE and have also taken a look at the broader microRNA biogenesis machinery. In most brain tissue samples we have analysed, the levels of Dicer, AGO2 and Drosha appear quite normal. But in the most damaged hippocampal tissue, where there is severe neuronal loss and gliosis, we have detected a curious change: a reduction in Dicer levels but elevation in AGO2[228] (Drosha was again unchanged). Where this was observed, we also found lower levels of many mature microRNAs. Precursor microRNAs appeared to be present at normal levels. This indicates a select failure of the microRNA system at the point of Dicer, an impairment in the ability of the remaining cells to generate the normal complement of mature microRNAs. We might speculate that the higher AGO2 level is some kind of a compensatory reaction, perhaps a way to maximise the available RISC loading of any mature microRNAs that do get made? Mice with TLE following kainic acid treatment also had reduced levels of Dicer in the most damaged part of the hippocampus, as well as elevated AGO2. The findings are evidence that the microRNA biogenesis system can be impaired in TLE. I wonder if delivering Dicer via a gene therapy approach might have therapeutic benefits in TLE? This has not been tried by anyone, as far as I know, and remains on my 'to-do' list.

A MicroRNA Controls Motor Seizures

In Chapter 5 we encountered structures in the central nervous system (CNS) and a microRNA that is important for control of movement: the specialised motoneurones that depend on miR-218 which are located within the spinal cord and the motor cortex of the brain. But there are other pathways in the brain that control movement. One of these systems is called the basal ganglia, which is a set of brain structures and nuclei that control, among other things, voluntary movement. One of these, located in our midbrain, is the substantia nigra and a subpart of this, called the pars compacta, is dense with dopamine-containing neurones. Signals from these neurones are required for movement and motor control. We know this, in part, because this is the region of the brain most obviously damaged in the brain of someone with Parkinson's disease. The dopamine-producing neurones run from the substantia nigra to a brain structure called the striatum. Here, they synapse and modulate GABA-releasing inhibitory neurones. These act on and inhibit neurones in a region called the globus pallidus, which has neurones that project to another structure, the thalamus. From there, we get activation of motor pathways and initiation of movement. We are skipping some details, but the take-home message is that dopamine pathways are important for motor control. But this brain network also has a strong connection to epilepsy. Experiments show that stimulating and blocking parts of the basal ganglia circuitry can modify seizures. One of the earliest studies on this came in a 1982 paper in *Science* by a team at Georgetown University in the USA.[229] They showed that injecting chemicals that act like GABA into the substantia nigra blocked generalised seizures in rodents. Conversely, injecting kainic acid into the substantia nigra of rodents triggered seizures. Since that time, evidence has accumulated in labs and in the clinic for this seizure-modulating role. For example, brain imaging studies in people with epilepsy have found increased activity in the basal ganglia during generalisation of seizures, when seizure activity jumps from one place to another as the seizure spreads through the brain. While the findings have not led directly to basal ganglia–directed therapies, there are implantable medical devices that control seizures by stimulating another part of this circuit. And the amygdala, which we encountered in Chapter 5, is connected to the basal ganglia and commonly involved in the seizure circuits in TLE. Indeed, researchers apply kainic acid into the amygdala in rodents as a way to trigger seizures and model epilepsy.

Against this backdrop, Schaefer's team explored what happened when a key brain-enriched microRNA, miR-128, was deleted from specific neurones that are innervated by the dopamine-containing neurones in the substantia nigra. Their findings, reported in *Science* in 2013, were a major advance in the field because they demonstrated that epilepsy could result, at least in mice, from the deletion of a single microRNA gene.[230] Schaefer's team began with a full knockout of miR-128 ($Mir128^{-/-}$). Mice deficient in miR-128 were born and seemed largely normal, for a while. But they did not survive beyond two to three months of age. By watching the mice over time, they noticed that they were dying because of severe seizures. The loss of miR-128 was making the mouse brain much more excitable. They decided to narrow down the region of the brain and the cell type causing the epilepsy. This led them to a surprising finding. Deficiency of miR-128 in just a subset of the dopamine-responsive neurones of mice, those present in the striatum, resulted in the same phenotype as the full-body knockout, that is, severe motor seizures that were life-shortening. These were epileptic in nature since giving mice the drug sodium valproate, a common ASM, prevented the seizures and extended the lifespan. When they looked at the neurones of miR-128-deficient dopamine-responsive neurones, they found that they had higher spine density. Electrical recordings from the dendrite area also detected increased excitability. The study went on to show that miR-128 controlled levels of more than 150 gene transcripts. This included sodium and calcium channels and downstream signalling pathways. The team finished by demonstrating that boosting levels of miR-128 in mice protected against seizures caused by kainic acid. The study stands out as providing the first genetic evidence that a single microRNA controls the pathways that in turn control the motor component of seizures. It revealed miR-128 to be a master controller of neuronal excitability, and linked this effect to the pathways of the basal ganglia. The high-profile publication also stirred the field more generally, and more researchers became interested in what microRNAs were doing in epilepsy.

Control the Potassium, Control the Seizure

Regulating the concentration and the movement of potassium is critical to maintaining the appropriate excitability of the brain. As was covered earlier, one of the simplest ways to provoke seizure-like activity in neurones is to bathe them in a high-potassium solution. This has the effect of changing the membrane potential of the cells, de-polarising them and triggering bursts of action potentials. The human genome contains about 80 genes for components of potassium channels; even a simple animal such as C. elegans has 40 potassium channel genes. Faults in potassium channel genes give rise to a number of epilepsies, referred to as potassium channelopathies. They also give rise to some genetic causes of heart disease. But not all potassium channel variants are equally bad. Carriers of genetic variants and mutations in potassium channels display a spectrum of severities. Mutations in the KCNQ2 gene, which codes for the Kv7.2 voltage-gated potassium channel subunit, give rise to a condition called benign familial neonatal convulsions, an epilepsy syndrome that typically resolves within a few months of life. At the other end of the spectrum, variants in the KCNA2 gene, which encodes the Kv1.2 channel that contributes to the resting membrane potential and how the membrane re-polarises after action potentials, cause severe and life-threatening seizures. The importance of potassium regulation has driven several teams to look for microRNAs that target the transcripts that encode potassium channels and transporters. If dysregulated, these microRNAs could represent potential underlying causes or risks for human diseases, including epilepsy. The first study to specifically link a microRNA to the control of a potassium channel appeared in the mid-2000s in connection with potassium channels that regulate heart function. Later, in 2013, the KCNA1 transcript that encodes the Kv1.1 voltage-gated potassium channel subfamily A member 1 was shown to be targeted by miR-129.[231] My lab joined the microRNA–potassium channel hunt briefly, as part of a collaboration with a US team based at Emory University in Atlanta. Led by Nina Gross, now at Cincinnati Children's Hospital, they began with a specific search for microRNAs that might regulate the *KCND2* transcript that encodes the Kv4.2 potassium channel, a major contributor to potassium currents via controlling dendrite excitability.[232] Although rare, *KCND2* mutations can give rise to epilepsy in humans. The team found that the transcript encoding Kv4.2 was present in AGO2 pull-downs from the hippocampus of the mouse, indicating active regulation by microRNA. Searches of the 3' UTR of the potassium channel transcript revealed a promising seed match (GGAUGC) for miR-324, a brain-enriched, moderately expressed microRNA. In further experiments, they found that manipulating miR-324 in neurones resulted in changes to levels of the Kv4.2 protein. For example, blocking miR-324 using antimirs increased the amount of the potassium channel on the surface of dendrites of hippocampal neurones. The team reasoned that this should dampen overall excitability and moved to test this in mice. Giving mice an antimir inhibitor of miR-324 resulted in higher levels of the potassium channel and, when exposed to kainic acid, they had less-severe seizures. The finding could have applications as an epilepsy treatment because delivery of the antimir into mice with chronic epilepsy resulted in about a 50 per cent reduction in spontaneous seizures. This led us and others to expand our thinking slightly. While microRNA-based targeting seems a natural fit for complex pathophysiology where you want to change many pathways, the basic mechanism by which it works could serve other purposes. You could, in theory, target a microRNA to restore levels of specific genes, including treating epilepsies where a single gene is at fault. We will return to this later in the chapter.

The search for microRNAs that regulate potassium channels has been productive. Recently, a Korean team based at Daegu Gyeongbuk Institute of Science and Technology used a slightly different search strategy to identify microRNAs that could regulate the *KCNQ2* transcript.[233] This encodes a slowly activating and deactivating potassium channel. The spectrum of epilepsy associated with mutations in this gene is wide, ranging from benign neonatal seizures to a severe epilepsy syndrome in which the brain becomes damaged by the frequent seizures (an encephalopathy). Notably, mice lacking the *Kcnq2* gene do not survive long after being born, suffering fatal epilepsy. The team searched three different databases for microRNA binding sites in the 3' UTR of the *KCNQ2* transcript. This search yielded a shortlist of five microRNAs common to all three databases. The researchers went on to confirm that at least one of these, miR-106b, could regulate levels of *KCNQ2*. For example, increasing the level of miR-106b in neurones reduced the specific potassium channel current gated by Kv7.2, the protein product of the *KCNQ2* gene, whereas inhibiting the microRNA produced the opposite effect. Specifically, inhibiting miR-106b moved neurones to a more negatively charged resting potential, making them less responsive, with delays in action potential firing. Together, these studies and ongoing work show that microRNAs regulate multiple potassium channels. By affecting their electrophysiological properties, these microRNAs fine-tune the excitability of neurones. The findings have potential applications in treating some of the genetic epilepsies and, since neuronal hyper-excitability is common to acquired epilepsies, perhaps TLE. Several questions remain to be explored. How is the correct amount of these potassium channel–regulating microRNAs set within the neuronal substructures? What system of feedback determines this? Get this wrong and it can profoundly alter neuronal excitability. So far, very few studies have linked specific transcription factors to these microRNAs and this needs to be done in the context of epilepsy. The fact that modulation of these potassium channel–targeting microRNAs can produce measurable effects on neuronal excitability strong enough to modify seizures demands carefully regulated checks and balances of the microRNAs. This is true not only for these potassium channel–regulating microRNAs, of course, and applies to the other examples in this chapter.

Calming the Flames of Inflammation

Control of neuronal structure and function is not the only way that microRNAs influence the excitability of the brain in epilepsy. Glia-produced microRNAs have important roles, by shaping how these cells respond to the injuries that can trigger epilepsy and the ongoing effects of seizures on brain tissue. Here, a lot of attention has been on microRNAs that influence inflammation. A link between inflammation and epilepsy has been known for a long time. Indeed, in the account earlier in this chapter of the treatment of the young woman with nocturnal epilepsy in the *Edinburgh Medical and Surgical Journal*, dated 1852, there is mention of a fever in relation to an increase in the frequency of her seizures. This was supported, upon autopsy after death, by evidence of a brain infection. Besides the shocking list of attempted remedies, the article mentions that a cold press was applied to the head, although this was unlikely to have been much help.

Epilepsy therapy has come a long way. Unfortunately for Janet Duncan, she died a decade before evidence-based research revealed that bromide had anti-seizure effects. Later we have phenobarbital, phenytoin and the modern era of ASMs. As mentioned, these mainly work by targeting ion channels and neurotransmitter systems. But some epilepsies respond to therapies that target the immune system and inflammation. These includes acute, infection-related causes and epilepsies that arise because the immune system launches an attack on one or more brain proteins, so-called autoimmune epilepsies. Autoimmune epilepsies are increasingly being found to account for new onset epilepsy. There is a growing arsenal of treatments that help treat epilepsies of an inflammatory and immune nature.[234, 235]

The inflammatory process serves a critical role in the brain as it does elsewhere in the body. At its simplest, the inflammatory process is how we repair damaged tissue and also how we defend against attack. There are two major divisions: the innate and the adaptive arms. The former represents the systems intrinsic to any cell that allows them to react to an event such as tissue damage, and launch the repair process. The adaptive arm comprises white blood cells such as B and T lymphocytes and their weapons, including antibodies, that recognise the agent of harm and mount a counter-attack. Both aspects are vital to health.

Brain cells have an innate capacity to activate an inflammatory response. In the healthy brain, however, many of the gene pathways that drive inflammation exist at low levels or are entirely 'off'. But cells express sensors of damage. This includes toll-like receptors (TLRs), which comprise a series of protein structures on the surface of brain cells, each configured to react to different classes of molecule. Some respond to viral nucleic acids, others to features unique to bacteria. These systems are ancient and highly conserved, with versions present in Cnidaria, those simple animals that evolved more than half a billion years ago. When infection or damage activates TLRs, cells rapidly mobilise gene signalling pathways. One of these is called nuclear factor kappa light chain enhancer of activated B cells (NFκB), a transcription controller that mediates key early phases of inflammation including production of releasable molecules called cytokines that coordinate the inflammatory response. One of the best understood cytokines is interleukin 1β (IL1β). We shall return to this molecule shortly.

When it comes to the brain, the wound-healing process is a bit of a tightrope. The cells of the immune system are normally excluded from brain tissue and their entry can spell trouble. Some of the molecules released by resident and incoming cells sensitise neurones and change the function of glia to reactive, hyper-vigilant states, and this can literally spark trouble for the brain. Work published in *Nature Neuroscience* in 2022 found that surgically removed brain tissue from treatment-resistant epilepsy patients contains significant numbers of immune cell types that are absent from control brain samples.[236] Using remarkable new molecular imaging techniques, they could visualise these immune cells physically contacting resident brain cells, locking receptors on to their surface and presumably exchanging signals that direct one or other cell to specific courses of action. Since we know that some of these immune cells have cytotoxic effects, this may include killing brain cells. But we also need the inflammatory process to repair damage when it arises. A 2014 study of traumatic brain injury published in *Nature* showed that blocking early inflammatory signals from glial cells resulted in leaky, porous blood vessels in the brain and interfered with immune cell responses.[237] Early inflammatory reactions are essential for the recovery process.

A good example of the two-faced nature of inflammation is what happens to microglia. Injury to the brain rapidly changes the structure and function of microglia and this profoundly changes what they do. Work by Schaefer's group has shown that microglia are normally continuously sensing neuronal activity, responding to changes in neuronal firing rates by complex changes in their inner molecular chemistry.[238] By coaxing microglia to fluorescence under a microscope and using powerful microscopes, it was possible to resolve new finer details of the structure of microglia. It turns out that microglia continuously extend and retract delicate processes to synapses. As neuronal activity ramps up, the probing towards synapses also increases. Microglial processes become more wedged and embedded among the neuronal circuitry. This happens because of receptors on their surface that sense ATP. Microglia also make an enzyme that breaks down ATP into adenosine, which acts to reduce the further release of neurotransmitters. A natural function of microglia appears to be to limit excessive excitation in the brain. That is, microglia locally produce a signal in response to rising neuronal activity that opposes further neurotransmitter release.

If microglia depart the synapse for any reason, the brain loses one of the endogenous mechanisms it relies on to keep things calm. Unfortunately, this is exactly what happens after a brain injury. A key job for microglia is moving to sites of damage and scavenging tissue debris. Since they must desert their posts on the synapse watch, this action comes at the expense of synaptic homeostasis. So, when there is brain tissue damage, we lose some of our natural inhibitory 'tone'. Other experiments have shown how important microglia are to setting the excitability of brain networks. Experiments where microglia were depleted from the brain saw animals become hypersensitive to stimulation. Exposure to a normally innocuous dose of kainic acid produces powerful seizures in mice lacking microglia. Even without an external stimulus, neurones around sites of the brain where microglia were removed begin to synchronise, a hallmark of epileptic networks. It is curious that microglia seem to depend on a constant signal to stay alive. This signal comes in via a receptor called CSF1R. If you block the receptor, even for a relatively short period of time, microglia disappear from the brain. A team led by Michael Johnson at Imperial College London and UCB Pharma found that blocking the CSF1R receptor that keeps microglia alive reduces seizures in animals with pre-existing epilepsy.[239] Targeting the receptor has also been reported to improve outcomes such as cognition in models of traumatic brain injury.

A protracted inflammatory state is strongly linked to the development of treatment-resistant epilepsy, but if we try to block inflammation and get the timing wrong, outcomes can be much worse. Anti-inflammatory drugs including steroids, immuno-globulins and small molecule inhibitors of inflammatory signalling have been used with varying degrees of success to treat childhood and infection-related epilepsies. Clarifying the causes and the players in persistent inflammatory tone in brain tissue from patients and animal models may improve the use of these drugs and lead us to new and more effective approaches. Progress is being made in how cytokines change the properties of neurotransmitter receptors and the ion channels that underlie neuronal firing. Cytokines can activate enzymes that then modify the chemistry of neurotransmitter systems. The response and the sensitivity of neurones to neurotransmitters directly change in an inflammatory environment, favouring increased excitability. Few parts of the neurotransmission system are spared. Indeed, the systems used to reabsorb or inactivate released neurotransmitters are also impaired by inflammatory cytokines. This means that neurotransmitters stay around synapses longer, producing stronger effects in some cases but leading to desensitisation in others. Cytokines also make the microvessels in the brain leakier. This provides a permissive environment that encourages and facilitates entry of immune cells. There are several mechanisms by which IL1β provokes hyperexcitability. In addition to effects on neurotransmitter components, IL1β is a potent activator of astrocytes, stimulating their expansion. This alters excitability in different ways, but a key mechanism is that astrocytes are the major repository of the enzyme that breaks down adenosine, called adenosine kinase (ADK). More ADK means faster clearing of the brain's natural anticonvulsant. This makes it more likely that a seizure can start and, once underway, harder to stop.[219] Any pathways that drive IL1β are therefore critical targets for an inflammation-based approach to treating epilepsy. Recent studies on miR-146a suggest that it functions to dampen down the IL1β pathway. Consistent with this, the infusion of miR-146a into mice with epilepsy was shown to reduce the occurrence of seizures.[240] So, microRNA control of the IL1β system offers new opportunities for therapies for epilepsy. Or, put another way, control the IL1β system and you control the epilepsy.

The link between microRNA and IL1β caught our interest. Back in 1998, I was looking at some of the proteins known to control cell death, a family of enzymes called caspases. I was interested in finding out whether blocking these might protect neurones from dying. A few members of the caspase family did not control cell death but instead were part of the pathway by which cytokines are produced. The first member of the family, Caspase-1, was originally called interleukin-1 converting enzyme. As its name suggests, the enzyme processes the precursor form of what will become IL1β. The team I was working with at the University of Pittsburgh had access to brain samples from epilepsy patients and had developed a technique to measure the activity of these caspases. All caspases are originally made in an inactive form called pro-enzymes. They must be cleaved to rearrange and form the active enzyme. You can monitor this by measuring a reduction in the amount of the heavy pro-enzyme form relative to an accumulation of the lighter active form. Looking at Caspase-1, we noticed a strong signal at the correct weight for the active form in the brain samples from the epilepsy patients. Caspase-1 was active, indirect evidence that IL1β was being produced in the brains of people with drug-resistant TLE.[241] Animal and later clinical studies by Annamaria Vezzani in Milan, Italy and collaborators would go on to test drugs that targeted this in the first human trials.

So, the machinery for making IL1β is sitting active in the seizure zone. Let's think upstream now. It is often a goal to find the earliest or proximal event in a cascade and to intervene at that level to have greatest impact. How or what activates the Caspase-1 enzyme? Put another way, what lies between ATP being released, that is, the damage signal, and Caspase-1 being activated? The answer was found in the mid-1990s, much of the detective work being led by the team of Klaus Schulze-Osthoff at Tübingen University in Germany. They studied the receptors for ATP, finding that some of these contained an ion channel. These would eventually be named P2X receptors (the 'P1' nomenclature is reserved for the adenosine-responsive receptors). Seven members of the P2X family have been discovered in the human genome, each built from three subunits and possessing a channel down the centre that opens upon binding ATP.[242, 243] This triggers a pulse of sodium and calcium entry into the cell and the efflux of potassium. The seventh member, P2X7, differs in certain aspects. In particular, only high levels of ATP can activate the receptor. This means that the P2X7 receptor is probably inactive under normal conditions. When tissue injury occurs or there is a strong release of ATP, the receptor becomes activated. In this way, the P2X7 receptor is tuned to respond to damage. The German team were key in pinpointing that the P2X7 receptor lies upstream of the IL1β release pathway, showing that cells lacking P2X7 receptors but containing all the other components do not release IL1β in response to ATP. The coupling appears to occur via a mixture of effects. As the P2X7 receptor opens, potassium effluxes from the cell and calcium enters, stimulating a pulse of oxidative stress that combines to drive the pathway. There has been some debate since on the role of Caspase-1 in this and there is evidence that IL1β can be released via P2X7 receptor activation without Caspase-1. Regardless, ATP activates the P2X7 receptor and this leads to IL1β release. There is also a long-running debate about what cell types make the P2X7 receptor in the brain. It is mainly present on the surface of microglia, less on other glia, and sits poised to react if injury occurs. Several studies suggest that it is also present in neurones where it might serve to modulate neurotransmitter release.

In the late 2000s around when we started our microRNA work, Tobias Engel, a postdoctoral researcher in my team, suggested that we look at the P2X7 receptor in epilepsy. This idea was nurtured by his former colleagues in Spain where he had conducted his PhD research; these included one of the pioneers in this field, M. Teresa Miras Portugal, who sadly died in 2021. They offered us some of the toolkit they had been using to study the receptor in other conditions. They had drugs to activate and block the receptor and genetically altered cells and mice that could help prove, one way or another, if the P2X7 receptor was doing anything important. We learnt quickly that, under certain circumstances and with the right doses, we could reduce seizures in mice by blocking the receptor. Tobias, working with Eva Jimenez-Mateos who was leading the miR-134 project, was to co-discover a microRNA that limits the amount of P2X7 receptor in the brain and, more broadly, acts as an inflammation dampener.[244] The route to this discovery came from searching for 'protective' microRNAs. We reasoned that, rather than always looking in the damaged hippocampus, we should pay some attention to the distant but connected *contralateral* hippocampus that was inside the other hemisphere of the mouse brain. The two hippocampi are physically connected and we knew from recording electrical signals within the contralateral hippocampus that bursts of action potentials passed through this region during a seizure. But the contralateral hippocampus did not display signs of neurone loss or much gliosis. Perhaps some sort of protective mechanism was being engaged in the contralateral hippocampus? In this way, our thinking linked back to work on tolerance, the idea that brief or sub-threshold insults awake endogenous programmes that, if given enough time to switch on, protect the brain. Might there be microRNAs in the contralateral hippocampus that serve such functions?

When we measured responses to ATP in cells in the damage zone, the ipsilateral hippocampus, we detected strong channel activity consistent with the presence of the P2X7 receptor. But we recorded only weak responses to high-level ATP in the cells on the other side. Levels of IL1β in the contralateral hippocampus were also negligible. Was something blocking the P2X7 receptor? We decided to check if the P2X7 receptor was a microRNA target. We extracted the AGO2 complex from the contralateral hippocampus and found that it contained the *P2rx7* transcript. So, microRNAs were targeting the receptor. But which ones? We used some of the usual search algorithms and found that the *P2rx7* transcript had 3' UTRs for quite a few microRNAs. We needed to narrow this down so we extracted more AGO2 from the contralateral hippocampus and this time analysed the microRNAs. We then put together a list of the ones that were there, but not in the ipsilateral equivalent, and had the required seed site for the *P2rx7* transcript. At the top of the list was miR-22. We set about finding out whether this was restricting levels of P2X7 receptors.

In subsequent experiments, we learnt that blocking miR-22 caused an increase in P2X7 receptor levels in the contralateral hippocampus. This was associated with more IL1β production and increased numbers of astrocytes. Epilepsy became worse than normal, with mice given the miR-22 inhibitor having more frequent seizures. This told us that miR-22 had been constraining inflammatory signalling in the contralateral hippocampus. By blocking miR-22 we had removed a critical molecular brake on inflammation. That is, miR-22 served to limit the extent of the epileptic network, acting to restrict the focus to one side of the brain and to curb, albeit incompletely, the epilepsy. Seizures were not the only aspect affected when we blocked miR-22, however. Inhibition of miR-22 made mice more anxious and less able to recognise moved objects in maze tests. Most of the effects could be prevented by treating mice with a drug that blocks the P2X7 receptor. A final experiment looked at what happened when a mimic of miR-22 was injected close to the hippocampus. This had the effect of slightly reducing the frequency of epileptic seizures in mice.

Eva and Tobias were curious about what controlled the controller. What was increasing miR-22 levels in the contralateral hippocampus? For that matter, what controlled the levels of the *P2rx7* transcript? Here we had a lead already. Our Spanish collaborators tipped us off that it might be a transcription factor called Specificity protein 1 (SP1). When we delivered SP1 into neurones, it stimulated them to make the *P2rx7* mRNA. It also increased levels of miR-22. Sitting upstream of both the *P2rx7* gene and the gene for miR-22 was a site for SP1 to bind,[245] a promoter, which explained why both could be controlled by SP1. So, this appeared to be a homeostatic loop. The same system that increases P2X7 receptor levels also adjusts the amount of miR-22. A checks-and-balances feedback loop that serves to control pathways. But if SP1 increases miR-22, why didn't this stop the build-up of the P2X7 receptor in the ipsilateral hippocampus? We found that high intracellular calcium interferes with the SP1 system. Perhaps the seizures hitting the ipsilateral hippocampus open calcium-permeable NMDA receptors, whereas on the contralateral side the lower seizure intensity failed to trigger such a calcium entry and SP1 could do its job raising miR-22 levels. This system of SP1 driving miR-22 to control the amount of the P2X7 receptor appears to act as a natural brake on inflammation in experimental epilepsy. But is it relevant to what is happening in human epilepsy? We have found that levels of the P2X7 receptor are increased in brain tissue from patients who had hippocampal tissue removed for the treatment of drug-resistant epilepsy. We do not know if the miR-22 system fails to act or perhaps is simply inadequate. Perhaps P2X7 receptor antagonists, if given at the right time, could be an approach to treatment. Alternatively, we could try to supplement miR-22 levels. Interestingly, P2X7 receptor antagonists are undergoing clinical trials for some brain diseases and perhaps should be tried in epilepsy. Chapter 7 will look at some of the potential ways we might move microRNAs into the realm of medicines.

Capturing It All

Shortly after our study on miR-134 was published, a research fund was announced in Europe for large-scale epilepsy projects. I had recently met a German neurologist, Felix Rosenow, who was interested in the topic and we drew together scientists that included, among others, Stephanie Schorge at UCL; Jorgen Kjems, an expert on small RNAs at Aarhus University; and the Dutch team led by Jeroen Pasterkamp, who had also become interested in microRNAs in epilepsy. Completing the team, we had Jochen Prehn, an expert in modelling complex pathways with mathematics and founder of a systems biology centre at my institute. One of the core parts of the project, named EpimiRNA, was to create a definitive atlas of microRNA changes in experimental TLE. We and others had performed various types of microRNA profiling study, but they suffered certain limitations. First, they invariably used samples from just one model. Whether such findings would extrapolate to other models, much less human epilepsy, was uncertain. Second, the methods used to identify the microRNAs had a limitation in that they did not take account of whether or not the microRNA was active. So far, everyone had been grinding up brain tissue and extracting the microRNA. While this captures the microRNAs, it cannot tell you if they are loaded into the RISC. A portion of your 'signal' will be from microRNAs that are not actually doing anything at the time you took the sample. A number of studies had shown that profiling the AGO-loaded microRNAs gives a more accurate impression of what microRNAs are active at a given point in time.[246] But there are downsides too. The method to extract the AGO is not completely efficient, meaning that some will always get left behind or lost, and some of the complexes may break open and their contents become dispersed. Nevertheless, the approach is an important tactic in the quest to record which microRNAs are functional. We had used this AGO2 analysis approach in our mouse studies on miR-22. We planned to scale this up and run across multiple time points in different models, sequencing *all* the bound microRNAs. We would document all the active microRNAs at each stage of the development of epilepsy.[247]

By performing an AGO2 sequencing analysis of three different animal models of epilepsy, we would be able to triangulate the results to discover which microRNA activities were shared across all the models and which changes were model-specific. Each model uses a different method to trigger epilepsy and so we knew we would find microRNA changes that were specifically reacting to, for example, kainic acid. We were also keen to take account of possible species differences. The final experimental design used two chemical models and one electrical model of epilepsy in two different mouse strains and one rat model. Samples of the hippocampus were generated by different teams to capture what might be happening at different moments during the process by which the brain became capable of generating epileptic seizures. We included a time point on the day when the animals had their first spontaneous seizure, to get as close as possible to the moment when the brain's circuitry finally generated a true epileptic seizure. There is no way to know the exact moment this is going to happen, so this time point is really picking up both the final period of conversion to an epileptic state and the consequences of a first epileptic seizure on the microRNA environment.

All the samples were packed and sent to Kjems and his postdoctoral researcher Morten Venø (who later started his own RNA company). They pulled out the AGO2 protein from all the samples and sequenced the bound small RNAs, eventually identifying more than a billion molecules. We had a remarkable dataset, a time-map of all the microRNAs that are active as epilepsy develops, and we had information on the relative abundance of every microRNA. This is important for reasons covered in the earlier chapters of this book. A low abundant microRNA is less likely to produce biologically important effects. With the database finished, a group of us pored over it. We were looking for three things. First, assurance that the experiment had worked properly. Before looking at what might be different in epilepsy, we wanted to be sure that it contained the expected microRNAs and in the right proportions. Were the levels of microRNAs we knew to be abundant in the brain among the highest levels in our own study? Were microRNAs that are not expressed in the brain absent? This was an important sense-check that the technique had worked. The AGO2 results fitted perfectly. When the top AGO2-loaded microRNAs were listed, we found all the usual suspects. The most abundant across the three models was miR-181a, the microRNA that had been the focus of Schuman's study in Chapter 5. The list contained many others, including miR-128 in fourth place and miR-9 in fifth. When we looked for microRNAs made in other organs in the body, such as miR-122 made in the liver, they were absent. So, the method had worked and, importantly, appeared to be faithfully representing the microRNA landscape that was known from other work. This dataset, particularly the levels at baseline, has become an important reference because it allows us to quickly look up and check whether a particular microRNA is expressed in the brain and at what level relative to others. This can be critical for influencing decisions on whether or not to pursue a particular microRNA. You might spot a new microRNA in a screen, but if its expression is very low, it might be better to keep looking.

Next, we wanted to check some of the microRNAs that had already been linked to epilepsy. We looked first for miR-132 and miR-146a because they were the two microRNAs first linked to epilepsy and they had come up in many studies since, including in our own early screening work. A rapid increase was seen in levels of miR-132 in all three models, fitting with other teams' findings and what would be expected for an activity-regulated microRNA. Levels of miR-146a also went up in each model, but with a delay relative to miR-132, consistent with it being produced when glia react to injury and initiate inflammation and repair processes. We then looked for other patterns across the models. We were surprised with just how similar the overall amounts of AGO2-loaded microRNAs were between the two mouse strains and the rat. As an example, the abundance in terms of reads per million on a log2 scale for miR-181a was 17.3 in the black mouse, 17.2 in the white mouse and 17.1 in the rat. For miR-26a the read counts were identical across all three rodent models, at 16.2. This reinforces how highly conserved microRNAs can be. Not only are the sequences of the mature microRNAs the same between these species but the amount of them in the brain is the same. Of course, this wasn't true of all the microRNAs; there was some divergence between the models, particularly when we looked at lower-abundant microRNAs.

Consistent with our predictions, several microRNAs showed the same change in all three epilepsy models, whereas others changed in two and some just changed in a single model. From here it was easy to identify which microRNAs were common to all models. Each phase of the process of epileptogenesis had a set of microRNAs that changed in all three models, meaning that there is a common signature of functionally engaged microRNAs in experimental epileptogenesis. The numbers of these common-to-all microRNA varied according to the time point. The lowest overlap occurred early, one hour after the epileptogenic insult had occurred. This suggested that early reactions to brain injury are most strongly shaped by the specific method of insult. The greatest overlap was seen at 24 hours. This is still an early time point in the epileptogenic process. It suggests that some core aspects of the process affect many of the same microRNAs. What were the microRNAs among the common-to-all list? At the early phases of epileptogenesis, we found multiple microRNAs we'd come across before, including miR-132 and miR-134. Interestingly, many of the microRNAs in the early phase list were not found later. Different sets of microRNAs emerged in samples taken during the later days and weeks after the insult. Only three of the same microRNAs seen in the early phase of epilpetogenesis were still changed at the later phase. This revealed that epileptogenesis has distinct 'waves' of microRNA changes. What these were doing is unclear, but since the early phase was enriched with the known neuronal microRNAs, that phase appears to be enriched with microRNAs that react to the intense periods of firing that accompany the early brain injury phase. That period likely also features significant changes to neuronal morphology and even neuronal death. This settles later on, with glia changes and repair-related microRNAs becoming more obvious. Consistent with this idea, we found that several of the up-regulated microRNAs during the 'second' phase of epileptogenesis were indeed ones known to be enriched in glia. Thus, we can actually trace waves of cell function change by tracking the peaks and troughs of microRNAs. The microRNA changes are therefore a biomarker of the cell contributions and changes that accompany epileptogenesis.

On the day of the first spontaneous seizure, we found an almost entirely different set of microRNAs that hadn't been active during the early phase and were also not regulated across the models in the chronic phase. This points to unique events occurring on this transition day, between a state in which spontaneous seizures do not occur to one where the epileptic circuit is now set. These are final molecular adjustments after which a new and permanent state of hyperexcitability exists. We also found a set of microRNAs shared between the models at the final time point, when spontaneous seizures had been occurring for some time. Again, this pointed to a common microRNA signature of established and, in these models, most likely drug-resistant epilepsy.

In addition to creating the dataset, we asked two more questions. First, do the same microRNAs change in the same way in human TLE? The answer was yes. Several of the microRNAs we found dysregulated in all three animal models were also changed in human epilepsy. This backed up the translational value of these models. They had generated leads relevant to human epilepsy. Second, did the changes in microRNA levels affect brain excitability? We had a set of eight microRNAs that were up-regulated in all three models at the last time point representing chronic epilepsy. Two of these were miR-132 and miR-146a, so we skipped them and focussed on the remaining six. We then deployed antimirs to block these and find out if that altered anything. Here, we were primarily looking for a change either in seizures or in something with clear relevance to the pathophysiology of epilepsy, such as neuronal death. Until this point, epilepsy researchers had hit individual microRNAs one at a time. Because of the teams of scientists that the EpimiRNA project had brought together, we could be more ambitious and decided to go for all six at the same time. After designing the targeting sequences and then testing them, we had our answer. Blocking three of the six new microRNAs reduced seizures in mice. This was a strong validation of the discovery approach and evidence of the practical applications of this type of large-scale profiling study. In addition, we learnt that the three microRNAs converged on a pathway that, among other things, controls how brain cells react to injury. **Figure 6.5** shows the overlapping networks of genes related to the transforming growth factor–beta pathway, controlled by the new epilepsy-associated microRNAs. Notably, genetic variants in one of the genes in this pathway causes epilepsy in humans. By inhibiting the microRNAs that suppressed this pathway, we may have enabled the signalling system to perform more effectively. This idea was backed up by the finding that when we inhibited the pathway as a way to simulate what the microRNAs were doing, using a drug this time rather than an antimir, the seizures got worse again. The study is a good example of how microRNAs exert strong effects by converging on multiple targets in a pathway. It is also an example of how 'team science' approaches can take on bigger challenges that generate rich datasets for the wider research community.

Treating Genetic Epilepsies by Targeting MicroRNAs

While microRNA-based targeting seems a natural solution for the complex pathophysiology of TLE where you need to hit several pathways at once, the ability to increase levels of genes by targeting their microRNA regulators has clear applications for treating other epilepsies. Genetic factors underlie, to a greater or lesser extent, many forms of epilepsy. Gene mutations can result in the effective loss of half the normal gene output. The impact this has depends on the gene. We can tolerate a drop in levels of some genes better than others. Activity of the unaffected copy of a gene may be sufficient to avoid a phenotype. If not, increasing the protein yield from the 'healthy' copy of the gene is a strategy to alleviate some genetic epilepsies. Since microRNAs naturally dampen expression of their target genes, blocking a microRNA that targets a gene that is faulty in epilepsy could be a way to increase, at least slightly, the level of the remaining output of the gene. Taking an example from earlier, inhibiting miR-324 in someone carrying a mutation in *KCND2* might be an effective way to restore enough of the encoded dendritic potassium channel to reduce hyperexcitability. The approach of using a microRNA inhibitor to increase levels of a gene in a genetic epilepsy has, of course, limitations. The levels of the other targets of the inhibited microRNA will also change, although there may be solutions for this, which will be discussed in Chapter 7. One other limitation is that this approach will be unsuitable for genetic conditions that affect the X or Y chromosomes and genetically imprinted diseases. If the mutated gene resides on the X chromosome, then, in males, there is no other copy of that gene from which to boost gene expression by removing the microRNA repression. In fact, since one copy of the X chromosome is also silenced in female cells, the problem is common to both sexes. A similar issue arises for a set of more than 200 imprinted genes in humans. Imprinting means that one copy of the gene, either the one inherited from the mother or the one inherited from the father, is permanently inactivated.[248] Only one copy of the gene ever contributes to protein levels in the cell. If a mutation is present in the

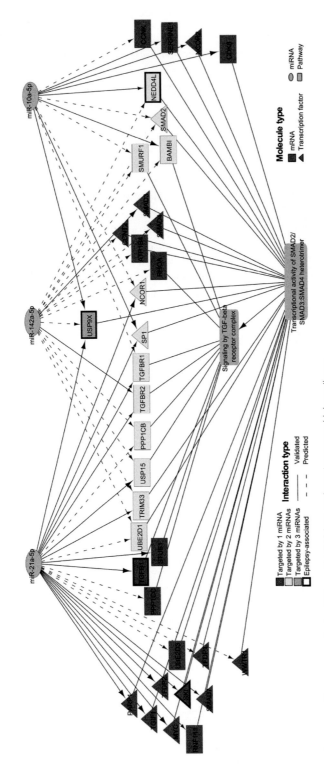

Figure 6.5 Convergence of microRNAs on the TGF–beta pathway in temporal lobe epilepsy

Wiring diagram depicting the experimentally validated and predicted mRNA targets of a set of three seizure-modifying microRNAs that converge on TGF (transforming growth factor)–beta signalling, illustrating the convergence of diverse microRNA targets at the pathway level.

Source: From Venø et al., *Proceedings of the National Academy of Sciences of the United States of America*, vol. 117, pp. 15977–88 (2020).[247]

one version of the gene that can be transcribed, then targeting a microRNA that controls that transcript will not help. You would just end up with more of a faulty protein. There are examples of epilepsies that both are X chromosome-based and affect an imprinted gene.

Are there microRNA-based approaches we could use for genetic epilepsies, either as a precision therapy, where deployment of the microRNA inhibitor would directly restore some amount of the protein deficient in a genetic epilepsy, or because there was another link between the microRNA and the pathways altered in the genetic epilepsy? Alternatively, if a microRNA inhibitor were simply a very potent anti-seizure molecule, that might also be useful. Many of the most recently approved drugs for rare genetic epilepsies are not at all targeted (e.g. cannabidiol for Dravet syndrome), yet they provide some patients with symptom control.

We have explored a microRNA approach for Angelman syndrome. It is not a classical epilepsy but a disorder of brain development in which drug-resistant epilepsy is often a serious problem.[249] Angelman syndrome is caused by mutations in the gene that encodes the UBE3A protein. The main symptoms are profound cognitive impairment, problems with movement, called ataxia, and drug-resistant epilepsy. The name of the disease comes from the doctor who first fully described the condition, Harry Angelman. The UBE3A protein is highly abundant in the brain, where it serves a number of roles, including helping cells break down unwanted proteins in a similar process to the one used to break down MOV10. The UBE3A protein is particularly important for the function of inhibitory neurones, regulating the various components they need at synapses. For certain reasons not completely understood, the lack of UBE3A in Angelman syndrome disproportionately affects the cerebellum and the hippocampus. Further, *UBE3A* is an imprinted gene. The paternal copy is normally silenced in neurones. This means that all expression comes from the maternal copy of the gene. Curiously, the imprinting occurs only in the brain, with the gene expressed from both maternally and paternally inherited genes elsewhere in the body. Patients with Angelman syndrome possess a fault in the maternal copy of *UBE3A*, effectively meaning that they can't produce any useful UBE3A protein because the paternal copy is silenced. There isn't yet a specific treatment for Angelman syndrome, with most medicines being used to simply manage symptoms. However, gene therapy approaches are being trialled that aim to interfere with the imprinting process and allow expression of *UBE3A* from the healthy but normally silenced paternal copy.

We picked Angelman syndrome because of a curious molecular link to microRNA dysregulation that had been discovered in 2015. The team of Schratt who first linked miR-134 to control of dendritic spines had found that one of the RNAs transcribed from the *UBE3A* gene contained a series of binding sites for microRNAs.[250] This is nothing unusual, of course. But what was unusual was that the *UBE3A* transcript in question could not generate a full-length protein. It was a so-called non-protein-coding RNA variant of *UBE3A*. The presence of microRNA sites was not going to serve the usual purpose of reducing the translation of the transcript into protein. What might the function of this non-coding transcript be? By manipulating the amounts of the *Ube3a* variant in rodent cells, the team found that it was important for synaptic structure. This in itself was a noteworthy finding because the human genome contains and generates large numbers of these types of non-coding RNAs but we still know relatively little about what they do, if anything at all. What caught their eye, and later ours, was that this unusual *Ube3a* transcript contained a seed site for miR-134, not only in the rodent, where most of the research was focussed, but also in the human *UBE3A* transcript. It also contained sites for many other microRNAs from the same cluster that miR-134 is expressed from. Could this *UBE3A* variant actually be working to control microRNA levels? Acting like a 'sponge' to keep a pool of microRNAs in check? If this were true, then in Angelman syndrome the levels of the sponge would be lower and the microRNAs that would normally be attached could be available to go off and bind to other targets. In effect, Angelman syndrome might create a state akin to what we had seen in TLE, where levels of miR-134 were higher. If this were the case, perhaps our microRNA inhibitor could help to treat the disorder? At a minimum, it might work against the epilepsy and perhaps it could correct one or two of the other core symptoms.

We set out to test this idea.[251] We began by measuring levels of miR-134 in brain samples from a mouse model of Angelman syndrome in which a mutation was introduced that disrupted the maternal copy of the *Ube3a* gene. The mice are quite a good model for Angelman syndrome as they display several hallmarks, including altered synaptic structure and function. Hippocampal levels of miR-134 were, however, normal, casting some doubt on whether the loss of the 'sponge' *Ube3a* transcript in Angelman model mice was sufficient to perturb miR-134 or other microRNA levels. We pressed on. When we checked the cerebellum, we detected a small elevation in miR-134 levels. This seemed to suggest that we were on to something after all. The cerebellum is an important structure that regulates multiple brain functions, including motor coordination. There is also evidence that the cerebellum exerts a strong influence on overall brain excitability and seizures. Esther Krook-Magnuson, now at the University of Minnesota, has performed elegant experiments showing that activating certain parts of the cerebellum can interrupt seizures in the hippocampus.[252] Since Angelman syndrome features both reduced mobility and epilepsy, any molecular changes in the cerebellum could be relevant. Of course, there could be other reasons why the level of miR-134 differed in the cerebellum rather than it being owing simply to loss of the microRNA 'sponge'. For example, we know that miR-134 is activity-regulated and perhaps this part of the brain was more excitable and therefore driving more miR-134, independent of the lost sponge defect. However, a quick check of the levels of some known activity-regulated genes, those which always switch on when there is high firing of neurones, suggested that this wasn't the cause of the elevated miR-134 in this part of the brain. The evidence for a disturbance to miR-134 in Angelman syndrome remained slim, however. We decided to take a look at the levels of the unusual *Ube3a* RNA. One of the reasons for this check was another study, published since the work by the Schratt team, that searched for the transcript and could only find it at extremely low levels. There was scepticism in the Angelman field that this transcript could really perturb microRNAs.[253] We looked for it ourselves, managing to detect it, both by sifting through published mouse and human brain data generated by other groups and by analysing our own mouse and human samples. Here, we had RNA from neurones that had been reprogrammed from blood cells from an Angelman patient. Levels of the *UBE3A* microRNA sponge were very low but were nevertheless detectable. So, the conclusion? The microRNA sponge is present in the brain, but perhaps not at a level that could really cause much disruption to microRNA levels. Perhaps functional studies would help resolve the debate. Since the cerebellum is a key structure in movement and locomotion, we first tested whether inhibiting miR-134 with an antimir would have any effect on movement. Mice with the Angelman mutation have a characteristic gait that is slow and they also tend to avoid open spaces, a behaviour interpreted as elevated anxiety. Treating Angelman model mice with an miR-134 inhibitor (antimir) resulted in them becoming more mobile in the test area, moving slightly more quickly and also crossing over into the centre of the field (see **Figure 6.6**). This suggested

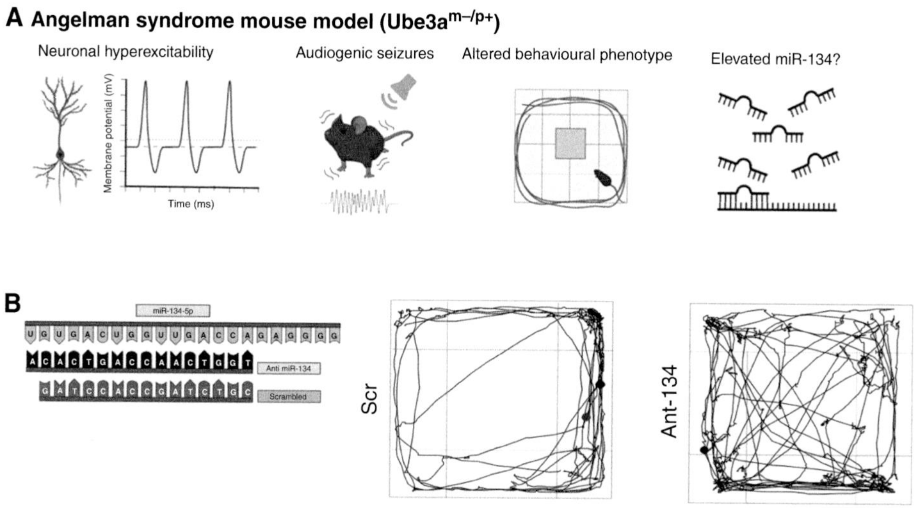

Figure 6.6 Reduced ataxia in Angelman mice after inhibition of miR-134

Panel A shows some of the phenotypes of Angelman model mice.

Panel B shows the antimir sequences and (right) representative track plots of juvenile Angelman model mice (*Ube3a$^{m-/p+}$*) moving around a test arena. Treatment with the inhibitor of miR-134 resulted in more exploring and centre crossings compared to a scrambled version of the sequence (Scr).

Source: From Campbell et al. *Molecular Therapy Nucleic Acids*, vol. 28, pp. 514–29 (2022).[251]

that at least two of the symptoms of the Angelman model mice could be corrected using this microRNA approach. However, there are other ways to interpret this data. Perhaps we had interfered with the animals' natural and protective aversion to open spaces? Perhaps the animal is now less aware of potential dangers or is even slightly confused and thus walking into areas that it would not normally enter? Figuring out which explanation is correct is not trivial and, as a lab focussed on treating epilepsy and ill-equipped to tackle interpretation of mouse behaviours, we were not able to separate these two possibilities and so moved on to the epilepsy question. Could inhibiting miR-134 stop seizures in Angelman mice? Unfortunately, this is where the mouse fails to copy the human condition. Our mice did not develop epileptic seizures. They were, however, sensitive to loud noises. Stimuli such as rattling a cage would cause the mice to have an audiogenic seizure. These are rare in humans, but there are people who have seizures in response to certain sounds and even music. We therefore tested whether blocking miR-134 could reduce audiogenic seizures in Angelman mice. It did. Angelman mice given antimirs against miR-134 developed less-severe seizures in response to a cage rattle, and it worked in both young and older mice. This was important because there was evidence that some of the features of Angelman syndrome cannot be corrected beyond a certain age. The hyperexcitability had been reported as one of those features. But we noticed some distinct differences in how the inhibitor performed in Angelman syndrome compared to our model of TLE. In particular, the anti-seizure effect didn't last very long. Retesting the antimir-treated Angelman mice just a week later revealed that they were no longer protected. This contrasted with the months-long effects we had seen in the TLE model. We think this is because of the enduring genetic basis for the hyperexcitability in Angelman syndrome. But it could also be around dosing. It could also be that the part of the brain driving the seizure susceptibility is not the same between these conditions. We would like to find answers to some of these questions in the future.

Is this approach worth pursuing as a treatment for Angelman syndrome in humans? Improvement in epilepsy and motor control would be a substantial therapeutic gain, but it would come with the need to undergo repeated injections of the antimir. It was time to look again at human samples to see if any of this would translate to patients. We did this in two ways. The first step was to see if we could modulate miR-134 in human neurones. We turned to our Angelman patient neurones and incubated them for a few days with the microRNA inhibitor. This nicely reduced the levels of miR-134 and caused a small increase in the levels of some of the known targets of miR-134. This told us that we could inhibit miR-134 in human neurones just as well as mice. We found that levels of miR-134 were no different in human Angelman neurones compared to control human neurones, questioning again the microRNA sponge hypothesis. We are still looking through some data to resolve this issue, having screened microRNAs across the mice, a set of donated brain tissue samples from Angelman patients and the human Angelman neurones. At the moment, it looks like the Angelman mouse hippocampus does express higher levels of some of the microRNAs for which binding sites existed in the *Ube3a* sponge transcript (but not miR-134). This does not appear to be the case for the human Angelman neurones. But does this mean that the mouse is a poor model of the human or that the human neurones we had were a poor model of the human brain? Culturing neurones and turning them into something akin to a mature brain circuit is not easy and such *in vitro* models lack many of the elements of the brain, including many of the non-neuronal cell types. But, actually, the human neurone microRNA profiles look similar to the human brain tissue. So, it looks like the microRNA sponge effect may be most relevant to mice. Why the species difference? We don't know and it could be something specific to this neurodevelopmental disorder. If this divergence holds for other neurodevelopmental disorders, it will have important implications for the translatability of mouse findings for such genetic conditions in humans. The answer may also lie elsewhere. The molecular defect in our mice and our human cells was not the same. The mouse model carries an error that only prevents the production of the UBE3A protein. In contrast, the cells we used were from a patient carrying a chromosomal *deletion*. In these, *UBE3A* was lost but so were several other genes. Perhaps this molecular difference will be important in understanding why the mouse and human profiles did not align better?

Another Roll of the Dice for Dravet

Midway through the Angelman study, we became interested in another genetic epilepsy called Dravet syndrome. First described by Charlotte Dravet in an obscure French journal in 1978, Dravet syndrome is also a rare disease, affecting about 1 in every 15,000 people. The condition has three distinct phases. The first is the presentation of a severe seizure in infancy, usually accompanying a fever. Shortly after recovering, seizures return and become more severe. This continues and often worsens. Sudden death claims many infants with the gene defect. The seizures are so frequent and severe that they directly damage the developing brain, often leaving lifelong impairments in cognition and movement control. Later in life the seizures may ease, but the cognitive impairments remain. In 2001, a series of three papers in the *American Journal of Clinical Genetics* identified mutations in *SCN1A*, a gene that makes a key protein component of sodium channels, as a cause.[254, 255, 256] At the start of the action potential, there is a brief opening of sodium channels which causes the membrane potential to flip to positive. Without the inward sodium current there can be no action potential. But why would a reduction in the firing properties of neurones cause a predisposition to seizures? Surely the opposite would happen, that is, reduced excitability? Experiments revealed that the channel encoded by *SCN1A*, called NaV1.1, is particularly enriched in inhibitory neurones.[257] It is critical for their high firing rates. A reduction in *SCN1A* levels meant reduced inhibition in the brain.

We had the idea of trying our miR-134 inhibitor in Dravet syndrome. Why? By this stage, we knew that targeting miR-134 could reduce seizures in younger mice and reduce seizures in at least one genetic model. Also, the work by Gross' team was proof-of-concept that microRNAs could be targeted to increase an ion channel in the brain. We wondered if miR-134 levels might be elevated in Dravet syndrome, since a Chinese team had found increased miR-134 levels in children with non-genetic causes of drug-resistant epilepsy. Finally, it was possible that other gene levels altered as a result of the *SCN1A* defect might be adjustable by a microRNA approach. Unfortunately, inhibiting miR-134 didn't protect mice deficient in *Scn1a* from seizures in two different tests and we found no evidence that miR-134 was altered in the Dravet mouse brains.[258] But negative findings are not always a wasted effort. The mechanisms that underlie the seizures in Dravet probably involve different neural circuits from those in TLE or Angelman syndrome. MicroRNA-based treatments need to take account of this and be tailored to the underlying molecular imbalances in an age- and aetiology-specific manner.

Targets of MicroRNAs in the Human Epileptic Brain

The first studies to profile the full complement of microRNAs in human TLE appeared in 2012: one from our lab and one from Pasterkamp's. This provides a good picture of what is 'up' or 'down', but it doesn't tell you which targets the microRNA is acting on. Studies have interpreted changes to target levels as driven by a change in a microRNA where the target-pair has been previously validated. But this cannot be assumed to be the case without more direct proof. In a given cell/tissue/organ, whether a microRNA binds to a specific target depends on them being co-expressed at the same time, in the same cell and, within that cell, coming into contact within a specific region of the cell. This is particularly important in the brain where we know that many microRNAs are actually shuttled out to distant dendrites to locally regulate synaptic structure and function. A microRNA could have the potential to regulate a target, but if it is not in the right place at the right time then no regulation will occur.

How do we find out what targets are controlled by microRNAs in human epilepsy? This challenge was posed at the start of the EpimiRNA project. Tackling this, Kjems, Venø and team used samples of the hippocampus from patients with treatment-resistant epilepsy and performed an experiment called individual-nucleotide resolution cross-linking and immunoprecipitation (iCLIP). The method glues RNAs to proteins, in this case the protein AGO2, the catalytic core of the microRNA silencing complex. The sequences of the RNAs can be determined and mapped against seed sequences for microRNAs. They were able to identify which mRNAs were being actively targeted by microRNAs. The result was a database of microRNA–mRNA interactions that allows anyone interested to look up the targets of any microRNA in the human epileptic hippocampus.[259] Or, if you prefer, look up a gene of interest and find out what microRNA(s) target it. You can now ask some interesting new questions. For example, do any microRNAs target the *SCN1A* transcript that is lost in Dravet? This gives you a potential set of microRNAs to block to help up-regulate *SCN1A* levels. The first question I asked was what is bound to miR-134 in the human hippocampus from these patients? We found 99 AGO2-linked mRNAs with seeds for miR-134 in the database. This was very exciting. It proved that this microRNA was very much a 'multi-targeting' molecule in the human brain. But what was missing was also interesting. Some of the known miR-134 targets, including *LIMK1*, were not on this list. This doesn't completely rule them out as being under miR-134 control because false negatives are always a possibility with this type of experiment, but it does give us pause for thought. Again, just how similar are microRNA targets between rodents and humans and what are the implications for trying to turn microRNAs or their inhibitors into therapeutic agents?

In addition to using this database to validate microRNA–target interactions in the human brain, the data can also be used to get a sense of the cell type making a particular microRNA. You can take the list of transcripts that were cross-linked to AGO2 and then cross-reference that list with a database of single cell sequencing data. Single cell sequencing and the microfluidics that accompany the technology make it possible to separate individual cells from a tissue and then sequence the mRNAs inside each cell. We now know what cell makes each mRNA in the human brain. If we know that a specific microRNA is targeting a specific transcript and we know what cells make that transcript, we have a good sense of what cell(s) the microRNA is working in. Taking, for example, the list of 99 mRNAs attached to miR-134 and checking it against single cell data revealed that the transcripts were expressed in either excitatory or inhibitory neurones, not glia. This is a neuronal microRNA and one probably used by both neurone subtypes.

A Single Letter Can Change Everything

In the final part of this chapter, we re-encounter the world of RNA editing. It turns out that microRNA sequences can be altered. In particular, one of the four bases, the A, can undergo a chemical modification. If that happens, the A is read as a different base. This was first shown to happen to certain protein-coding mRNAs transcripts, but it was later found to also occur to non-coding RNAs, including microRNAs. What purpose does this serve? The answer lies with increasing the repertoire, the diversity, of a given RNA.[260, 261] Most often, this results in introducing a different amino acid from the one originally encoded by the gene. The ability to make changes to any RNA transcript independently of the DNA creates flexibility and efficiency. As we will see shortly, the effects of even a single base change can be quite remarkable.

The editing of RNA is a post-transcriptional process, meaning that it relates to the insertion and/or deletion of nucleotides within an RNA molecule, as well as conversion of nucleotides. Credit for the discovery dates to 1986 when discrepancies were noted in nucleotides between the genomic sequence and the RNA sequence of a mitochondrial protein.[262] The most common form is A-to-I editing, which is mediated by a group of enzymes called ADARs (adenosine deaminase acting on RNA). These enzymes use a molecule of water to alter the amino group in the carbon ring of adenosine.[263] This hydrolytic deamination event results in inosine in place of adenosine. Now comes the important part. Inosine is structurally very similar to guanine. The cell machinery reads an I as a G, so the original A is now behaving as a G, forming Watson–Crick pairs with cytidine instead of uracil, adenine's normal binding partner. So, if ADARs act on an RNA, they introduce one or more inosine which would later be read as a G. When an altered base encounters the protein synthesis machinery, we can get a new amino acid in a protein. This can have dramatic effects, particularly when it is close to the active site of an enzyme or performs key gating functions. One of the best-understood examples in the brain is the editing of the *GRIA2* transcript, which encodes part of the AMPA (α-amino-3-hydroxy-5-methyl-4-isoxazolepropionic acid) receptor for the neurotransmitter glutamate. The AMPA receptor serves as the workhorse of excitatory transmission in the brain. When glutamate binds the receptor, it opens and you get a brief pulse of sodium entering the cell. This drives the cell towards firing an action potential. Unusually, the transcript coding for the protein is almost entirely edited under normal conditions in the brain. Without this editing, the AMPA receptor is too permeable to calcium. Unwanted calcium entry can trigger neurodegeneration, and mice engineered to prevent the editing from happening develop epilepsy and die prematurely. Deletion of the ADAR enzymes produces a similar result. Thus, the brain depends on RNA editing. There are other effects of A-to-I editing. For example, if it occurs close to a splicing site, this can result in changes to the inclusion or exclusion of exons. This can produce even more extensive changes to a protein. And ADARs seem to know whether and where to edit based on key sequences of nucleotides within RNAs which attract them. They also prefer double-stranded RNA. Thus, we have an elegant system in our cells for dramatically scaling up the possible outputs of a gene, creating diversity in a highly efficient manner.

Editing of microRNAs was first spotted in 2004.[264] Later studies found more and more examples. The brain was a particularly rich source, with edited microRNAs showing up in different brain regions at different times.[265, 266] Hundreds of RNA editing sites have now been mapped for brain microRNAs and most of the editing appears to be carried out by ADARs. But microRNAs are not read and translated into protein. So, why edit them? Editing microRNAs produces several effects. The most obvious is that editing a site in the mature microRNA can change its alignment to its targets. This could result in loss of affinity for one mRNA and gain of affinity for another. This redirection of a microRNA's targets has been implicated in several human diseases. But it doesn't end there. MicroRNA editing can affect the stability of the RNA, by altering how much 'wobble' the molecule makes. Also, RNA editing can make an RNA more or less likely to be degraded. Editing can also affect biogenesis of microRNAs, for example by altering the recognition and processing steps that are used by Drosha to process the pri-miRNA.

We suspected that microRNA editing would be different in epilepsy and became interested as the EpimiRNA project ended. Kelvin Lau, a PhD student, began by checking for the presence of ADARs in human hippocampal samples from patients with treatment-resistant TLE. Levels were quite similar to controls and, using single cell data and other techniques, he found that they were most abundant in neurones. The search for editing took advantage of a dataset of brain samples from the Amsterdam group; having finished an analysis of microRNAs, the group passed sequencing data to us to check for editing.[267] By comparing sequences in the samples to the reference genome, we were able to estimate the number of microRNAs that were edited. In total, 45 microRNAs showed some amount of editing, which varied from less than 1 per cent of the overall amount of a microRNA upwards to nearly 90 per cent. Thus, as was seen for protein-coding mRNAs, there are some microRNA that are normally heavily edited in the brain. This tells us that whatever the original use of the microRNA, it has changed. The brain has co-opted a previously evolved microRNA for a new task. So, what is that task, and does having epilepsy change that?

We were surprised when we compared patients with controls. The amounts of editing hardly differed between the groups. Despite all the disruption to normal brain function and all the changes in cell number and structure, the brain's ability to keep on editing microRNAs seemed to be preserved. This contrasted with what we knew about microRNA abundance. Hundreds of microRNAs showed differences in their levels in human epilepsy tissue when compared to controls. The microRNA editing system seemed undisturbed. But we did find one change that was significant: miR-376a carried a nucleotide change at position 6, right in the seed, and the editing levels of this microRNA were lower in patients. Although the drop in editing was small, it could be important. First, because brain levels of this microRNA are quite high, which is important as we've discussed in earlier chapters. Second, miR-376a was among the most highly edited in the brain, about 85 per cent of the total amount. Would the change in editing do anything? Computer model predictions showed that it would not affect the structural stability of the microRNA but it should affect the target pool. Plugging in the unedited and edited versions of miR-376a to a target prediction algorithm revealed that the targets were almost completely different. Despite only a single base difference, the two versions of the microRNA had only 22 targets in common out of about 500 predicted. This meant that this single base had dramatically changed what the microRNA targeted. Perhaps the edited version was regulating different genes within its normal pathways. Or maybe the microRNA was regulating entirely different pathways. If that was the case, then the change in epilepsy could be quite important.

We looked at the genes and pathways under the control of the two forms of miR-376a. When plugged into a program that predicts affected pathways, the targets of the edited form included pathways involved in neurotransmission and synaptic function. Compared to the unedited form, some of the signalling pathways differed, with what seemed like a switch between neurotransmitters. This suggests that at some point the value of the original microRNA for the brain declined. By using editing, a single base change generated a 'new' microRNA that had a use. Again, the efficiency is striking. The cell has to make only a single base change to a single microRNA and it has a completely new tool, ready to ensure that the gene expression landscape is balanced. Now some of this had been lost in epilepsy, where the level of editing was lower. Would this have consequences?

To prove this required functional studies. We proceeded to test what happened when we lowered the editing level in neurones. This was achieved using antimirs. Reducing the edited form in a way that mimicked the situation in epilepsy resulted in dramatic changes in the levels of protein-coding mRNAs, specifically, increased expression of more than 250 genes in human neurones. This reinforced that the editing of this microRNA is a biologically important event in neurones. The types of pathway that were changed in neurones brought a further surprise. Multiple genes linked to cellular energy control were increased. Many of the transcripts encoded proteins that allow mitochondria to do their job, generating ATP for the cell. This could have the effect of altering how neurones generate energy in epilepsy. This is useful, perhaps, because the majority of the energy (fuel) used in the brain is spent just on keeping the neurones excitable. Energy is expended to run the sodium–potassium pumps and to store and release the neurotransmitters at the synapse, which are packed with mitochondria. We know from brain imaging studies that seizures produce a surge in energy and substrate demand. So, when we tweak the target pool of this microRNA, neurones might be adapting to the prevailing situation and keeping the cellular energy tank full. But could this come at a price? Sustaining higher-than-normal metabolism is unlikely to be without a downside. At a minimum, you burn up more fuel so other things such as glucose supply and oxygen need to be ramped up. This high-energy state might also affect resilience to brain insults. Indeed, down-regulation of energy-hungry pathways had been discovered to be a way the brain naturally adapts when faced with a crisis.

Back in the early 2000s, Roger Simon and colleagues at the Oregon Health and Sciences University in Portland had been looking for ways to protect the brain from stroke, such as caused by a blocked blood vessel. They marvelled that hibernating animals could tolerate prolonged periods of low blood flow in the brain without adverse effects. One of the ways the animals survive is by shutting down metabolic processes. Without a demand for energy, the brain fares pretty well with extremely low blood flow. The researchers learnt how to mimic this hibernation state by briefly interrupting the blood supply to the brain of mice. When the mice were exposed to a full stroke a few days later, the brain was almost completely protected from damage.[268] What was the forewarning event changing in the brain to make it react so differently when later hit with a stroke? It turned out that multiple energy-hungry pathways were being switched off. So, gene turn-off could provide a sustained period of protection from harm. Going back to our microRNA editing example, if we are ramping up energy for the brain to deal with seizures, could this be at the expense of neuronal well-being?

It seems that it could. Critically, the other genes that stood out as changed when we reduced the amount of edited miR-376a were linked to degenerative diseases. Pathways including Alzheimer's, Huntington's and amyotrophic lateral sclerosis (ALS) came up. Reducing the amount of the edited form of miR-376a appears to switch on something else, processes that could be harmful if unregulated. So, it is possible that the adaptation to provide more fuel for the hyperexcitable brain is at the expense of long-term neuronal survival. Could this cause deterioration over time? Brain imaging studies suggest that there is some brain atrophy over time in drug-resistant epilepsy.[269] Nothing like what is seen in neurodegenerative diseases, but nonetheless significant over time. This raises a final thought. Could this be turned into a therapeutic? Could we force a change to the amounts of this edited (or unedited) form of miR-376a to adjust back the altered balance and switch pathways? Perhaps raising the level of the edited form could be protective, or lowering the amount of the unedited form would trigger a compensatory rise in the edited form? I hope to explore this idea with my lab in the future.

Reflections

This chapter has covered the emergence of microRNA links to the pathophysiology of epilepsy. We've seen that substantial changes occur to the microRNA landscape in response to brain injuries that cause epilepsy. Models of epilepsy each display unique microRNA fingerprints in the brain, but there is also a common set of microRNAs that undergo similar changes at every stage of the process from insult to the first spontaneous seizures and on into the chronic period of epilepsy. This has generated interesting possibilities for targeting specific microRNAs as a way to interrupt or reverse that disease process. There are several microRNAs strongly linked to epilepsy, including miR-134, and there may be prospects for them as therapies. We have also seen how microRNAs make potential targets for the genetic epilepsies and neurodevelopmental disorders in which epilepsy is a major co-morbidity. Changes to microRNA levels in these models may contribute to how a gene mutation affects brain network function, excitability and behaviours. We have also begun to learn more about the microRNA system in the human brain, through analysis of tissue and modelling in iPSC-derived neurones. In many cases, the rodent models have been quite successful in generating microRNA profiles that match the human. But we have seen examples when this is not the case.

What are some of the next important questions in the area of epilepsy and microRNA? My own priorities and interests lie with learning which processes are controlled by which microRNAs in the disease setting, and applying this knowledge for therapeutic development. Which pathways are actually controlled by microRNAs in the human epileptic brain and which are not? Not all transcripts harbour suitable sites for regulation by microRNAs. Within microRNA-controlled pathways, which targets are the most regulated? What are the implications of enrichment of microRNA control for transcripts in particular pathways?

We need comprehensive cellular resolution of microRNA expression in healthy and epilepsy brain. There is some cell type–specific data on microRNAs in the human brain, but what is needed is a way to systematically map this, to learn which cells produce which microRNAs and how this changes, if at all, during the development of epilepsy and on into the chronic stage of the disease. Coupled with this, we need to understand better how a given microRNA represses a given set of targets in that cell.

Which targets are affected most (or least)? Building up this kind of knowledge will help us prioritise how therapeutic approaches might best be achieved. Going deeper into the cells, do inhibitory and excitatory neurones depend equally on the microRNA systems? Is the extent of perturbation similar between these cell types? What about cell subtypes? We can identify, either electrophysiologically or molecularly, multiple subtypes of GABA interneuron. What is the state of the microRNA system between these subtypes and does that help explain in any way the specific vulnerabilities of these cells or their particular function in epileptic networks?

Last, we need to bring some of the molecular tools that have been developed to study microRNA activity in real time into the epilepsy field. Can we see microRNA activation switching on and off in the epileptic brain? At which synapses? Does this follow or even precede an episode of seizure activity?

Chapter 7

MicroRNAs Become Medicines

Wherever the art of medicine is loved, there is also a love of humanity.
Hippocrates

The top 10 human diseases account for more than half of the more than 50 million deaths per year around the world. Heart disease is the biggest killer, followed by stroke and lung disease. Supporting our healthcare systems in tackling this enormous burden are an armamentarium of thousands of approved medicines. Nearly 500 of these are deemed by the World Health Organization (WHO) to be essential medicines. The most effective and safe anaesthetics, antibiotics and drugs for high blood pressure. But the drugs we have are not evenly distributed among the diseases or available in proportion to disease burden. For example, we have a number of good drugs to control blood pressure and manage cholesterol. We have some very effective treatments for cancer. But for other diseases we have next to nothing. For dementias such as Alzheimer's, number seven on the list of global killers, we have basically nothing that works. Stating the obvious, there remains plenty of need for new medicines, but a lot of the low-hanging fruit has been picked and we find ourselves with some very difficult diseases that urgently need medicines. Many of these are brain diseases. The reasons for this are complex, but one is that the causes of many brain diseases have yet to be fully solved. Without understanding what causes the disease it is very difficult to design a drug to stop it.

As we have seen in the previous chapters, microRNA levels are disrupted in several important human diseases. They are, therefore, viable targets to develop medicines against. We have already been introduced to some of the ways drugs can be designed against microRNAs, including using antimirs, a form of antisense oligonucleotide (ASO). Some ASOs have already been approved for the treatment of certain diseases. So, the groundwork is done. We can develop microRNA-based drugs. Will they be safe? One of the key strengths of microRNAs is also their biggest weakness. They are multi-targeting molecules. While this might offer advantages over the 'single bullet' approach of going after just one gene, they have effects on many targets, making off-target effects likely and difficult to predict. That can be a hard sell to a drug company, knowing already how hard it is to get any medicine into humans. Unknowns are not much liked. But, as we will see, microRNA-based medicines can be developed and have been given to humans.

The development of new medicines is built on pharmacology, the discipline I studied as both an undergraduate and a postgraduate. Fittingly for the subject of this book, it is the ultimate multi-tasker subject. Pharmacologists pick and borrow from several different disciplines including biology, chemistry and physiology. Pharmacologists are interested in how drugs work, what happens to the drug when it enters the body – the sub-discipline of *pharmacokinetics* – and what it does within the body – the sub-discipline of *pharmaco-dynamics*. Any time an advance is made in our understanding of a biological process, particularly one that happens in humans, there is an opportunity to ask can we make a drug out of this? Developing a new drug begins years before clinical trials ever happen. There needs to be extensive preclinical testing in non-human species, checks for safety and establishment of the manufacturing processes that will be used to produce the product. If that all goes well, the drug can begin human testing. Phase 1 is to test in healthy volunteers. Here, the regulators are looking only at whether or not the drug is safe. The next step is a Phase 2 trial. This is the first exposure of a patient to the drug and usually involves a small number of subjects. Again, safety and tolerability are the main things, but these studies are also on the lookout for some measure of potential benefit, a sign that the drug is doing what it is supposed to do. If the drug is found to be well-tolerated this will usually lead on to a further, large recruitment of patients and expanded testing.

At the time of writing, a search of the clinical trials database clinicaltrials.org with the terms 'microRNA' and 'interventional' returns more than 500 hits. If you just use the term 'microRNA' you get more than 1,000 hits on the trials register, the larger number being mainly studies that are monitoring microRNA levels as a surrogate of the disease process or to track the effects of a drug. It is largely biomarker work, which we will cover in Chapter 8. This gives an indication of the trajectory of practical applications in the biomedical field. The interval of time between when microRNAs were first discovered in humans at the turn of the millennium and the start of efforts to develop a drug based on targeting a microRNA was just a few years. The field went from discovering microRNAs in humans to testing a microRNA drug in humans in a single decade. The seeds of this can be traced to the discovery of microRNAs unique to specific tissues. The finding of a molecule that is highly enriched in one tissue or organ gives a strong indication that it is required for the function of that system, and if it is required in health then it may change in a disease affecting that system. A change in disease is an opportunity for a treatment, either replacing it in the case of it being deficient or blocking it if there is too much.

While fast, the road to microRNA drugs has not been smooth. Some of the companies involved in developing microRNA-based therapies have closed or abandoned parts or all of their microRNA programmes. There is not yet a standard-of-care treatment for a patient group that employs a microRNA-based approach. But other companies have sprung up and efforts continue around the world. The human diseases for which a microRNA therapy is being considered are remarkably diverse, spanning from a common cause of liver disease to the progressive neurodegenerative disorder ALS, as well as work by several teams, including my own, in the field of epilepsy. And there is not just one type of microRNA drug. As we have seen already, microRNA loss as well as microRNA gain or up-regulation represent viable therapeutic targets. There are ways to deliver a microRNA where its insufficiency is to blame as well as ways to block a microRNA that is in excess. In this chapter, we will encounter examples of both approaches that have entered clinical trials. We will look at the broad diversity of diseases being targeted and some of the targeting approaches. Finally, we will look to the future, to ask what are the prospects going forward and what techno-logical breakthroughs will help to continue to drive this exciting new area of therapeutics.

A MicroRNA Therapy Gets a Clinical Trial

The idea for the first microRNA-based drug has its inception in one of the early studies by Tuschl's team. They had been searching for microRNAs in different mouse tissues, including the heart, parts of the digestive system and the brain. They noted that miR-122 was a liver-only microRNA.[20] By their estimate, miR-122 accounted for more than 70 per cent of all the microRNA molecules in liver samples, an estimated 50,000 copies per cell. Thus, miR-122 was produced at scale and likely important for liver cells, called hepatocytes, to function. Since then, we have learnt many other things about this particular microRNA. It is highly conserved, being present in all vertebrates, and comes from a single locus in the genome. Levels of miR-122 are carefully tuned by transcription factors that ensure that appropriate amounts of miR-122 are made. As might be expected of such an abundant microRNA, it is involved in multiple aspects of liver function, beginning with how the liver develops and on through to its function in the adult liver. Some of the many natural targets of miR-122 have been identified. The work to map these began in 2005 by a team at Rockefeller University in New York. They showed in *Nature* that when mice were given an inhibitor of miR-122 there was an increase in 363 liver gene transcripts.[270] Not all changes went in the same direction, however, with a number of liver genes being down-regulated by the same treatment. This emphasises the complex systems-wide effects of perturbing microRNA function. As expected, among the list were multiple genes involved in liver development and function. Some of the transcripts that increased after blocking miR-122 were from genes that should not be active in the adult liver. For example, one of miR-122's targets is a transcription factor called cut-like homeobox 1 (CUX1). Suppression of this gene is required for developing liver cells to stop dividing and then differentiate, to turn into mature cells. In fact, experiments have shown that if you block miR-122 then precursor liver cells cannot mature properly. A key function of miR-122, therefore, is to tune the transition to an adult liver and then make sure it stays that way. Another function of miR-122 is to regulate cholesterol levels by targeting some of the enzymes in the pathways that underlie the generation and processing of cholesterol, a key function of the liver. In a later experiment in the same paper, the team showed that plasma cholesterol levels dropped by 40 per cent in mice treated with an antimir against miR-122.

As important as miR-122 is for the control of gene expression in the liver, you can live without miR-122. At least mice can live without it. Studies published in 2012 revealed that mice in which the gene for miR-122 was deleted were viable.[271, 272] But they were far from healthy and, as might be expected for a regulator of the development of the liver, mice lacking miR-122 developed several problems. These matched the features of a number of liver diseases in which low levels of miR-122 had by this stage also been reported. That includes liver cancers; alcoholic steatohepatitis, that is, fatty deposits in the liver caused by alcohol consumption; and liver cirrhosis, which is scarring and severe decline of liver function. The findings confirmed that mammals need miR-122 and implied that replenishing miR-122 might be an option for treating certain types of human liver disease. It might be a surprise, therefore, to learn that the first microRNA medicine to reach patients was a molecule to block miR-122. That molecule, an antimir, was named miravirsen. The time that elapsed between the discovery of miR-122 in humans and the first tests of a treatment targeting miR-122 in a human was less than a decade. This is an astonishing timeline. How this came about is a fascinating example of taking a basic science discovery and recognising the potential it has for translation to the clinic.

Miravirsen was developed to treat hepatitis C (HCV).[273] Hepatitis or inflammation of the liver is a global health problem and HCV is a major cause.[274] An estimated 58 million people are living with HCV infection. Based on 2015 data, 1.75 million more cases get added every year. An HCV infection causes chronic liver disease and it is in the sights of the WHO to be eliminated by 2030. This is achievable, in theory, with sufficient screening, diagnosis and access to affordable treatment. We will have to wait and see how close we get to the target. Gloomily, back in 2018 only 12 of the world's 194 countries were on track to achieve the WHO target.

So, what is HCV, how do you get it and why does it cause liver disease? Let's take the middle question first. The most common way to get infected with HCV is by direct exposure to the blood of someone infected. This can be through a blood transfusion, by injection via another healthcare-related procedure or by intravenous drug use. A substantial number of people with HCV are co-infected with human immunodeficiency virus (HIV). Anyone can get HCV, but in reality half of the people who get HCV live in just six countries – China, Egypt, India, Nigeria, Pakistan and Russia. The high rates in these countries come down to a mixture of unsafe medical practices and rates of injected drug use. Acute infection with HCV is often not accompanied by any signs or obvious liver-related symptoms such as jaundice, the medical term for which is anicteric. Your body fights back, but this is not always successful. If you have a chronic HCV infection you are at risk of liver failure and liver cancer, the risks of which vary with factors such as age, concurrent infections and general liver health at the time of infection, and sex; males are more at risk than females. Having HCV infection, at least in Western countries, is the leading reason for someone needing a liver transplant.

But HCV is actually a group of viruses.[274] There are currently eight major subtypes of HCV and a further 86 subtypes have been genetically identified (see **Figure 7.1A**). Type 1 accounts for nearly half of all infections. Viruses carry either a DNA or an RNA cargo, and HCV is an RNA virus, more specifically a subtype of RNA viruses called a positive-strand RNA virus. This means that the virus contains a strand of RNA, not DNA, which can be directly read and translated into protein by the host infected cell. There are some nasty cousins of HCV that are also positive-sense single-stranded RNA viruses, including SARS-Cov2 and West Nile virus. Their genomes are tiny. The entire instruction manual for HCV is contained in just 9,600 nucleotides. Once the RNA is released inside the cell, it gets translated into a single, long polypeptide before being cut up into smaller parts that are the individual functional proteins. A lot is packed into a small space, with both structural and non-structural proteins generated. It gets to work doing what viruses do so well – making more copies of the virus. Replicating. New viruses are assembled based on the instructions, creating new infectious particles.

The exclusive expression of miR-122 in hepatocytes had been noted early by micro-biologist Peter Sarnow at Stanford University in the USA. A key interest of his was mechanisms of viral replication. He and his team set about exploring if there were any potential links to HCV.[275] They began by testing a set of different tissues and cells for miR-122. When they ground up a piece of rat or human liver and extracted the RNA, they could detect a strong signal for miR-122, confirming what Tuschl's team had reported for mice. Then they switched to human cell lines. They found no signal for miR-122 when testing extracts from HeLa cells consistent with their origins as cervical cancer cells. Testing extracts from liver cell lines, including a line called Huh7 cells, gave a strong miR-122 signal. And then something interesting happened. They got almost no signal for miR-122 in

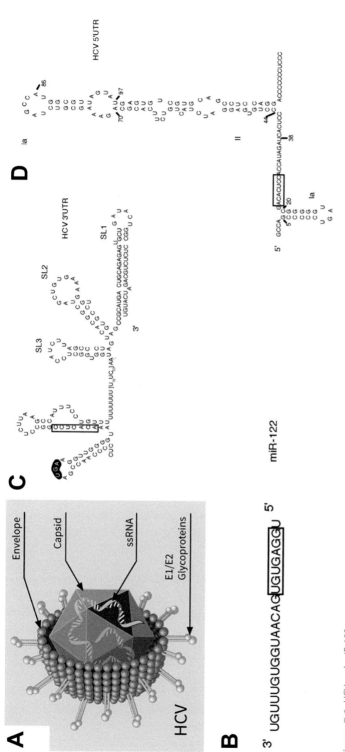

Figure 7.1 HCV and miR-122

Panel A shows the basic structure of the HCV virus.

Panel B is the miR-122 sequence (seed is highlighted in the box).

Panels C and D show the secondary structure of the non-coding regions of the HCV (miR-122 sites in boxes).

Source: Panel A illustration courtesy of www.hegasy.de. Images in Panels B–D reprinted with permission from Jopling et al., *Science*, vol. 309, pp. 1577–81 (2005).[275]

a human liver cell line called HepG2. This was noteworthy because it was known that HCV could replicate in Huh7 cells but not in HepG2 cells. This was one of those 'lightbulb' moments. Was it possible that miR-122, the liver's most important microRNA, was actually helping HCV to work?

The team began looking for potential sites in the viral genome where miR-122 might bind. They found two regions with suitable seed complementarity, both in the non-coding region of the HCV's long RNA. The first one was at the 3' end of the RNA, a traditional spot for a microRNA to bind. The other site was at the other end of the viral RNA, the 5' end, which at the time had not been thought to mediate microRNA-target interactions in human cells (see **Figure 7.1B–D**). Both sites for miR-122 were present, that is, conserved, in all the HCV genotypes. To find out what miR-122 was doing, they designed an antagomir to the mature miR-122 sequence and incubated this with the Huh7 cells, the ones where HCV could replicate and that normally express high amounts of miR-122. Blocking miR-122 reduced the replication of HCV by 80 per cent. This was a stunning discovery. When new HCV infections were performed in liver cells, the antagomir dramatically reduced the ability of the virus to infect liver cells. This meant that miR-122 was somehow helping HCV to replicate. To complement this, they performed experiments introducing either the native form of miR-122 or versions of it with altered nucleotide sequences to cells and showed that the native but not mutated forms supported HCV replication. With some final experiments they concluded that miR-122 was most important in the replication of the viral RNA, perhaps by affecting the folding of the RNA in the replication complex. The final sentence in the *Science* paper was a speculation on the potential therapeutic implications. With such poor treatments for HCV at that time, could targeting miR-122 provide a possible anti-viral drug?

Double-Blow: A Second Mechanism for How miR-122 Helps HCV

Sarnow's team had uncovered key principles about miR-122 and HCV. The presence and direct interaction of miR-122 with the RNA of HCV increased the amount of viral RNA. That is, more miR-122 resulted in more viral RNA in liver cells. But this was not the only way the virus took advantage of the liver's favourite microRNA. As other groups picked up on the discovery made by Sarnow's team, further discoveries were to be made and another key mechanism of action of HCV was uncovered in 2008. The virus had a second use for miR-122. A team based in Giessen, Germany revealed that HCV also used miR-122 to increase translational efficiency.[276] The virus' long RNA is translated into an amino acid sequence which is then chopped up into smaller pieces that comprise the various functional proteins the virus needs to create more virus. Remarkably, miR-122 was increasing the amount of the virus RNA *and* making sure as much of the protein as possible was made. An insidious solution to how to replicate and spread an infection in this organ. It was during the experiments to prove this second mechanism of action, promoting viral protein production, that a second miR-122 site was uncovered in the 5' UTR. The virus actually held three sites for miR-122. The extra 5' site comprised a six-nucleotide rather than the more common seven-nucleotide seed match for miR-122, but it was enough and, as it turned out, key to the translation-promoting action of miR-122 for HCV. The German team stripped out the two 5' miR-122 site sequences from the viral RNA and created artificial assay systems to test how they affected translation. They found that both sites contributed to the protein production-boosting effect of the virus, and showed that the 3' UTR site for miR-122 had no role in this part of the virus replication mechanism. Without these two 5' sites, the addition of miR-122 molecules into their test system had no effect on the translation rate. Together, the two sites boosted translation 12-fold. The team went on to show that binding of miR-122 to the HCV RNA promoted formation of the ribosomal 48S initiation complex. This is the first step in protein manufacturing, the moment when an mRNA is picked up by the large RNA engine called 40S and scanned for the necessary sequences to make a protein. When miR-122 was present, more of these 48S complexes formed. In essence, miR-122 had been co-opted to add workers to the assembly line at the HCV viral production factory.

AGO2 Gets Roped In to Help HCV

Research also shows that the microRNA binding sites contribute to stabilisation and survival of the virus in the infected host cell, working to protect the genome against attack by host cell RNA-degrading enzymes. Work to resolve more details of how the HCV genome hijacks the microRNA system to succeed continues and new breakthroughs keep coming. One of the most recent was a study led by MacRae's team at the Scripps Research Institute in La Jolla, California.[277] The team wanted to better understand how the interactions between viral RNA, miR-122 and AGO2 occurred and how this process was stabilised as part of the virus life cycle. To do this, they first created purified crystals of human AGO2 bound to miR-122 and then used X-ray crystallography to visualise how the protein and the RNA interacted. They found that when miR-122 is bound to AGO2, it protects the 5' UTR end of the virus genome from RNA-degrading enzymes. This effect occurred at the miR-122 'site 1' binding region because when this site was replaced with a different, non-miR-122-binding sequence, the virus' RNA was no longer protected. That is, when AGO2 is sitting with miR-122 on the site 1 part of the virus' genome, the viral RNA is protected from attack by the host cell's RNA-degrading machinery. The virus' 5' UTR also has a unique stem-loop structure that works to separate some of the potential base pairing between miR-122 and the viral RNA and this also contributes to how the docked AGO2-containing miR-122 protects against degradation and promotes stabilisation and longer life expectancy of the viral RNA in the host cell. Using the crystallography approach, they could visualise the conformation of AGO2 with both the viral RNA and miR-122 together. This showed that miR-122 becomes threaded through the central cleft of AGO2. They could also see that the HCV RNA forms multiple contact points with AGO2 including an unexpected nucleotide of the HCV RNA that bulges out and forms an important contact with a pocket in AGO2. It was also possible to see that, with AGO2 locked in this three-way embrace, the very end of the viral RNA was shielded from enzyme attack. Thus, by drawing AGO2 to itself via its miR-122 site, the viral RNA keeps its tail away from the bite of the host cell enzymes and survives longer inside the cell. The team made a further discovery about the importance of site 1 for protection from degradation. It altered AGO2's ability to shunt along RNAs, a process termed lateral diffusion. Effectively, the structure in the viral RNA was acting like a car handbrake, altering AGO2's conformation and anchoring AGO2 more firmly than normal to the RNA. Once again, this helped keep AGO2 sitting on top of the vulnerable-to-degradation end of the viral RNA. It seems likely that microRNA binding sites in other viral genomes work in similar ways, recruiting proteins and altering their movement in ways that increase the survival of the foreign genetic material in the infected cell and ultimately help the virus succeed. Indeed, HCV is not alone in hijacking the microRNA system for nefarious purposes. Viruses and their hosts are relentlessly battling each other. Several other viruses are known to exploit aspects of the microRNA system for replication. This even includes microRNAs encoded within viral genomes. In 2007, a team from Duke University in the USA reported in *Nature* that the genome of Kaposi's sarcoma-associated herpes virus contained a microRNA that mimicked human miR-155.[278] The virus' microRNA suppresses various targets of this microRNA in B lymphocytes and is implicated in the tumour-causing effects of the virus. In 2017, a team from the University of Utah made new discoveries, also reported in *Nature*, about Herpesvirus saimiri, another virus that can cause leukaemia and lymphoma.[279] The virus produces small non-coding RNAs that bind to two microRNAs in host cells. But rather than inactivating the microRNA or affecting their abundance, the viral RNAs work by recruiting the two natural microRNAs to suppress key apoptosis-regulating proteins. This effectively disables the host cell's ability to kill itself, leaving the door open to unchecked replication. This reveals a new 'microRNA adapter' function of viral small non-coding RNAs, expanding our understanding of the diverse and ingenious (or insidious) mechanisms that viruses have evolved that involve the microRNA system in how they replicate or cause disease. Moreover, while the focus here is on HCV, there are other RNA viruses that have also been found to directly recruit host microRNAs, including the Zika virus genome which contains RNA sequences that can interact with miR-21. Erik Miska's group at Cambridge University found that the virally encoded RNA contains a sequence match for miR-21 and AGO-bound miR-21 docks to the RNA, which enhances its replication efficiency.[280]

On to a Medicine

Let us shift away from the work to link miR-122 to HCV replication and infection and on to the research that would eventually provide the medicine to target miR-122 and treat HCV. Two companies had the miR-122/HCV story in mind for their RNA-targeting antisense drug platforms. These were Regulus in the USA and Santaris in Denmark. Both began work with the same goal in mind: developing an miR-122 inhibitor to treat HCV. While the target, miR-122, was the same, the two companies would use different chemistry. In the end, Santaris won a key race, getting to a clinical trial first. At the time of writing, however, Regulus is still in business, whereas Santaris no longer exists, having been subsumed into a large Pharma. The Regulus chemistry was based on a formula for creating stable ASOs that Ionis developed. The Santaris chemistry used another approach, called locked nucleic acid (LNA). This involved modifying the ribose group in an oligonucleotide by creating an extra 'bridge' that connects the oxygen molecule at the 2' position to the carbon at the 4' position. This had actually been invented in the late 1990s, independently, by the Japanese team of Takeshi Imanishi and Jesper Wengel, a chemist in Denmark. Antisense oligonucleotides had been around for many years at this stage, but chemists were forever working on ways to tweak these to improve potency, stability, safety/biocompatibility or all three.[281] And LNA chemistry was one of the key breakthroughs that improved ASOs for targeting microRNA. The microRNA inhibitors my own research has used all include LNA modifications.

One of the scientists at the centre of getting LNA-designed ASOs to target miR-122 was a Finnish scientist, Sakari Kauppinen. Now running the Center for RNA Medicine at Aalborg University in Denmark, at the time of the miR-122-HCV breakthroughs in 2005 Kauppinen was working at the University of Copenhagen. He had undertaken his PhD in molecular biology from that university, after which he moved to industry where he began work on methods to detect gene activity, spending time in Novo Nordisk and Novozymes before a move to Exiqon in 2000. It was at Exiqon where he worked to improve the technology used to design probes to detect gene expression changes, the microarray technology covered in Chapter 2. To precisely detect and measure the abundance of RNAs required the ability of probes to stick on with absolute fidelity. Mismatches between the probe and the RNA could give false positives and an inability to stick to the right probe a false negative. These types of gene array were being used by academics and industry to profile the gene activity that changed in a particular model or disease and were of great interest to diagnostic companies who wanted to use these as tests for health and disease. Kauppinen's time at Exiqon seeded interest in synthetic methods to detect short RNAs such as microRNA. Because of their small size, detecting microRNAs en masse had been proving difficult and various researchers were working on a fix that would create the probes to more reliably measure short RNAs. A key breakthrough was taking advantage of LNA technology. The extra chemical bridge on the DNA base created a less flexible structure, a stiffening rod running down the length of the molecule. When synthetic RNA-modified sequences or 'probes' were designed which incorporated some of the LNA-modified bases, they worked much better than before, with fewer mistakes and false readings. The same technology, it turns out, made for exceptionally good ASOs to target microRNAs.[282] The LNA-based ASOs were precise and stable, resistant to the enzymes in our cells that naturally break down nucleotide sequences. The first papers to use LNA technology to design microRNA inhibitors to treat a disease appeared in 2005. One of these studies, reported in *Science*, used an LNA-based microRNA inhibitor to demonstrate that miR-32 protected against certain viral infections.[283]

After five years at Exiqon, Kauppinen moved back to academia at the University of Copenhagen. It was here that he began to use some of the technology that had worked to detect microRNAs and turn it into a tool that could target microRNAs. He was not to stay long. Within a year he moved back to industry, to a new company, Santaris Pharma, where he began work on an miR-122 drug. Santaris was a relatively new company at that time, having been founded in 2003. It had formed through the merger of two pre-existing companies that had microRNA targeting chemistry. Santaris owned the patent to LNA technology and would use the chemistry to design various LNA-based inhibitors to RNAs of interest. Although it also had mRNAs in its sights for the treatment of certain cancers and metabolic diseases, it began a microRNA programme in 2005 with miR-122 its target. By 2007, its preclinical lead, SPC3649, had already reached testing in non-human primates and then entered human trials as miravirsen in 2010. An impressive feat in the drug development field. The results of the clinical trial, the first ever for a microRNA drug, were published in the *New England Journal of Medicine* in 2013. By 2014, the company no longer existed.

The first studies from Kauppinen's team at Santaris began with designing a suitable antimir and then testing it in mice, using the known effect of blocking miR-122 to decrease blood cholesterol as a convenient pharmacodynamic read-out of it working. The antimir they designed contained 16 nucleotides that targeted the first 16 bases of the mature miR-122 molecule. Every third base was LNA modified, for a total of five bases (indicated in capital letters): 5-ccAttGtcAcaCtcCa-3. This was not the only tinkering that was done to create a more drug-like molecule. The backbone of the molecule, a sugar–phosphate chain, was also modified to phosphorothioate. This worked as a mask, first improving stability and second altering surface charge. As we learnt in Chapter 5 on neurones, cells generate a negatively charged interior by pumping ions back and forth across the membrane. Neurones are not the only cells to do this and other cells create their own membrane potentials to control the movement of substances in and out. The negative charge repels nucleotides trying to get inside. By modifying the backbone of the antimir, designed molecules are able to stay under the radar of the body's DNA breakdown defences and can pass into cells more easily. The Santaris team also synthesised a control version of their antimir, with a mixed-up version of the base sequence that contained the same number of LNA-modified bases, but with one half of the molecule having a different sequence of bases that would prevent it binding to miR-122. They ran tests in liver cell lines first, checking that the sequence really was specific for miR-122, and then gave intravenous injections to mice. Within a few days of the injections, they found that mice given the antimir had much lower levels of miR-122 in the liver, and the drop in miR-122 matched the amount of antimir given, a reassuring dose–response relationship. No changes to miR-122 levels were found in the mice injected with the mismatch version and the antimir-122 did not change the levels of other microRNAs in the body. So far, so good. Further experiments suggested that the way the inhibitor was working was by forming a very stable duplex with miR-122. Similar to the 2005 *Nature* study which first tested an miR-122 inhibitor in mice, but with different chemistry, the Santaris team found that blocking miR-122 increased levels of more than 100 gene targets of miR-122 in the liver, several of which were for liver enzymes now confirmed as having been under miR-122 control.[284] The team confirmed that the antimir reduced plasma cholesterol and found no signs of liver or other toxicity, which had been a concern with some of the earlier ASO chemistry. Last, they noted that a single dose of their antimir produced effects lasting for weeks in mice.

Antimir-122 Makes It to Trial

The use of non-human primates in medical research and drug development is controversial and opposed, often violently, by certain groups. But for some human diseases, testing in non-human primates is necessary, either because the risk of jumping from rodents to humans is too great, for example when there is not enough experience with the compounds to be sure they are safe, or because aspects of the disease in question only fully manifest in non-human primates. By the end of 2007, not even a full year after the mouse tests, the Santaris team submitted findings on their antimir-122 in non-human primates, specifically African green monkeys.[285] They used a 15-mer antimir design, meaning that the sequence contained 15 nucleotides that perfectly matched to the miR-122 sequence. Intravenous injections were given and the team used the known cholesterol-lowering actions of the antimir to indirectly monitor whether it was working. These studies also helped guide the right dose, with an injection of 10 milligrams per kilogram bodyweight producing a strong and sufficient reduction in cholesterol that perfectly matched the dose that had done the same in earlier mouse tests. Cholesterol levels remained lower for a remarkable three months after injections, suggesting that the antimir worked for longer in non-human primates than it had in mice. This would suggest that treatment in humans might not need to be as often as would have been expected based on the rodent studies. Blood tests from the monkeys showed no signs of toxicity from the injections. Liver function tests, general tests of coagulation and microscope work looking for cell damage all came back fine. But measuring a surrogate such as cholesterol could only go so far in assuring that the microRNA inhibitor was doing what it was designed to do. More direct measures were needed and that required liver biopsies from the monkeys. Liver sample analysis backed up the cholesterol tests, showing that the antimir had potently reduced the levels of miR-122 in the monkeys' livers. The conclusion was that SPC3649, as Santaris' lead compound was known at the time, was a well-tolerated drug that worked exactly as had been expected in non-human primates. They were ready for human testing.

Testing a completely new type of drug for the first time in people with a deadly liver disease is a risk. You want to pick the best clinicians to run these trials. Santaris chose Harry Janssen to lead the clinical trial that would inject people suffering from HCV infection with their antimir to miR-122. Janssen is the world's top expert on hepatitis infections, running the Toronto Centre for Liver Disease, the world's largest liver research and trials centre, in Canada. Originally from the Netherlands, his credentials to lead the trial were impeccable. After medical school he undertook a PhD focussed on use of immunotherapy to treat hepatitis B infections. From there he specialised early in hepatology, the science and medicine of the liver, including time at the Mayo Clinic in the USA. At the time of writing, he has more than 600 publications. A good pick for the person to lead a clinical trial of an experimental medicine for liver infection.

The human trial of SPC3649, or miravirsen as it was now called, included 36 patients with HCV infection gathered from across seven international liver specialist treatment centres.[286] There were specific enrolment criteria. These included no previous exposure to other anti-HCV treatments and a minimal viral load at the time of enrolment. Recruitment began in 2010 and ran for a year. Incredibly, just five years had passed since the discovery that miR-122 was involved in the HCV infection mechanism. The trial was run as a placebo-controlled double-blind trial. Some patients got no miravirsen and neither the patients nor the clinical team treating them knew what was being given to whom. Three different doses of miravirsen – 3 mg, 5 mg or 7 mg per kilogram body mass – were tested, with the treatment given under the skin in weekly injections over a month. Patients returned for check-up visits and blood tests for several months. At these check-ups, the clinical teams confirmed which subtype of HCV each patient was infected with and measured their viral load in the blood. They also checked for signs of any toxicity and asked patients about their general health and well-being. Miravirsen worked as expected. It reduced HCV viral load in the treated patients and this happened in a dose-related way. That is, the reduction in HCV was highest in the patients given 5 mg and 7 mg per kilogram injections; there was less of an effect in the 3 mg per kilogram group (**Figure 7.2**). The patients in the placebo arm showed no change in infection levels. The onset effect of miravirsen was fast, obvious within the time of active dosing, and the knock-down of the viral load lasted weeks beyond the last injection, with viral loads just beginning to recover around the 15th week after starting treatment. For five patients in the study, miravirsen worked so well that at times the medical teams could no longer detect HCV in the blood, signs that for some patients this could potentially be a cure. Adverse events were reported, not uncommon in any trials, but none resulted in patients having to drop out of the trial. There was some local skin irritation at the injection site which later cleared up. Blood tests showed that miravirsen had reduced serum cholesterol, as expected, but also had some effects on liver enzymes, reducing levels of three enzymes that help the body break down proteins, albeit keeping within a clinically safe range. So, miravirsen seemed safe.

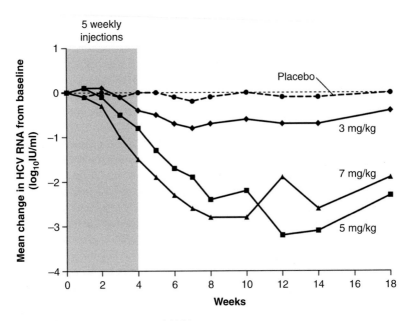

Figure 7.2 Effect of miravirsen in patients with HCV

Graph shows the change in HCV levels from baseline after treatment with miravirsen. Shown are the average HCV RNA levels in the plasma of patients in the trial that received one of the three doses.

Source: Reprinted with permission from Janssen et al., *New England Journal of Medicine*, vol. 368, pp. 1685–94 (2013).[286]

What Happened to Miravirsen?

So, the first ever clinical trial of a microRNA-based drug in a patient with a disease was a considerable success. It had done what it was designed to do, lowering HCV levels, and it had managed this without causing too many side effects. This was a breakthrough in any sense of the word. But miravirsen never made it to the pharmacy shelf. What happened? Competition is the main reason. Now, HCV infection is mainly treated with what are called direct-acting antivirals (DAAs).[274] There is more than one option and the choice comes down to factors such as HCV type as well as cost and availability. In combination, DAAs can be highly effective at blocking the HCV enzymes that drive the formation of new viruses, resulting in elimination of the infection. The combination and orally available HCV treatments that were being co-developed around the same time were both more effective, essentially offering a cure, and could be taken as a pill rather than an injection. This represented a double-blow to miravirsen. Other factors almost certainly played a role. Roche bought Santaris, principally to acquire the LNA platform which was still under patent, to drive its own RNA medicine programme. That didn't include HCV. Work has continued on an anti-miR-122 treatment, led by Regulus in the USA, but at the time of writing there is no sign of that entering the medicine cabinet.

Two other discoveries in relation to HCV and microRNA control are worth a mention. While miR-122 promoted HCV replication, not all microRNAs were so accommodating. In 2007, a team at the University of California in San Diego discovered that host cell microRNAs were mobilised to defeat HCV.[287] One of the molecules the immune system produces in response to a viral infection is called interferon-beta and interferon treatment was known to reduce HCV infections, although the mechanism of how this worked was unknown. The team found interferon-beta switches on a set of five microRNAs that could target the HCV RNA, reducing HCV levels by 80 per cent. This was a potent and natural protection against viral infection. The sites for these microRNAs were conserved across all the major HCV genotypes. We have, it appears, evolved strategies within our genome to fight this and other viruses, deploying microRNAs as a frontline defence by directly sticking onto the viruses' own RNA to reduce replication. In effect there has been co-evolution, a molecular arms race between HCV and our liver cells: HCV co-opted our most highly expressed liver microRNA as part of its means to boost its own production. We counter-attack, deploying other microRNAs within our arsenal to suppress HCV.

A second important addition to the miravirsen story appeared about a year after the *New England Journal of Medicine* trial reported the phase II findings of miravirsen for HCV. A team based at the ETH in Zurich discovered an additional mechanism of action of miravirsen that might have added to its effectiveness.[288] At the time, the main therapeutic effects were assumed to derive from the ability of miravirsen to bind miR-122 and block it from working. The Swiss team added something further to miravirsen's already powerful armamentarium. They found that miravirsen also reduces the production of miR-122 itself by the liver.

Miravirsen is the trail-blazer drug in the microRNA field, but many other programmes are active and for a variety of diseases. The list is extensive and includes a large heart disease–related microRNA therapy programme that is targeting miR-132. This is being led by Thomas Thum and Cardior Pharmaceuticals, based in Germany. The programme spun out of a discovery made in 2012 reported in *Nature Communications* that miR-132 regulated two mechanisms that contribute to heart failure.[289] The over-growth of heart cells is called cardiac hypertrophy and a process called autophagy involves removal of some of the internal contents of cells and is one of the ways heart cells use to protect against stress. Transcripts that drive both processes were found to be targeted by miR-132 and its close relative miR-212, and blocking miR-132 using antimirs helped protect mice in a model of heart failure. The study was followed up by refining the drug candidate and tests in a large animal pig model. The anti-miR-132 is now in a phase II trial, NCT05350969, for patients with reduced left ventricular ejection fraction after having experienced a heart attack.

MicroRNAs as Medicines for Epilepsy

Targeting microRNAs could represent a new approach to treat epilepsy. This would be a major departure from current anti-seizure medicines, which are small chemical compounds that mostly act on the channels and receptors on the surfaces of neurones. New approaches are essential, however, because one in three people with epilepsy live with uncontrolled seizures. This amounts to perhaps 20 million people globally. This is not to minimise the success of drug development for epilepsy. Compared to many brain diseases, it has been a spectacular success. New drugs for epilepsy had been appearing at intervals ever since phenobarbital (1912) and phenytoin (1938) were discovered. That pipeline became organised in the mid-1970s, with the establishment of a screening programme in the USA funded by the National Institute of Neurological Disorders and Stroke (NINDS). For the first time, any company or researcher could bring forward their potential treatment and have it screened through a number of standardised models for anti-seizure effects. In the years that followed, more than 30,000 compounds were screened and there was a surge in new epilepsy drugs.[290] The programme, based at the University of Utah and led by Karen Wilcox, is now called the epilepsy therapy screening programme (ETSP) and has recently been re-funded.

But we have big gaps. In addition to the drug-resistance problem, we know the drugs we have, even when controlling seizures, are not disease-modifying. This means that if you stop taking the medicine, seizures will almost certainly return. The circuits that gave rise to seizures in the first place have not substantially changed, despite often years of treatment. The treatments we have for epilepsy also have no ability to prevent epilepsy in an individual at risk. We have no drug* we can give that can stop epilepsy emerging in an individual who is at risk, for example owing to a traumatic brain injury (*there is some evidence that treating genetic epilepsies caused by mutations in the mammalian target of rapamycin, or mTOR pathway, might have lasting effects that suggest that the underlying pathophysiology has been changed[291, 292]). So, we have a triple problem: resistance to current drugs, lack of disease modification by current drugs, and lack of anti-epileptogenic effects of current drugs. The multi-targeting actions of microRNA offer something new. Well, they do *if* there is a microRNA out there that regulates the right set of transcripts or pathways to shift or adjust brain networks in epilepsy. Some combination of ion channels and transmitter changes, gliosis, neurodegeneration, restructuring, brain-immune cell interactions . . ..

A Dog's Tale: A MicroRNA Therapy for Epilepsy Gets a Large Animal Trial

The search for the 'right' microRNA for epilepsy is still at an early stage. **Figure 7.3** lists some of those targeted to date which resulted in altered seizures in preclinical models. The list is already long and continues to grow. As covered in Chapter 6, an inhibitor of miR-134 is among the most advanced, proving effective at reducing seizures in five out of seven tested models.[293] Some of the best anti-seizure medicines work in only one or two rodent models. The most powerful effect, an almost complete prevention of TLE, was observed in mouse studies that began as a result of asking questions about how we might, one day, be delivering these molecules in a clinical trial. Why this question? Despite the potency and the long-lasting effects of antimirs seen in our studies and others, there are some major obstacles ahead. Antimirs are large, bulky molecules. When given systemically, for example, via an injection into the bloodstream, they do not pass into the brain. This is because the brain is separated from the circulation by the blood–brain barrier, an exclusion zone comprising specialised cells in the blood vessels of the brain that are tightly packed together to exclude many components of the blood from entering the brain. This is essential for healthy brain function as it prevents the passage of blood-based substances into the brain that would be neuroactive or neurotoxic. That includes large, bulky and charged molecules such as antimirs. The blood–brain barrier can be bypassed by injecting directly into the cerebro-spinal fluid that circulates in the brain, but this requires a lumbar puncture injection into the spine of the patient. This is not uncommon in clinical practice as it is how local anaesthetics are given during labour/childbirth, but this is a major departure from how people receive treatment for epilepsy. It's a long way from swallowing a pill once or twice a day. Once injected, antimirs last a long time, but you're probably still looking at repeat spinal injections every few months.

Studied miRNA	Alteration	Method	Effect of manipulation on excitability/seizures	Target and/or pathway affected
miR-22	Knock down	Antagomirs	Increase	P2X7 receptor, inflammation
miR-23b	Over expression	Mimics	Reduction	Unknown
miR-34a	Knock down	Antagomirs	None	Apoptosis
miR-96	Over expression	Mimics	Not measured	Autophagy
miR-124	Over expression	Mimics	None	Epigenetic
miR-128	Knock down	Genetic	Increase	ERK signalling
miR-129	Knock down	Antagomirs	Reduction	RBFOX1 signalling
miR-132	Knock down	Antagomirs	None	Apoptosis
miR-134	Knock down	Antagomirs	Reduction	Cellular structure
miR-135a	Knock down	Antagomirs	Reduction	Synaptic function
miR-146a	Over expression	Mimics	Reduction	IL-1R1 or TLR4, inflammation
miR-155	Knock down	Antagomirs	Reduction	BDNF signalling
miR-181a	Knock down	Antagomirs	Not measured	Caspase signalling
miR-184	Knock down	Antagomirs	None	Apoptotic signalling
miR-199a	Knock down	Antagomirs	Reduction	SIRT1–p53 signalling
miR-203	Knock down	Antagomirs	Reduction	Glycine receptor signalling
miR-204	Over expression	Mimics	Reduction	TrkB-Creb signalling
miR-210	Knock down	Antagomirs	Not measured	GABA signalling
miR-211	Knock down	Genetic	Increase	Cholinergic signalling
miR-219	Over expression	Mimics	Reduction	NMDA receptor signalling
miR-324	Knock down	Antagomirs	Reduction	Potassium channel $K_v4.2$

Figure 7.3 MicroRNAs targeted in preclinical epilepsy models

The table summarises preclinical studies manipulating microRNAs in rodent models of epilepsy.

Key: BDNF, brain-derived neurotrophic factor; Creb, cAMP-responsive element binding protein 1; ERK, extracellular signal-regulated kinase; IL-1R1, IL-1 receptor type 1; miRNA, microRNA; N/A, not applicable; P2X7R, P2X purinoreceptor 7; RBFOX1, RNA-binding fox 1 homologue 1; SIRT1, sirtuin 1; TLR4, Toll-like receptor 4; TrkB, neurotrophic tyrosine kinase receptor type 2.

Source: Brennan & Henshall, *Nature Reviews Neurology*, vol. 16, pp. 506–19 (2020).[10]

However, the permeability of the blood–brain barrier can change. In particular, injuries to the brain can cause it to open more, with gaps wide enough for certain molecules to squeeze through. While thinking about how we might one day deliver antimirs to patients, we came across a new brain imaging study by a team at the University of Bonn.[294] They used a scanning technique that made it possible to detect leaks in the blood–brain barrier. When they rushed some of their patients into a magnetic resonance imaging (MRI) scanner shortly after having a seizure, they found there was a time period when the barrier was open. For us, this was literally a window of opportunity. If we timed a systemic injection (e.g. intravenous) of antimirs with the blood–brain barrier opening, some of it should pass through the gaps and into the brain. We could avoid the spine or the direct brain injection

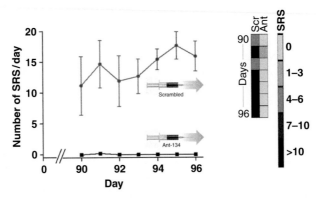

Figure 7.4 Potent anti-seizure effects of inhibiting miR-134

Intraperitoneal (abdomen) injection of antimir timed with the opening of the blood–brain barrier arrests epilepsy development in mice. The graph shows difference in counts of EEG-detected spontaneous recurrent seizures (SRS) recorded three months after treatment. The chart on the right shows daily counts of individual animals.

Source: Reschke et al., *Molecular Therapy*, vol. 29, pp. 2041–52 (2021).[227]

routes. And the antimir might only pass into the brain precisely at the spot where the seizure was occurring, concentrating it right where it was needed.

We decided to test this using the kainic acid model we worked with back in the 2012 study. We checked when the blood–brain barrier became leaky using the brain imaging method, and then gave mice a systemic injection of the antimir via a fine needle into the belly area, a common way to deliver drugs in dosing studies called intraperitoneal, and one that is vet approved.[227] We then tracked the development of epilepsy in the mice. Over a period of several months of monitoring, the mice given the systemic injection of antimir had 99 per cent fewer spontaneous seizures than the controls (**Figure 7.4**). We had nearly eliminated experimental epilepsy. This research continues, led currently by a talented researcher called Omar Mamad who is testing a new generation of microRNA inhibitor to this target.

The results with antimir-134 in mice have prompted us to think about moving towards a clinical trial, but we are conscious of the gap between rodents and humans. Is there a step in between we could take to de-risk this? On 29 July 2019 (I still have the email), I was contacted by a veterinary neurologist at the University of Glasgow. Dr Rodrigo Quintana explained that he cared for some very sick dogs with epilepsy. Would I be interested in working together to test the microRNA therapy? Here was an offer to move to a large animal study, an ideal midway point on the road to human trials. And if it was safe and worked in the dogs, then it could have the twin benefit of becoming a veterinary medicine. We first met in January of 2020. Rodrigo explained that epilepsy occurs at a similar frequency in canines as in humans, and in some breeds the rates are much higher. Some dogs also display a syndrome similar to TLE. His team even use an MRI to scan the brain and support diagnosis. For other dogs, the cause often remains unknown and one or more genetic factors are suspected. Therapy is similar to humans and many of the same ASMs work in dogs. But, like with many humans, seizures remain difficult to control in a sizeable proportion. If severe enough, owners and their veterinary carers are faced with the decision to humanely end the life of the dog. Rodrigo suggested we ask owners of dogs with severe, life-threatening seizures if they would consider enrolling their pet in a clinical trial of the antimir-134 therapy. And then the Covid-19 pandemic struck . . ..

Unsurprisingly, Covid-19 was highly disruptive to research. In some cases, it accelerated it to warp-speed, giving us vaccines in a few months. For many other teams, including my own, research became severely restricted. Labs were closed for weeks and, when reopened, had to operate under severe restrictions. Fewer people could work at the same time owing to spacing requirements and lab productivity dropped by at least half. Supply chain interruption also meant that certain reagents for experiments became scarce. Access to patient samples in the hospital was almost impossible. Rodrigo and I kept in touch, using the downtime to design the trial and figure out a way to pay for it. Clinical trials, even veterinary ones, are costly, and making enough of our antimir drug was going to be expensive. This would require new money and we agreed to co-apply to governments and non-profit grant-funding agencies. Midway through 2020, we spotted a USA-based charity looking for projects that would accelerate the development of new disease-modifying therapies for epilepsy. We wrote to them, explaining the study and the trial design. They were interested, but wanted to see some firm evidence of a link between the microRNA and the dogs with epilepsy. Rodrigo sent me some blood samples from his dogs and we measured levels of miR-134, finding that they were elevated in the samples from dogs with drug-resistant epilepsy. He also sent some autopsy brain tissue from dogs and we confirmed that miR-134 was present in neurones in the canine hippocampus. We reported back to the agency and were awarded funding to pay for the trial in 2021. After submitting paperwork to the regulator of veterinary trials in the UK, we were approved to proceed with METriC in late 2022. This would be a placebo-controlled blinded trial. Rodrigo would not know whether he was giving his patient the real drug or a salt solution. The first 'patient' was enrolled and received an injection on 15 March 2023. Fingers crossed.

MicroRNA Therapies Go Viral

Antimirs are not the only way to 'medicinise' microRNA. Where low levels of a microRNA are the root problem in a disease, delivering a microRNA may be the therapeutic solution. And there are some limitations with using antimirs. One of the problems is that antimirs, indeed any ASOs, are blind in terms of the cell types they enter. Once they reach a tissue, they will be taken up by whatever cells they encounter, and this may vary depending on the particular surface chemistry of the cell. This can result in blocking a microRNA in the wrong cell type. A microRNA might target quite different transcripts in two different cells. If you want to change microRNA actions in only one cell type, then introducing the microRNA into another could produce unwanted effects or even counterbalance the actions you are trying to achieve. We considered a hypothetical version of this problem in Chapter 5. Blocking miR-134, for example, in inhibitory neurones might produce opposite effects on excitability compared to blocking it in excitatory neurones.

When microRNAs encounter targets in the wrong cell type, it can spell trouble. A former PhD student and now professor at University College Dublin, Gary Brennan, observed such an 'invasive species effect' during studies on miR-124 with Tallie Baram at the University of California, Irvine.[295] He had noticed that levels of miR-124, one of the most abundant, neurone-enriched microRNAs in the brain, decline in the hippocampus after injuries that cause epilepsy. This led to an effort to try to restore brain levels of miR-124 by delivering the microRNA back into the brain. But when miR-124 was injected, in the form of precursor duplexes, it triggered widespread inflammation around the injection point. This was traced to a reaction of microglia, the brain's resident immune cells. The microglia in the region of brain that was exposed to the extra miR-124 became supercharged, pumping out an excess of inflammatory cytokines. Bringing the microRNA into contact with cells that normally do not make it had triggered an unexpected firestorm. An important lesson was learnt. If you plan on tinkering with microRNAs, particularly delivering a microRNA, you need a way to control the amount delivered and to ensure that it doesn't end up in the wrong cell.

There have been efforts to modify the chemistry of ASOs to steer them towards specific cell types, but the challenges are significant and far from solved. Fortunately, there are other ways to deliver a microRNA therapy to the right cell and at the right time, namely, viral vectors. Until quite recently this might have been seen as impossibly futuristic, but the Oxford-Astrazeneca Covid-19 vaccine used a virus as the delivery vehicle for the spike protein antigen. Gene therapy is now being given to children with spinomuscular atrophy, via zolgensma, a virally delivered gene-replacement treatment. A great advantage of viral vectors is that you can add promoter sequences to the instructions for making the cargo such that it will switch on only in certain cells. The virus may enter other cells but will not be active and will sit dormant. Many viruses also have natural tropism towards specific cell types, meaning they are better at getting inside some cells than others.

Viruses are incredible machines for gene delivery. They evolved that way, fine-tuned by evolution into simple and effective gene-injection devices for hijacking cells. Virally delivered genes are one of the leading approaches for gene therapy. Ever since mutations and missing genetic material was understood to cause disease in humans, people have had in mind that restoring, repairing or delivering the missing genetic information could be the best way to treat or cure the disease. The phrase 'gene therapy' refers to a medical product that contains a nucleic acid sequence to repair or restore function and where the effects of the product depend on a specific sequence. The origin of gene therapy can be traced at least as far back as the 1950s, when experiments by Joshua Lederberg, who would later receive a Nobel prize, discovered a new mechanism of genetic transfer that was credited to bacteriophages, that is, specialised viruses that infect bacteria.[296] In the following decade, a key study by Waclaw Szybalski using a modified human cell line proved that a genetic defect could be restored by delivering functional DNA from another source. In the same decade, Howard Temin's work on the Rous sarcoma virus demonstrated that foreign genetic material from a virus could be stably inherited by infected cells. In the second half of the 1960s, Edward Tatum proposed the use of a virus to deliver genetic material to treat human disease. This would spawn the idea of co-opting viruses to spread genetic material, the blueprint for modern gene therapy. The first human trial of a gene therapy happened in the early 1970s. An attempt was made to use Shope papilloma virus to restore a gene in two children who lacked an important enzyme needed by the liver. The team behind the study believed that the virus contained this gene, but unfortunately the virus didn't carry the gene and the trial failed. Gene therapy stalled for a while, mainly because of the lack of tools needed to engineer viruses, to remove the parts that were not wanted and to insert the sequence for the gene that was needed. The first successful gene transfer trials in humans were published in the early 1990s by Steven Rosenberg's team at the National Cancer Institute in Bethesda, Maryland. They used Moloney murine leukaemia virus to infect immune cells, beginning with a tracer gene and then using the approach to deliver a therapeutic gene called tumour necrosis factor. The trials were a success, proving that human cells could be virally transfected with a therapeutic gene, resulting in a human health benefit. The mid-1990s also saw gene therapy trials for genes missing in rare metabolic conditions in small numbers of patients, but with mixed results. Then, in the late 1990s, another high-profile failure, when a US trial involving a high dose of a virus to deliver the liver enzyme ornithine transcarbamylase resulted in the death of a patient. Beginning in the 2000s, the first clinically approved gene therapies appeared on the market, mainly for cancer. There have now been thousands of trials of various types that have used vectors and other approaches to deliver therapeutic genes and gene sequences to treat human disease.

Picking a Virus for a MicroRNA

The viral vector tools available in most neuroscience labs are safe versions of the original wildtype viruses in which sections of the original genome have been removed. For example, deleting the genes that allow them to reproduce in the cell renders them replication-defective. This means that the virus enters the cell and delivers the gene to just that one infected cell and does not spread farther. There are a number of decisions that need to be made when picking a virus to deliver a gene. The three major viruses that have emerged as front-runners in the area of CNS gene therapy are adeno-associated virus (AAV), lentivirus and herpes simplex virus.[297] Each has strengths and weaknesses. Some like to infect certain cells better than others. Even within the same virus, variations in the surface chemistry of the virus affect the infectivity of specific cells, so-called serotypes. Each virus also has a different payload capacity, the amount of genetic material it can carry. Some will deposit their genetic information directly into the host cell's DNA, the integrating viruses. In theory, this could mean a 'parent' infected cell could pass the viral genome on to any daughter cells. This may be less of a concern in neuroscience because there is relatively little cell replication in the adult brain. Non-integrating viruses make use of the host replication machinery but without incorporating their genetic material into the host DNA. Each different virus class also varies in the stability and the longevity of the expression of the inserted gene. So, which to pick? How do you narrow the list? The herpes simplex virus can carry the largest payload of the three, but microRNA genes are small. The AAV and lentivirus have space only for small payloads, but AAV is winning the race because of safety and a better toolkit for delivery to different brain cell types. There are now private companies that offer to make AAVs as a service, complete with the gene of your interest and a choice over what cell types it will home in on to express its payload. This has democratised the field in the sense that anyone's lab can use gene therapy in their research.

The idea of using AAVs for a microRNA-based epilepsy therapy is at a very early stage, but there has been striking progress in other brain diseases. In two cases, teams are using artificial microRNAs to control excess production of toxic proteins and this has already reached patients. The first example is for ALS. As we covered in relation to miR-218 in Chapter 5, ALS is a progressive, fatal neurodegenerative disease.[298] The first gene linked to the disease was superoxide dismutase 1, or SOD1.[299] Coincidentally, this discovery was in the same year, 1993, that Ruvkun/Ambros discovered lin-4. The job of SOD1 is to break down oxygen free radicals, a highly reactive by-product of metabolic reactions inside the cell. Left alone, free radicals cause damage to the insides of cells, wrecking just about anything including mitochondria, the protein trafficking and turnover systems, and activating cell death pathways. Unchecked free radical production is implicated in various human diseases including neurodegeneration, but SOD1 renders these free radicals harmless. About one in five people with inherited forms of ALS carry a mutation in the *SOD1* gene. The mutant form is toxic and research has been focussed on how to reduce levels to treat ALS. In 2016, a team from the University of Massachusetts Medical School designed an artificial microRNA to do this job, incorporating a guide strand sequence (ATGAACATGGAATCCATGCAG) into an AAV9 vector.[300] This specifically targeted a region on the *SOD1* transcript. The vector was injected into the brain of mice that had been engineered to carry a human *SOD1* mutation and that develop many of the clinical signs of ALS. The AAV9-delivered anti-*SOD1* microRNA worked, reducing by half the levels of the mutant *SOD1* in both brain and spinal cord motoneurones. The lifespan of the mice nearly doubled because of preserved neuromuscular condition and respiratory function. Based on the successful mouse studies, the team moved on to tests in non-human primates (macaques).[301] Here they compared different promoters to optimise the knockdown of *SOD1* and checked the distribution of the vector using a green fluorescent tracer also coded into the AAV payload. The primate studies were also a success, showing that the AAV9 delivered the artificial microRNA with minimal off-target effects on other genes and knocked down *SOD1* in the spinal cord by 30 to 60 per cent. This opened a path to human trials and, in 2020, preliminary results of these were reported in the *New England Journal of Medicine*.[302] Two volunteers carrying inherited mutations in *SOD1* received intrathecal injections of the AAV9 carrying the artificial *SOD1*-targeting microRNA. The first patient entered the trial six months after being diagnosed. While well-tolerated, the treatment did not appear to affect the course of their disease. Consistent with the rapid progression of this form of ALS, the patient died just over 15 months following treatment. About a year after the first patient was treated, a second patient carrying a *SOD1* mutation received the AAVs. At the time of reporting, the patient was stable with no signs of deterioration and disease progression. However, the *SOD1* mutation in that patient was associated with a much slower course of disease so conclusions on efficacy may be premature. The study was mainly intended to assess the safety of the treatment, however. Here it flagged immune/inflammatory responses to the treatment that would, in future studies, require immunosuppression. While perhaps not the cure that was hoped for, this study represents an important advance towards the use of microRNA-based medicines for this and perhaps other devastating human diseases.

And ALS is not the only neurodegenerative disease for which an artificial microRNA is moving towards clinical trials. The field of Huntington's disease has also been exploring a similar approach. Huntington's is a rare, inherited and fatal neurodegenerative disease.[303] The main symptoms are progressive loss of motor control called chorea, in which movements of the body become rapid, jerky and involuntary, and are accompanied by severe cognitive and psychiatric disturbances. The most affected neurones are the GABA-releasing cells of the striatum, the cells that receive input from the dopamine-releasing neurones of the substantia nigra. The disease is caused by expansions of nucleotides in the huntington gene (*HTT*). Specifically, a CAG sequence in the first exon. Any more than 39 of these repeats in your copy of the gene and you will develop the disease. There is also a type of genetic dose–response relationship with higher numbers of repeats causing an earlier and more rapid progression of the disease. The mutant protein aggregates in cells, triggering toxicity via a multitude of pathways including some of the same as seen with the *SOD1* mutation in ALS. The trafficking of molecules around the cell, protein degradation and mitochondrial function are all impacted, ultimately resulting in degeneration of neurones. Therapeutic strategies have been focussing on blocking production of the mutant protein.

Beginning in 2005, researchers showed that RNAi could be used to knock down the mutant *HTT* transcript and this improved outcomes in mouse models.[304] Over the years, this strategy progressed on to large animal and primate studies. This has yet to be successfully translated to the clinic, however. An artificial microRNA-based approach is also in development. This has not yet reached human trials, but a study in *Science Translational Medicine* in 2021 reported the results of an AAV carrying a mutant *HTT*-targeting microRNA sequence in genetically engineered pigs, a large animal model of Huntington's disease.[305] The findings were encouraging in terms of safety and efficacy. That included long-term detection of the artificial microRNA and a lowering of the level of mutant *HTT*. Further studies and assessment of clinically relevant outcomes will be needed. However, along with other approaches, this microRNA-based strategy may represent a clinically viable approach for this and other neurodegenerative disease.

Triangles Help Circle In on a New MicroRNA for Gene Therapy

We continue to look for additional microRNAs that could be targeted for epilepsy. This recently brought us into the viral vector business. The microRNA in question, miR-335, had been found using a search strategy that we hoped would offer some advantages over earlier approaches.[259] We and others have used 'triangulation' methods to zero in on microRNAs across several datasets, finding what is common among them. This approach had led to finding that miR-106b controlled a key potassium channel.[233] Hermona Soreq's team, based at the Hebrew University of Jerusalem, identified a new epilepsy-relevant microRNA using a triangulation approach.[306] They mined the microRNAs associated with AGO2 in neurones and cross-referenced these with microRNAs known to regulate synaptic proteins and microRNAs that changed in rats upon seizures induced by acetylcholine receptor super-activation in the brain. Lying at the centre of those three datasets was miR-211. The team went on to show that when levels of miR-211 are reduced in neurones in the brain, it results in hyperexcitability, including spontaneous seizures in mice. Strategies to upregulate miR-211 may have therapeutic applications in epilepsy.

Having had success with triangulation approaches ourselves, we began to think of the next way to discover a microRNA for epilepsy and here two trains of thought were converging. First, we were thinking that rather than just identifying microRNAs that changed in a particular model or after a particular treatment and then looking for their targets, we should have particular targets in mind. Perhaps we should even be using a 'reverse engineering' approach, picking target genes that would be important and relevant for epilepsy and then finding the microRNA(s) that controlled them. The targets we had in mind were sodium channels. But why these?

First, we had seen the success that came from finding potassium channels under microRNA control in epilepsy. We had every reason to expect that sodium channels would also be regulated by microRNAs (despite our failure in the Dravet studies to get a result with antimir-134). Sodium channels also aligned with some of the skills of Gareth Morris, the electrophysiologist who had earlier been working to elucidate the mechanism of action of the antimir targeting miR-134. Gareth had joined my lab in Dublin after the EpimiRNA project ended; he knew how to isolate just the parts of the electrical recordings that come from the movement of sodium ions in and out of neurones. By doing a bit of detective work, we could look at recordings from cells and know whether there had been a change in the sodium channel properties. It was this skill set that would be critical later.

Sodium channels are also common targets of anti-seizure medicines.[307] Many epilepsy drugs adjust the opening and closing times or the amount of current that can pass through. While we lament the lack of effective treatments, sodium channel drugs do provide seizure control for millions of people. These drugs include phenytoin, carbamazepine, lamotrigine and zonisamide. They work for focal seizure syndromes, which includes TLE and general-ised epilepsies that tend to have a genetic component. Sodium channel blockers also work for some of the epileptic encephalopathies such as Lennox–Gastaut syndrome. Each drug has its own particular mechanism of action. Phenytoin seems to work by causing a voltage-dependent block of the sodium channels. By binding to the channel, phenytoin promotes the channel to remain in an inactivation state. This relates to how, fractions of a second after opening to allow sodium through, the channel pore is blocked by part of the channel's own protein. This 'inactivation gate' needs the membrane to return to negative before it reopens and the cell can fire another action potential. Because of this, phenytoin reduces the ability of neurones to fire as fast, which is very useful in stopping seizures while not interfering too much with normal transmission in the brain.

Effective as they sometimes are, however, these drugs are still a rather crude way to treat epilepsy. Sodium channel blockers prevent the very rapid firing of neurones, but they reduce this ability in both excitatory and inhibitory neurones. So, while you are able to curb firing rates in excitatory neurones, you will also reduce the inhibitory neurones from doing the same. This is probably a reason why sodium channel blockers don't work for everyone and why people who take them often complain about a lot of unpleasant side effects. It's a 'block them all' approach. In theory (and leaving aside the inconvenient evidence from some labs that find that inhibitory neurones undergo extreme bursting behaviour immediately before seizures), you might develop a better sodium channel blocking drug if you could direct its effects just at excitatory neurones. Reduce their ability to fire while sparing the inhibitory neurones. Small molecule drugs can't do this. They wash into a neural network and get jammed into whatever channel they find and do not discriminate. Gene therapy suffers no such limitation. If you have a gene you want to deliver or an RNA sequence you can use to block something, then you can use molecular tricks to switch it on only in certain cell types (we will come back to this later in this chapter). Sodium channels are therefore very interesting as potential targets for epilepsy. If you could find a microRNA that targeted sodium channels then you could dampen down excitability. If you found one that was only in excitatory neurones, you might have a way to be even more selective. If inserted into an AAV as a gene therapy, a microRNA could be delivered in a sustained way, thus avoiding the need for taking pills every day.

But we don't always want to block sodium channels. As we saw earlier, some epilepsies arise because of a fault in a sodium channel.[308] In that setting, there is insufficient sodium channel function. This includes Dravet syndrome where the fault lies with a sodium channel that is particularly important for inhibitory neurones to fire quickly. Thus, lower levels of this sodium channel impair the brain's inhibitory 'tone', the equivalent of removing the brakes on a car. Blocking a sodium channel–targeting microRNA could be a way to treat those types of epilepsy. For these reasons, we would keep an eye out for anything sodium channel–related among the targets of new microRNAs.

The second idea for how to improve or change our search for new microRNAs was to include human microRNA data. This was an element missing from most previous triangu-lation approaches. Human data can be messy, of course. Sources of variability that can be controlled in a lab animal cannot be controlled for in humans, so there is inevitably more noise in the data. Variations exist in overall health, age, sex, diet and medicines, each of which can produce changes to microRNA levels in the body. We also wondered about including data on microRNA changes in response to epilepsy drugs. Perhaps having human and drug data would lead us in a new direction. The final search strategy would feature three quite different but nonetheless epilepsy-relevant datasets. We figured that if any microRNA made it through that mix then they had to be worth a hard look.

The first of the three datasets came from the EpimiRNA project that finished in 2018. We had managed to separate the rat hippocampus into its three major subparts, the cornu ammonis (CA) areas 1 and 3 and the dentate gyrus. These are the three key parts through which information flows through the hippocampus. We had run AGO2 sequencing on the three individual sub-fields and so had lists of microRNAs that were up- or down-regulated in each sub-field. Several on the list were new to us. For our second dataset we wanted a list of microRNAs that had been altered by a treatment for epilepsy that had a link to sodium channels. Here, we took the chance to look at one of the new drugs on the market for Dravet syndrome called cannabidiol, better known as CBD.[309] This is an extract from the *cannabis sativa* plant. The history of cannabis and epilepsy is an interesting one and there is also an Irish link. Anecdotal reports of the benefits of cannabis extracts for a variety of conditions, including epilepsy, go back centuries. But the modern era of the medical use of cannabis can be traced to William B. O'Shaughnessy. He was a physician who finally applied the scientific method to the testing of extracts. The medical uses later ran into legal restrictions owing to the psychoactive aspects of cannabis. The modern era began in the 1970s, testing cannabinoids for potential anti-seizure effects. This work mainly used rats and tested the effects of dosing animals with extracts and then testing their responses to chemical and electrical stimulation. Overall, CBD worked quite well, including when combined with conventional anti-seizure drugs. Then things went quiet again. The US government had classified cannabis as a substance of abuse with no medical value and this effectively shut down research because most academic teams have to apply to the government for funding. No funding meant that no one could work on it. This contributed to a gap in research between the early 1980s and the early 2000s. The laws relaxed in the 2000s and academic research ramped up again along with some commercial interests. This included a UK-based company called GW, which saw that there could be a market for a properly controlled form of medical cannabis for epilepsy. Working with academics, it published convincing evidence of the anti-seizure effects of CBD in well-controlled, sufficiently powered preclinical studies. This eventually led to the first placebo-controlled, blinded clinical trials of CBD.[310] The results of those trials proved that CBD had real anti-seizure effects in Dravet syndrome patients and the epilepsy community had its first CBD-based medicine, Epidiolex.

I began to follow these developments after I had hired a postdoctoral researcher, Tom Hill, who had undertaken his PhD in the lab that had been working with GW. We discussed experiments we might perform to try to understand the mechanism of action. Specifically, we wondered if CBD might have effects on microRNAs in the brain. The research became part of studies by a new PhD student in my lab, Mona Heiland, funded through FutureNeuro, a new national research centre focussed on chronic and rare neurological disorders. The basic plan was to dose mice with CBD and look for microRNA changes in the hippocampus. Tom and Mona also had the idea to compare this to two other phytocannabinoids, molecules with very similar structures to CBD but with different or no effects on seizures. We found that CBD caused more extensive changes to microRNA levels in the mouse brain than other phytocannabinoids. Several of the CBD-altered microRNAs had links to brain function and excitability. This suggested that some of the actions of CBD might be owing to altering gene expression via changes to microRNAs.

The third, human dataset was an analysis of microRNAs that were altered in blood samples from patients with drug-resistant epilepsy.[311] This was part of a broader effort to see if we could diagnose epilepsy or a recent seizure by measuring microRNAs in the blood. We will return to this idea in more detail in Chapter 8. The dataset contained a list of blood microRNAs that were different in people with epilepsy compared to otherwise healthy controls. We brought together the three datasets. The data on the microRNA changes in the different sub-fields of rats that had developed epilepsy, the microRNA changes in the brain when mice were treated with CBD, and the microRNAs in the blood of people with drug-resistant epilepsy. A single microRNA was at the centre of all three datasets: miR-335.

miR-335

We set about finding out what miR-335 might regulate, keeping in mind our sodium channels. To look for the targets of miR-335, we started with target prediction databases. What came out of the lists immediately looked relevant for epilepsy: a long list of targets with roles in brain excitability, including genes that encode proteins involved in neurotransmission, calcium signalling, GABA and glutamate receptors. And we spotted, lying at the centre of this spiderweb-like network, a set of sodium channels: SCN1B, SCN2A, SCN3A, SCN3B and SCN9A. We also plugged the sequence of SCN1A into an algorithm and found that there was quite a good match for miR-335, even though the other tools hadn't picked it up. Here was a microRNA that fell at the centre of a series of datasets relevant to epilepsy and that was predicted to control sodium channels. A validation of our slightly unusual search strategy.

Next up, we asked if miR-335 is expressed in neurones. The usual way to determine this is by in situ hybridisation. An ASO-like sequence complementary to a region of the microRNA is labelled and then added to a tissue section. The ASO, carrying a tag, floats around and eventually sticks onto the target. You can then use the shape of the cell to determine the type, or counter-stain your tissue with a marker gene. We had done this before, to show that miR-134 is present only in neurones, and, in another study, we had seen miR-22 in multiple cell types including glial cells. But my lab no longer had anyone with hands-on experience with the in situ technique for microRNAs; Eva Jimenez-Mateos, the previous expert, was now a professor at nearby Trinity College Dublin. Then we realised that there was another way to learn which cells made miR-335. We dipped back into our iCLIP database to find the cross-linked RNAs that were inside the AGO2 complex in brain tissue from TLE patients. This contained a sub-list of mRNAs loaded into the RISC that held seed sites for miR-335. That was then cross-referenced with single cell data. In early 2022, there were several datasets listing what genes were expressed by every cell type in the human brain. Using marker genes known to be specific for cell types (e.g. genes that are only ever 'on' in, say, neurones) you can find out what other genes are made by that same cell type. Albert Sanfeliu, a postdoctoral researcher in my team, agreed to try this. Comparing the list of transcripts we had found with miR-335 seed sites in the human brain with the list of transcripts in different cell types generated a wonderful map in which we could see what cell types the targets of our microRNA were normally expressed in. The result was clear-cut. Virtually all the transcripts bound to miR-335 in the iCLIP database were expressed in either excitatory or inhibitory neurones. This told us that miR-335 was almost certainly made in neurones rather than glia and this tallied well with the predicted target profiling we had done. We also learnt that miR-335 probably functioned in both inhibitory and excitatory neurones. This could be a potential issue when it comes to manipulating the microRNA. If miR-335 is actively targeting sodium channels in both major cell types, we could end up with a cancelling-out effect of modulating miR-335. An antimir, for example, introduced into the brain would enter both excitatory and inhibitory cells, lowering miR-335 levels in both cell types and adjusting the sodium currents and thus the excitability of both cell types. The net effect might be no real change to the excitability. We will return to this issue shortly.

Linking miR-335 to Sodium Channels

To learn more about miR-335, we asked two new questions. First, does changing the level of the microRNA in the brain change the levels of some of the sodium channels and, just as important, does it leave alone some of the channels which are functionally similar but do not contain sites in their transcripts where miR-335 could bind? Second, can we show an effect of changing the level of the microRNA on sodium channel properties? Can we actually detect a change in things like action potential properties when miR-335 is modulated? Sodium channels are the key element driving the 'up' phase of the action potential, so if we increase the amount of these channels, do we see a steeper or larger up-phase of the action potential? We set about answering these questions before moving on to test whether the microRNA was able to influence seizures. We turned to antimirs to manipulate miR-335. By now, we knew the designs and doses that would block about 70 to 90 per cent of the active microRNA, and we knew how long to wait for it to have an effect. Also, by using antimirs we were blocking the endogenous microRNA. We were really asking what does it do normally? By lowering amounts of the brain's own supply of miR-335, we could estimate with some confidence how strong a hold it had over these channels. The opposite strategy, over-expressing miR-335, was a more ambitious ask for us. It would require a viral vector and at the time we had no experience with this approach. We settled on two experiments. First, measure sodium current–related properties in neurones after treatment with an antimir and second, in parallel, test brain samples from mice treated with the antimir for the levels of certain sodium channel levels. If miR-335 was really acting to suppress sodium channel levels then we should see changes to the rising phase of the action potential and we should see small increases in the levels of some of the sodium channels such as *SCN2A*. Gareth Morris took on the electrophysiology work, performing studies using a current clamp method. This is ideally suited to detect changes in neurone excitability that result from changes in ion channel activity. A known amount of current (ions) is injected into the cell and the change in membrane potential is recorded. Injecting positive current into a cell mimics synaptic events. If the overall membrane potential moves sufficiently towards –50mV then an action potential will occur in that cell.

If there are more sodium channels being made, and this was the prediction if we block miR-335, and if they get inserted into the outer membrane of neurones, then the membrane potential changes will be slightly different from normal. The experimental method allows recordings from only one cell at a time so we picked CA1 pyramidal neurones. These are very easy to spot under a microscope and arranged in a very orderly pattern. They are a very common cell type for 'output' functions, meaning that they are excitatory and when they fire they convey inputs on to the next cell(s) in the network. The architecture of the CA1 region of the hippocampus is highly conserved, being very similar between mouse and human. The activity of these neurones is linked to how memories of specific events are formed, as well as to how those memories get stored (consolidated) and retrieved (remembered). If you have damage to your CA1 region, you can experience memory problems. This region is often found to be damaged, with a loss of neurones, in brain tissue samples taken from patients operated on for drug-resistant TLE. These patients often experience memory problems such as forgetfulness (although ASMs may be as likely to blame). It is also common for people with TLE to experience a déjà vu sensation at the onset of their seizure. This is thought to be because seizure activity is building up or passing through the memory centre in the brain. As much as the organisation and the function of this region of the hippocampus are similar between mouse and human, similar does not mean the same. There are differences. In Chapter 5, we saw how the dendritic spines of mice injected with the miR-134 inhibitor were slightly fewer in number but larger in volume, experiments we performed with Javier DeFelipe. Using a version of their technique to study the complete structure of neurones, DeFelipe and his team recently filled and imaged dozens of CA1 neurones from the mouse and human brain, a monumental feat of patience and technical skill.[312] The result was the ability to measure all sorts of features of the neurones in addition to the dendrite number and size. In particular, look at the complexity of the dendritic tree. Since these extensions are how the cell receives inputs, they give an insight into the connectivity of a neurone. More expansive and elaborate trees enable the neurone to receive more inputs and from different cells and perform more complex computations. DeFelipe's team discovered that the CA1 neurones in the human hippocampus are actually slightly different in their shape from the equivalents in the mouse. The cell body itself was much larger in humans, more than twice the surface area. The diameter, length and area of the dendrites were also greater in human neurones. But the human version was not simply a bulked-up or stretched version of the mouse. The structures of human dendritic tress were also more complex, showing more branching. The findings have direct implications for the function of these neurones. If the input collection sites differ as well as the output (axon), the computational power of the cell will be different. The axons of the human neurone were actually thicker than the mouse. Since the thicker the diameter of an axon the faster it can send action potentials, this is a further performance enhancement that we see in humans. Together, the findings indicate that the human CA1 neurone is capable of performing a larger number of computations; it has more processing power. The neurones are capable of being more connected in the human brain than in the mouse. It must be noted, of course, that the experiences of a laboratory mouse are likely to be far less rich than those of a typical age-matched human and we know that experiences result in physical changes to neuronal morphology. So, it is just possible that, with a little more environmental enrichment, the physical differences between mouse and human would be less obvious. That remains to be determined.

Let us return to the experiment. Since the specific channels under the control of miR-335 open during action potentials, the action potential itself would be predicted to be slightly larger in terms of membrane potential change or to possibly happen slightly faster than normal. This is exactly what we saw. The action potentials recorded when a set amount of current was injected into a neurone after blocking miR-335 had a larger amplitude and the 'rising slope' was steeper. The steeper rise of the recorded membrane potential change was consistent with there being more sodium able to enter at this point. Together, the two measurements strongly suggest that we had changed the amount of voltage-gated sodium channels in the membrane of these neurones. We also found that the frequency of action potentials that fired for a given amount of current injected was higher in the neurones in which miR-335 was blocked. The results were consistent with a relatively specific effect on voltage-gated sodium channels. We felt confident that this microRNA was normally acting to suppress the number of sodium channels in neurones. The effect size, the amount by which we had modified the properties of the neurones, was also consistent with a microRNA effect. It was a small but nevertheless functionally detectable change in the excitability of these neurones that appeared to be largely owing to a change in sodium channel properties. So, miR-335 fine-tunes sodium channel levels in neurones. The experiment had also answered, indirectly at least, some other questions we had about this microRNA. It seemed that these targets, voltage-gated sodium channels, were among the most important in terms of what miR-335 was doing in the cell. Most of the effects we saw when blocking the microRNA could be ascribed to sodium channel changes. It is likely that the microRNA controls other transcripts, but at least here we seemed to see the major effect converge on the sodium channels. As we've seen in other settings, microRNAs are generalists. They act on transcripts across pathways. But some pathways or targets are more constrained by a microRNA than others, at least in terms of what we can measure functionally.

Were the findings relevant to humans? To determine this, we would need a source of human neurones. There are two options. You can try to make recordings from human brain tissue removed after surgery or you can try to grow human neurones in a dish. In theory we had the option to do the former. Epilepsy surgery operations are performed at the national neurosurgery unit in Beaumont Hospital in Dublin and we were approved, with the consent of the patient, to collect and keep brain samples to enable us to perform electrical recordings and measure the molecular effects of experimental treatments outside the brain. But the roadblock we ran into was how long we could keep the slices alive for. We knew it would take many hours and probably a day or more for antimirs to produce a measurable change in the levels of the microRNAs' targets. At the time, we hadn't figured out how to keep the slices alive that long. So we used neurones derived from iPSCs. The results lined up well with what we had seen in the mouse neurones, with larger sodium current densities in neurones that had taken up the microRNA inhibitor. We had human evidence that this microRNA was controlling sodium channel activity. We now needed to see if the molecular evidence would line up with the electrophysiological recordings. Do sodium channel levels change when we block miR-335? To answer this, we extracted RNA from brain tissue samples after injection of the microRNA inhibitor. Levels of *Scn1a*, *Scn2a* and *Scn3a* were all increased by inhibition of miR-335 in mice. We obtained the same result with the human neurones. Blocking miR-335 increased transcript levels of *SCN1A*, *SCN2A* and *SCN3A* in human iPSC-derived neurones (see **Figure 7.5**). We were now ready to find out if changing the levels of miR-335 would affect the excitability of the brain. Does it increase or decrease the chances of having a seizure?

A Brief History of Seizure Models

For this next phase we would need to pick a model to test the effects of changing levels of miR-335 in the brain. We decided to screen the effects of manipulating miR-335 using the pentylenetetrazol (PTZ) model. In mice, injection of PTZ causes the rapid onset of a generalised seizure. If your treatment is anti-convulsant then it will delay or prevent the seizure. So, you can measure the delay to onset of a seizure and if a seizure does occur, score

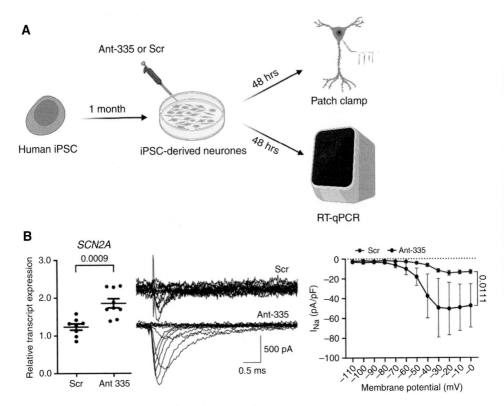

Figure 7.5 miR-335 targets sodium channels in human neurones

Panel A is a schematic of the experimental design. Human iPSC-derived neurones were treated with an antimir targeting miR-335 (Ant-335) or a scrambled sequence (Scr) followed by analysis of neuronal properties and gene expression.

Panel B shows (left) higher levels of *SCN2A* mRNA in iPSC-derived neurones given the miR-335 inhibitor (*SCN1A* and *SCN3A* showed a similar increase); (middle) traces of voltage-gated sodium currents; and (right) current density summary at different membrane holding potentials.

Key: I_{Na}, sodium current; pA/pF, pico amperes per pico farad.

Source: Heiland et al., *Proceedings of the National Academy of Sciences of the United States of America*, vol. 120, e2216658120 (2023).[259]

it in terms of severity. In many ways, the epilepsy field is fortunate to have models of the disease that have high predictive value for detecting drugs that work in people. This is not true for the majority of other brain diseases. There are various reasons for this. In some cases, it is simply very difficult to fully model the human disease in an animal. Psychosis and schizophrenia, for example, are thought to be caused by a complex mix of genetic and environmental factors. This alone makes it challenging to recreate them. Then we have symptoms such as hallucinations and altered thinking, which are hard to measure in a common laboratory rodent. In other cases, we have been able to model the primary brain disease well, but for various reasons this hasn't led us to new medicines. This includes stroke. It is possible to either permanently or reversibly occlude blood vessels in the brain of lab rodents; this produces regions of dead brain tissue caused by lack of blood flow that are similar to the ischaemic infarcts seen in human stroke. Despite this, none of the hundreds of experimental therapies tested over the years have gone on to show any benefits when given to humans. So, we can count ourselves lucky in the epilepsy field that we have models that predict efficacy in humans. There are a large number of epilepsy models, so the choice of which to use in any given study comes down to a number of decisions. What type of seizures am I interested in testing its effects on? How many drugs or doses do I need to test? Does the model need to reflect any particular pathology, such as hippocampal damage, or can the drug be tested in otherwise normal animals? Triggering a seizure is easy enough. Either you block the brain's inhibitory systems, primarily GABA signalling, or you super-activate the brain's excitatory systems, such as by injecting a compound that mimics the actions of glutamate. There are differences in the results, however. Generating seizures by boosting glutamate, such as by kainic acid, usually causes some toxicity in the brain. This may be what is sought if you are trying to find a drug to treat TLE. To block GABA, there are a number of choices, each with certain advantages and disadvantages. For example, some work quicker than others; others produce particular sequences of seizures. The PTZ model seems to trigger seizures through more than one mechanism. It has been found to block the main GABA receptor that is responsible for fast inhibitory transmission in the brain. Another effect of PTZ is boosting sodium and calcium ion channel opening. This would also tend to increase excitability. Regardless, PTZ has proven a useful method to screen for anti-seizure drugs as a first-pass approach. The standard experiment is to dose with your test drug and then inject PTZ shortly after, recording the seizure and noting whether it was reduced compared to your placebo control. It is nearly 80 years since PTZ was first used successfully by Everett and Richards to discover an anti-seizure drug called tridione.[313] The drug turned out to be useful for treating absence epilepsy and the PTZ model was found to pick out different properties of compounds with anti-seizure effects from those identified in the earlier maximal electroshock model. This had been made famous by Merritt and Putnam, who discovered phenytoin's anti-seizure effects using that model. The PTZ model became one of the standard tools used by the Utah epilepsy therapy screening programme. The PTZ test has also had some notable failures, that is, drugs that it missed. Levetiracetam is the most famous of these. Levetiractem had no detectable efficacy in either the PTZ model or the maximal electroshock model.[314] It works in some other models, however, and had it not been for the dogged determination of Henrik Klitgaard and others at UCB we might have missed what has been one of the most effective treatments for epilepsy. So, the PTZ model has a track-record for identifying molecules with anti-seizure effects, although it will miss a few. It is quick and easy to use and the result, whether the seizures are altered, is apparent within minutes. So, we settled on using the PTZ model, at least for now, to see if altering miR-335 levels in the brain would affect seizures.

Changing Seizures by Changing miR-335

Using the antimir we had designed, we ran our first studies to see if blocking miR-335 would have any effect on seizures.[259] We were expecting that seizures might be worse. If neurones can fire faster, it stands to reason that seizures might develop more easily or, when they occurred, spread more quickly. This is what we found. The onset of seizures after injection of PTZ was faster by just over 5 minutes – evidence that miR-335 acts as a kind of 'buffer' against brain over-excitation. We hadn't exactly removed the brakes on the car, but we had taken the foot off the brake a little. The strength of the effect was rather modest, however, probably because the inhibitor was making its way into both excitatory and inhibitory neurones. We might be seeing a bit of a cancelling-out effect. While our inhibitor would be boosting action potentials in excitatory neurones, which would likely increase seizures, it could be doing something similar in inhibitory neurones. Boosting the excitability of both cell types would effectively cancel each other out. We also learnt something important when we analysed brain samples at the end of the experiment. Measuring levels of miR-335 and plotting these against the seizure onset times showed a clear relationship. The animals in which the seizure had begun the fastest had the lowest levels of miR-335. As levels of miR-335 get higher, the excitability of the brain gets lower. The existence of this type of relationship could have diagnostic applications, for example monitoring microRNA levels to determine risk of a seizure (see Chapter 8).

Of course, increasing the brain's excitability doesn't have a medical use in epilepsy (although I wonder if it might in certain circumstances, such as coma?). But if the antimir increased seizures, could delivering more of the microRNA protect against seizures? It was time to embrace gene therapy approaches and use a viral vector to deliver the microRNA and try to reduce seizures. This was an exciting departure for us. For a decade we had used antimirs alone to study and understand the microRNA system and its relevance to epilepsy. This approach had served us well, but science rarely rewards treading water. Progress requires us to embrace new methods and that is what we did. We had to upskill ourselves fast about gene therapy tools, then pick a virus and figure out how to get miR-335 to be produced by it. We chose AAV9 as our microRNA carrier as it has a strong affinity for infecting neurones over other cell types in the brain. To control the amount of miR-335 produced, we used a human promoter for the synapsin1 gene (*SYN1*), which encodes a protein broadly involved in neurotransmission where it coats the outside of neurotransmitter-containing vesicles. It is ubiquitous in neurones and always 'switched on', so if you insert the promoter for this gene into the AAV you ensure that your microRNA is always on in neurones. The final design was an AAV9 containing the miR-335 sequence under the control of the *SYN1* promoter. Upon receipt of the AAVs, our first job was to check if it worked. Would an injection of the AAV carrying miR-335 under the *SYN1* promoter actually increase the amount of miR-335 present? We performed microinjections of the virus in mice, targeting them to three sites in the hippocampus. Then we waited. Gene therapy delivered via a viral vector takes time. The virus has to enter the cell, deliver its payload and then the cell has to start cranking out the new gene. It is usually a couple of weeks before full production is underway. Measuring levels of miR-335 in the injected hippocampus revealed that expression was increased by more than 10-fold. Of course, we didn't know if this was the 'right' amount. Too little and the extra miR-335 in the cell might not produce a change. Too much and we could hit targets too hard or overload the system. Indeed, experiments years earlier reported that if you swamp the RNAi pathway it can be toxic in the brain. We next focussed on whether it had gone where we wanted. We'd included a tracer gene added to the recipe for the viral vector. A short sequence encoding a green fluorescent protein meant that wherever the virus was actively producing miR-335, it could be seen under a microscope. The glowing tag could be seen in patches of cells with the exact location and appearance of neurones in the hippocampus. It was time for the final test. We injected additional mice with the virus and then waited for it to build up in the brain. After a two-week wait, we began the injection of PTZ. It worked. Hardly any of the AAV-335 mice developed severe seizures. By increasing the levels of miR-335 in the hippocampus, we had produced an anti-seizure effect.

What's Next?

What we have is really a proof-of-concept that miR-335 is a master regulator of excitability, mainly through actions on sodium channels. Our tools are far from optimised. Since finishing the initial study, the team gathered and kicked the tyres on what we might do next. What controls miR-335 and how does this relate to ongoing neuronal activity? We don't know much about what sets the normal amount of miR-335 in the brain or what drives any increases or decreases. This is clearly important. We showed that relatively small changes in the resting 'tone' of miR-335 in the brain can affect levels of various sodium channels which, in turn, then affects the firing properties of neurones. Clearly, a watchful eye is needed when it comes to putting out the right amount of miR-335 in the cell. What is controlling that? What systems do cells use to decide the correct amount? We think that miR-335 is mainly working in neurones, so what is stopping it being made in glia? What would happen if it started to be made in these cells? In theory, this shouldn't happen with a neurone-specific promoter, but damage to cells can lead to unexpected consequences. Perhaps in the damaged, epileptic zone of the brain, the specificity of certain promoters changes? Next, we might try to map the full repertoire of miR-335 targets. Just how many of the hypothetical hundreds of targets does miR-335 actually act upon? Here we could apply a couple of the investigative tools introduced previously. We could block or enhance the microRNA and then use single cell sequencing to measure what happens to the levels of different targets in different cell types. This might tell us if specific sodium channels under the control of miR-335 change more or less, depending on the cell type. It is possible that the effects of miR-335 differ between neurone types. That is, it may have a greater or a lesser influence on targets in different cells. We could push the insights further by staining for the actual microRNA itself, where it lies in a cell. There are methods for doing this and for staining for neighbouring mRNA or proteins that can tell us which cell type the microRNA is working in. We could also think about studying how deep brain networks change upon introducing an miR-335 manipulation. For all its usefulness, EEG is a crude tool that provides at best a reflection of the activity of neurones near the brain surface, quite far from the hippocampus; it is a signal made up of the collective actions of many neurones. But neurones have individual as well as group behaviour. The development of new electrode materials and surfaces now allows the implantation of ultrafine electrodes deep into the brain where they can record what individual neurones are doing during the awake state. How fascinating to track in real time the changes to neuronal circuit behaviour upon introduction of the microRNA! We're also thinking about what will be the next steps with our gene therapy. Near the top of the list is to re-engineer the viral payload and place the miR-335 under the control of a cell type-specific neuronal promoter. We could re-run the experiments but now boosting miR-335 levels only in excitatory cells. That would, in theory, reduce sodium channel levels in excitatory neurones, reducing their excitability while leaving unaltered the firing properties of inhibitory neurones. That should create a more potent anti-seizure therapy. While running these types of experiment, we can also ask questions about safety and impacts, if any, on other brain functions. Does the introduction of this therapy affect memory, planning or emotion? Viral vector approaches enable microRNA therapies to be delivered just to the cell type we want. However, once switched on, most gene therapies will continue to produce their cargo indefinitely. This might not be a problem in the case of a genetic disease where you'd always like the gene to be getting produced. However, in other disorders you might want the gene to switch off once levels are back to normal. This has got people thinking about whether a switch could be added so that a gene therapy turns on and off 'on demand'. MicroRNAs might be a way to control this switch. I will speculate on the opportunities for such an approach below and in Chapter 9.

A Breath of Fresh Air for CF

With all this attention focussed on AAVs, we have rather neglected antimirs. Here, there remains an exciting opportunity to create a different therapy based on the same microRNA. Loss of sodium channel activity is the cause of Dravet and several other rare epilepsy syndromes. With some fine-tuning, an miR-335 antimir might be an option. For example, what if you could interfere just with the binding of miR-335 to the one transcript of interest, for example *SCN1A*? This can be done in theory using target site blockers (TSBs). These are similar to traditional antimirs but designed to block only one target of a specific microRNA. This has not been attempted in the epilepsy field, but it has been demonstrated to work in other diseases. In fact, colleagues of ours have been trying just this approach for the rare disease cystic fibrosis (CF).[315] Ireland has the highest rates of CF in the world. There are about 1,400 people with CF at any one time and another 33 cases each year. It is a multi-system disease, but the primary problem is with the lungs.[316] Caring for patients requires multidisciplinary support from a variety of health professionals. One of the leading teams in the world is based at my institute and has been pioneering new treatments. It was part of the clinical trials that saw the first precision treatments for CF get approved for use in patients. The cause of CF is mutation of the cystic fibrosis trans-membrane conductance regulator gene, *CFTR*. The gene encodes a channel that allows the movement of chloride and other anions across the outer membrane of epithelial cells. These are cells that cover the surface of the body and line the airways. It is there that the faulty gene causes the most problems. Water movement is affected and CF patients develop thick, sticky mucus in their lungs, which severely restricts the passage of gases and promotes a microenvironment that favours repeated infections. It nearly halves the life expectancy of the affected individual. The most common type of mutation causes mis-folding of the protein and a defective passage of the protein up to the cell surface where it is needed. Most of the CFTR protein ends up being retained inside the cell and eventually destroyed. But a small amount does make its way to the surface. New treatments are trying to promote the amount of this protein that reaches the surface. The team at RCSI found that a set of microRNAs normally target the *CFTR* transcript. That sparked the idea that if these could be blocked, more of the transcript would be freed to be translated into protein. However, the specific microRNAs that were found had a number of other targets besides CFTR; thus, interfering with them broadly would be likely to have undesired side effects. To avoid this problem, the team, led by Catherine Greene, used the TSB approach, realising that a more selective approach would be only interfering with the microRNA recognition sites on the *CFTR* transcript. Five different microRNAs are capable of targeting *CFTR* and present in various models and human CF samples. The *CFTR* transcript has several sites for the five microRNAs, suggesting that the transcript is normally under strong and broad microRNA regulation and thus is a good candidate for the TSB approach. The team ended up designing nine different TSBs to cover as many of the microRNA sites as possible. They screened these for their ability to increase CFTR protein and found that two of them, which blocked sites for miR-223 and miR-145, produced a detectable increase. They then carefully checked the specificity of these TSBs, ensuring that changes to the sequence of bases that they were designed to block prevented their effects.

They went on to test these two in a series of models that report channel function in CF models, showing that the TSBs increased ion channel function. They finished by enclosing the TSB sequences in nanoparticles designed to improve uptake by lung cells, to mimic how a drug might be given, in an aerosol similar to an inhaler.

The study is a step forward for microRNA targeting therapies and a promising approach for CF. It indicates how this type of more selective approach to microRNA modulation can work. If anything was missing, it was perhaps that there was no direct comparison between a standard antimir blocking these microRNAs and the TSB versions. Were they equally efficacious? More importantly, would an RNA sequencing analysis of cells treated with the TSBs and standard antimirs have shown a difference? That is, would there be fewer or no off-target effects with the TSBs compared to a standard microRNA inhibitor?

Could the TSB approach work to selectively enhance *Scn1a/SCN1A* or some of the other targets of miR-335? It might offer a complementary or alternative approach to raising sodium channel levels in rare genetic epilepsies. We need to continue to find mechanism-based treatments for Dravet syndrome. For example, it is unclear whether the effects of CBD have anything to do with the root cause of Dravet syndrome. The microRNA approach would, instead, complement other precision and gene therapies in trial for Dravet that are intended to increase *Scn1a/SCN1A* levels. One of these trials is testing a drug called STK-001. This began after a 2020 study published by a team led by Lori Isom at the University of Michigan.[317] The team found that a small amount of the *SCN1A* gene mRNA is normally non-functional. It contains a sequence equivalent to a spelling mistake; as a result, some of the mRNA is destroyed rather than being made into protein. The team realised that if they could mask the error, the message would be skipped and more protein would be made. The technique was named targeted augmentation of nuclear gene output (TANGO). The team designed an ASO to hide the error message, like a genetic Tipp-Ex, and showed that when this was introduced into cells, those cells made more NaV1.1, the protein encoded by *SCN1A*. Having proven this, they turned to Dravet mice. The team injected the TANGO treatment into Dravet mice and reported an increase in survival of 74 per cent and a dramatic reduction in the number of seizures the mice had. They found that the treatment worked best when injected at an early age but was still very effective in older mice. The results of the ongoing clinical trials are still unknown at the time of writing.

So, if this works so well, will we need other approaches? Probably. We don't know how efficacious the TANGO or other approaches will be in Dravet patients. We don't know how well they will be tolerated. Or how long each treatment lasts. Or how affordable they will be. We don't know how well the drug will work at different life stages or whether it can improve co-morbid aspects of the disease such as cognition and ataxia. And we don't know how well it will mix with the other drugs that patients may continue to need to take. So, yes, we should keep looking for alternatives.

Listening to Patients to Make Sure They Want Your Therapy

This chapter has taken a look at some of the microRNA discoveries that are closest to becoming medicines. Some are much closer than others. Perhaps by the time this book appears, we may have an approved microRNA therapy on the shelves. Before we close, a point of reflection. One of the voices often missing from the push to develop the next medicine is the voice of the patients and their families. When it comes to gene therapies, this is particularly important. We're talking about medicines that may need to be given through spinal injections, or that may remain active in the body for months, maybe years after injection. A lot of research is performed separated from the issues this raises. When I attend a scientific meeting, I talk to researchers and we share ideas and build relationships that often spill into plans for the next set of experiments or the next target. And I have collaborated over many years with clinicians, the neurologists and neurosurgeons who care for people with treatment-resistant epilepsy. While we certainly have different priorities, we are generally aligned on what is needed and we try hard to think of experiments that might generate useful things for doctors who care for patients. There is rarely a connection between scientists and the people with lived experience of the disease. We know they would like a cure, to have fewer or no seizures, to have better medicines, to know when their next seizure might come. But like most basic scientists, I do not have contact with actual patients; I have no means to hear what it is they would really like us to work on. No way to ask them if the experiments we are doing really matter to them. And we miss the opportunity for insights that come from living with a condition 24/7. But the wall between scientists and patients can be removed. Public–patient involvement (PPI) is a growing movement within the basic sciences to ensure that research involves patients from inception through to trial and beyond. This goes beyond simple notions of participation in research which, and I was guilty of this in the past, begins and ends with asking a patient to sign a consent form to donate a blood or tissue sample. True involvement in research is quite different. My introduction to PPI came as a result of the mandate from the funder of FutureNeuro, Science Foundation Ireland, to run an education and outreach programme at our centre. At the time we started, in late 2017, most of us interpreted that this would mean occasionally going into schools to tell teenagers that a career in science was great, or doing our best to get a news outlet interested in our latest paper. This mindset changed a few years in. While there was nothing wrong with what we were doing, it was generic. Replicated many times by other research centres. If we were serious about performing research that would have an impact for patients, then we should be involving them in our research at the earliest stages and this should continue throughout the programme. This idea was not foreign to everyone. The team that led our digital health research was very familiar with PPI, having been involving patients in the design of connected health solutions for years. This had culminated in the co-creation of a patient portal, an app-based system that allows patients to directly upload information about their condition and remotely consult with their clinician. This was a literal life-saver during the Covid-19 pandemic when travelling to hospital for appointments was not an option. The remote connections that digital technologies had enabled were transforming patients' lives. But among basic scientists working to discover new genes and treatments, we had no connection to patients or awareness of what they wanted. We brought in an expert in PPI who contacted patient organisations to ask who might be interested in working with the basic scientists. The result was a panel of patients and carers of people with lived experience of several brain diseases, including epilepsy. Our first meeting was virtual as this was all happening in the middle of the pandemic. We met each other and relaxed into a discussion of what both groups were looking for. We outlined what we were working on and why and began to forge a bi-directional relationship that would eventually feed into the design of the research we planned for the next six years. Gene therapy was one of the focusses of the PPI panel discussions and where we learnt a lot about patient views that we had not considered up until that point. If we were going to take this seriously and focus more on gene therapy, we needed to listen to their thoughts, concerns and advice and incorporate that into what we did next. Otherwise, we ran the risk of developing something that no one would want to take. Indeed, by involving patients at every step in the research pathway, you increase the chance of the research being taken up at the end. So, what did our PPI panel think about gene therapy? First, there was strong excitement that this could herald a cure. But even a significant reduction in the frequency of having to take medicine would be valued by patients. That is, patients valued the idea that a gene therapy would mean not having to repeatedly dose yourself at specific times of the day, indefinitely. But we also heard that, for some, gene therapy would never be acceptable. Keeping that in mind, a balanced portfolio would need to include traditional drugs too. We were then asked, what happens to the gene therapy if the gene therapy cures me? Is there a way to stop a gene therapy when it is no longer needed? Great question. A related issue was whether there was a way to ensure that the gene therapy worked only in the part of the brain that needed it. Could we somehow engineer the vector so that it would respond to signals generated within the brain and turn on or off in response to locally produced signals. For example, a drop in levels of miR-335 would be an ideal way to couple an miR-335 gene therapy to the need for the molecule. Besides the design-input from our PPI group, there is another benefit to both sides that is important. Patients learn that someone cares about their condition and is trying to help. You might be surprised what an impact that can have. They know their neurologist cares deeply for their health, but to know that there are scientists in their local community working hard to try to make a difference actually matters. This works in both directions. Seeing first-hand that what you are doing matters to people is enormously beneficial as a scientist. It reminds you to keep going when you are struggling with an unrelenting workload filled with more failures than successes. My advice to any researchers is that if you haven't embraced some PPI yet, go out and do it.

So, could we engineer switches that register the need or lack of need for a microRNA therapeutic? A paper published in *Science* in late 2022 by a team at University College London showed that a potassium gene therapy could be placed under the control of an activity-regulated gene, *c-Fos*.[318] This meant that the potassium channel was produced only in cells that had undergone a period of hyper-excitability. Uninvolved, surrounding tissue remained untainted by the gene therapy. These ideas of on/off gene therapy control have resonated with one other project I am working on called PRIME (Personalised living cell synthetic computing circuit for sensing and treating neurodegenerative disorders). This is funded under the EU's future and emerging technologies programme. Unlike many research awards, the feasibility of these awards was balanced with a high-risk, high-gain mentality. The PRIME project is certainly that. The idea was based on a discovery that our team and colleagues had made a few years earlier. We found that fragments of transfer RNAs were elevated in blood samples in TLE patients.[319] What was surprising was that the higher levels were found in the samples we took just before a seizure happened. Once the seizure occurred, the levels dropped back towards the baseline before rising up again ahead of the next seizure. This had all the hallmarks of a seizure warning system. The idea behind PRIME is to engineer an implant that uses this signal as the prompt for the release of a neuroactive substance that would then stop a seizure occurring. Perhaps a microRNA could be used in a similar fashion? A sense and response system, incorporated into a viral vector that expressed miR-335? We haven't tried this yet, but there are examples of something like this. A Japanese team based in Kyoto has been working on synthetic biology, including artificial nucleic acid sequences, and described a system that places a gene's activity under the control of ambient levels of a microRNA.[320] The way the system worked was to use an RNA binding protein called L7Ae. This protein has an affinity for a 'kink' in particular RNA strands. When it spots one, it shuts down production of any gene contained on the strand. The way to turn this into a microRNA-based sensor is to place microRNA binding sites as part of the sequence encoding the L7Ae protein. That way, when the particular microRNA that can bind the sites is present, the L7Ae can't be made and the gene transcript with the kink in it is free to be translated. If the levels of the microRNA drop then the L7Ae increases, binds the kink and switches off the gene. In theory, a system like this could be engineered so that the system triggers 'on' or 'off' according to ambient levels of a microRNA. While still very much at the design stage, this is the type of thinking that could create on-demand 'on'/'off' switches in the next generation of gene therapies. It might give our patients reassurance that gene therapy won't always be on.

This chapter began with the remarkable story of the first microRNA drug to reach human trials and ended with how we might engineer sophisticated gene therapies that meet the demands and expectations for safe and effective medicines for brain diseases. We've seen a first microRNA-based medicine for ALS. We saw some of the recent progress on microRNA-based drugs for epilepsy. As I write, the large animal veterinary trial with an antimir targeting miR-134 is underway, for the treatment of drug-resistant epilepsy in dogs. Will it work? We will see. If it does, it may enable us to push on towards a first-in-human trial.

Circulating MicroRNAs Provide a Diagnosis

Don't deny the diagnosis; just defy the verdict that is supposed to go with it.

From Head First: The Biology of Hope, *by Norman Cousins,*
a journalist, world peace advocate and professor of ethics
and medical literature (E. P. Dutton, 1989, pp. 239, 258; see also p. 76)

Shortly after microRNA genes were discovered in the human genome, their RNA was found to be present in blood samples. During the intervening years, a branch of microRNA research has emerged that has the potential to transform medicine because it can answer a question that many healthcare professionals are asking themselves right now, in a hospital, in an emergency department, in a care home or a general practitioner's office... What is wrong with my patient? Measuring microRNAs might tell you.

Knowing what is wrong is a priority in medicine. Diagnosis, the art or act of identifying a disease from its signs or symptoms, is the cornerstone of healthcare. Assuming you can establish what is wrong, you may be able to treat your patient using a medicine, medical device or lifestyle intervention. Knowing the cause, the *aetiology*, is also extremely valuable. If we also know what is causing the problem, we have a better chance of choosing the right course of care. Sometimes the cause is obvious and sometimes it is not. Getting to the root of a patient's condition usually begins with taking the history from the patient and a clinical examination. A series of carefully posed questions and simple physical assessments are the first stage of finding out what is wrong. Supporting this in most modern healthcare settings is an array of diagnostic tools. We can measure blood pressure and test blood samples for variances in electrolytes, glucose, red and white blood cells and so on. We might be able to take a tissue sample – a biopsy – and have a pathologist look for cell anomalies under a microscope. We have machines to detect the weak electrical signals of the heart (electro-cardiogram) and brain (electroencephalogram). Powerful imaging systems such as MRI permit us to look inside the body, at the structure and function of organs.

But our system for diagnosing many diseases is inadequate. Some tests are slow, technically complex or laborious to administer or to analyse. Valuable time may be lost. The findings from the investigations may be inconclusive. In lower-income settings, the tools simply may not be available. Or they are available but not for many hours because they're in use and resources are stretched thin. Using the example of the brain disease epilepsy, here are some examples of the diagnostic challenges (see **Figure 8.1**). First, the primary symptom of the disease, a seizure, is rarely witnessed by the physician. A diagnosis must often be reached without seeing a seizure. Brain scans and EEG recordings frequently appear negative. Genetic testing is becoming more common, but it yields a conclusive result

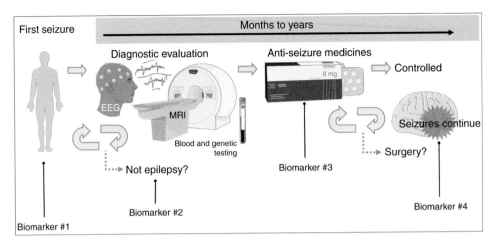

First seizure

Months to years

Diagnostic evaluation

Anti-seizure medicines

Controlled

EEG

MRI

8 mg

30

Seizures continue

Blood and genetic testing

Surgery?

Not epilepsy?

Biomarker #3

Biomarker #2

Biomarker #4

Biomarker #1

Figure 8.1 A diagnostic journey

Using epilepsy as an example, the patient presents with a first seizure. A clinical history is taken supported by a variety of diagnostic tools. The patient may then be placed on a first anti-seizure medicine (ASM). A cycle of adjusting dose and drug may continue until seizure control is achieved. Some patients may be candidates for clinical trials, surgery or alternative therapies. Examples of where circulating molecular biomarkers would be useful are depicted: #1, an epilepsy or seizure biomarker; #2, a biomarker of seizure mimic; #3, drug choice or monitoring biomarker; #4, drug-resistance biomarker.

Source: Schematic created using images from Servier Medical Art. Servier Medical Art by Servier is licensed under a Creative Commons Attribution 3.0 Unported License (https://creativecommons.org/licenses/by/3.0/).

less than half the time. An accurate diagnosis is much more likely if patients are admitted to a specialist epilepsy monitoring unit. Here, patients can undergo round-the-clock video and EEG monitoring. But the availability of beds in such units is usually very low and the resources used are very high. Such in-depth diagnostic work is time- and resource-intensive. Notably, during such intensive monitoring a portion of patients are found not to have epilepsy at all. Instead, they are diagnosed with psychogenic non-epileptic seizures (PNES). The cause is often psychiatric in nature. But by the time this is discovered, a patient may have believed that they have epilepsy for months or years and been treated accordingly with ASMs. These would have made little difference to their condition while imposing all the usual side-effects we learnt about in Chapter 7. So how can we improve this situation?

One of the most sought-after diagnostic supports is a *biomarker*. A biomarker is any characteristic that can be objectively measured, such as a molecule, something present on a scan, a bioelectrical signal, as an indicator of health or disease.[321, 322] Biomarkers are a subcategory of medical signs. There are all sorts of different categories of biomarker. A *diagnostic* biomarker would confirm the presence of disease or a condition ('you have epilepsy'). A *risk* biomarker would identify someone who is at an increased chance of developing the disease or condition, such as drug-resistance, in the future. A *monitoring* biomarker would be used repeatedly to assess the status of the disease, to check if seizures are becoming more frequent. A *prognostic* biomarker would be used to assess the risk of disease recurrence in someone who has the condition. A *pharmacodynamic* biomarker would tell if a drug is having the expected effect in the patient. This last example would really help with clinical trials which, for new epilepsy therapies, rely on patient self-reported seizure diaries. These are notoriously unreliable because seizures can occur without a patient being aware. So a biomarker of a seizure not only would be useful for diagnosis but could also transform future clinical trials. Biomarkers can also be used as surrogate endpoints. Rather than waiting for a disease to appear or change in an individual, a characteristic is measured as a proxy. Research continues to identify and improve how such biomarkers are used and to combine them with sophisticated data from other sources. Biomarkers are not an assessment of how a patient feels.

There are already diseases for which we have biomarkers, for example blood glucose levels in diabetes and measuring low-density lipoprotein cholesterol as a way to predict risk of heart attack. For other diseases we are getting quite close to clinically validated and accepted biomarkers. For example, there are some positron emission tomography (PET) tracers that light up parts of the brain where there are amyloid deposits to support Alzheimer's diagnosis. These are now being used in clinical trials to pre-select patients and then monitor whether or not the experimental medicine is having an effect. But there are many diseases for which we do not have clinically validated biomarkers, and epilepsy is one of these, unless you consider a seizure to be a biomarker of epilepsy, which is a bit of a tautology. We have no biomarker that can be used to provide a definitive diagnosis of epilepsy or confirm that a seizure has occurred. Various efforts have been underway for many years and progress is being made. Among the leading biomarker categories, as you might expect, are EEG signals. These are typically high-frequency and high-amplitude events above the normal background that are a telltale sign of hyperexcitability or abnormal synchronicity. But they are not always found, or not present during the period of time when the EEG was recorded. Of note, recent work is using artificial intelligence approaches such as deep learning to find signals 'hidden' in EEG to accelerate diagnosis. Brain imaging can identify structural or functional abnormalities which are thus biomarkers, but, again, many people with epilepsy have normal MRI scans. Not to mention, both EEG and brain scanning is complex, requiring highly skilled healthcare providers to administer and interpret the tests. Brain scans are also expensive. Another common situation is a patient arrives, perhaps into the emergency department, unresponsive or unconscious. They may be accompanied by a witness who may or may not be able to provide an accurate description of what happened. Was it a stroke? A faint? A seizure? If it was a seizure, was this epileptic in nature or caused by drugs or alcohol? Faints and cardiovascular problems can trigger sudden loss of consciousness, which can be confused with a seizure. Another issue is whether the event is still happening. A seizure that doesn't stop is life-threatening. If you don't know a seizure is happening because it is non-convulsive, then you don't know to stop it. Having a test that anyone with limited technical skills can administer to inform a diagnosis in this setting would be transformative. A cheap and reliable biomarker of epilepsy or recent seizure, such as a molecule present in a biofluid such as blood, would offer a powerful tool alongside the other parts of the clinical toolkit. While I will use epilepsy as the main focus in this chapter, similar needs exist for many other brain diseases and non-brain conditions, and research is actively pursuing these. Could microRNA be a solution to the search for biomarkers?

Why MicroRNAs as Biomarkers?

MicroRNAs have three important features that meet the demands of a biomarker. First, many microRNAs are expressed in specific tissues, at precise times of development and maturity. And within those tissues, specific microRNAs are made in certain cells. MicroRNAs are intrinsically linked to function in health and disease. Diseases can be caused by changes to levels of certain microRNAs in certain cells and diseases in turn cause further changes to microRNAs in certain tissues and cells. If a microRNA made only in the brain, for example, is found circulating in the blood, this is an indication that some kind of disease or damage is present. If different brain diseases feature varying contributions of cellular stress and injury response across neurones, glia and vascular cells, then a signal of this, made up of a set of circulating microRNAs derived from the cell mix, could be an accurate diagnostic. There is good reason to think that this would be found. While there are processes common to most brain diseases, such as inflammation, this varies, as does the role of metabolism, degenerative aspects and hyper- versus hypo-excitability. So, testing for changes to the composition of microRNAs in a biofluid such as blood has biomarker potential. But there are tissue- and cell-specific mRNAs (and proteins) that would presumably also satisfy this same profile, so why not use them? One argument is the longevity of microRNAs. They are inherently more stable than mRNAs, lasting longer in the circulation before being extinguished. We will return to why shortly. Another factor is measurement. This is an important consideration in the adoption of any biomarker. Simple/easy, reliable and cheap are all green flags for biomarkers. MicroRNAs can be measured using various existing technologies, including a polymerase chain reaction (PCR). It takes only a few hours to extract and measure RNA. You can compare the amounts of microRNAs between patients and controls and even count exactly how many molecules of an RNA you have per volume of body fluid. A standard lab anywhere in the world can do this work. No need for brain scanners or applying electrodes and analysing complex bioelectric signals.

There is another argument in their favour. As we saw in Chapter 7, controlling microRNA function is an avenue to therapeutics, for example using antimirs. This offers the tantalising prospect that you could deliver a microRNA therapeutic and use circulating microRNA profiles to monitor its engagement with the target and its effects on the disease. Now you have a specific link between the microRNA, the disease and the treatment. A strong basis for a biomarker. All told, microRNAs look very promising and with advantages over some of the competition.

The microRNA field was not the first to think of circulating RNAs as biomarkers. Researchers had reported detecting RNA in the non-cellular portion of the blood as long ago as 1948.[323] The fluid portion of blood can be easily separated from the cell component by spinning in a centrifuge. This results in a sediment of cells at the bottom while the resulting fluid on top is the plasma sample. Plasma is routinely prepared to measure electrolytes, glucose and indicators of kidney and liver function. Another way to collect the fluid portion of blood is to first allow the blood to rest after collection. Blood clotting begins, and the cells clump and stick together and settle to the bottom. After half an hour you can spin the tube and siphon off the liquid on top, which is referred to as serum. The two share similar chemistries, but serum has the added effects of time and clotting reactions, which can make a difference to some measurements, including of microRNAs. Indeed, studies comparing the two fluids generally find plasma to provide the more reliable readings. But in a busy hospital setting, the time flexibility of collecting serum has advantages. Also, because of the use of serum for many routine lab tests, it tends to be easier to access banked samples of this biofluid. A typical plasma sample contains between 1 and 10 micrograms of RNA per millilitre of plasma. Not much, but enough with modern, sensitive amplification and detection methods, a field that continues to improve in using ever smaller quantities of fluid for RNA analyses. It is possible, and we have tried this ourselves, to identify and quantify specific RNAs using the fluid from inside a single cell.

Returning to the history of this field, there were scattered reports in the 1970s and 1980s suggesting that extracellular and circulating RNAs served functions in short- and longer-range communication in the body.[324] Studies in the 1990s used plasma and serum to detect RNA from infections. Then, in 2004, a study by a University of Pittsburgh team found encouraging evidence that circulating RNAs were more stable than expected.[325] This overturned certain dogma that RNA in blood is immediately degraded. It is technically correct; if you add 'naked' RNA to blood, it is degraded within as little as 15 seconds by resident circulating ribonucleases. But some of the RNA naturally present in plasma was longer-lasting. Somehow protected from degradation. This cloak could be voided by adding detergents to the sample or passing the sample through a filter that blocked the passage of small membrane-enclosed bodies. This suggested that a portion of circulating RNA was inside something, a vesicle or protein complex. The longer your signal can last, the better your chance to detect it. Longer-lasting RNA meant the promise of a circulating biomarker.

The idea of circulating microRNAs as biomarkers came from work in the cancer field. Studies as early as 2002 reported finding altered levels of microRNAs in certain types of blood cancer. But the seminal biomarker paper in the microRNA field came in 2008. Teams working in Seattle, USA, showed that human plasma contained many small RNAs and a strong concentration of RNA measuring ~22 nucleotides in length.[326] When probed, more than 90 per cent of those sequences were microRNAs. So, microRNAs were present *outside* of cells in the blood. Not only were microRNAs extracellular but they were abundant. One of them, miR-16, was present at more than 100,000 copies per microlitre of human plasma. Buoyed by this, the team subjected plasma microRNAs to biomarker 'stress tests'. Leaving plasma out of a freezer at room temperature for a day or re-freezing it did not degrade the signal, meaning that plasma microRNAs were very stable. This contrasted with what happened when they spiked in a synthetic microRNA to plasma. In that experiment, the RNA was degraded within a few minutes. Clearly, plasma microRNAs such as miR-16 were not naked. Something like the vesicle/protein cloaking system also existed for naturally circulating microRNA. The team then turned to whether circulating microRNAs could be useful biomarkers. To test this, they implanted mice with human tumour cells. This is called a xenograft and is a common method to study tumour growth and responses to therapies. The implanted cells contained a set of microRNAs not made by mice. This gave them a way to find out if tumour cells release microRNAs into the circulation. After allowing the tumours to grow for a few weeks, they found a strong signal of the human-only microRNAs in the plasma of the mice. Furthermore, mice with larger tumours tended to have higher counts of the circulating human microRNAs. They then turned to a human scenario, using previously collected serum samples from patients with prostate cancer. There was a multi-fold enrichment of prostate cancer–related microRNAs within the serum samples and a solid correlation to levels of prostate-specific antigen, the gold standard biomarker for prostate cancer. The findings would spark a major expansion of the microRNA universe. It seemed possible to both detect the presence of disease, for example a tumour, and have a sense of the burden of that disease-causing agent by measuring plasma microRNAs.

The results caused a major stir. Were there combinations and levels of microRNAs in the blood specific to health states? How and why were these microRNAs being released? There followed intense global efforts to find and develop microRNAs as biomarkers of disease. In addition to cancer, research has identified circulating microRNA biomarkers of heart disease, diabetes, lung conditions, skin diseases such as psoriasis and infectious disease. Also, brain diseases and disorders of mental health – stroke, trauma, Alzheimer's, anxiety and depression, schizophrenia and epilepsy. But in most cases, this remains early days, with some promising candidate circulating microRNA biomarkers but a need for replication, larger cohorts and exploring whether results can survive in the hospital and 'real-world' setting. Most of the work has, appropriately, been conducted under rigorous and carefully controlled conditions in laboratories. But the clinical environment can be busy and bordering on chaotic at times. Will differences in levels of microRNAs still be detectable if samples are left too long before being processed? Or stored slightly differently, or processed in batches? This type of late-stage validation testing can be the make or break for biomarkers. There are, however, promising signs from outside the brain field. More than a decade ago, Rosetta Genomics launched miRview lung, a microRNA-based test for lung cancer. More recently, Gastroclear, a microRNA-based blood test made by a Singapore-based company, has been released for detecting early stomach cancer. So, circulating microRNA biomarkers have made it from discovery to a diagnostic test. In some cases, this happened within a few short years.

How do microRNAs find their way into the circulation? Research shows that it is a mixture of passive and active release mechanisms.[324] The break-up of dying cells and physical damage to tissue cause the rupture of membranes and the release of cellular contents, which includes the host cell's repertoire of microRNAs. The released microRNAs will be in a number of different forms. Some presumably midway along the biogenesis pathway while other portions, the mature form, may already have been loaded into AGOs. A second mechanism is via release within vesicles, which are tiny membrane-enclosed sacs of cellular contents. This type of release occurs via controlled cellular pathways and is thought to be a method of intentional short- and long-range signalling within and between cells.[327] Since most tissues are richly innervated by a vascular supply, including the brain, the released contents are quickly picked up, moved along and incorporated into the circulation. With brain-derived microRNAs, there is an additional impediment to reaching the circulation in the form of the blood–brain barrier. As we have seen, however, the integrity of this barrier is often compromised in brain disease, allowing passage of material between brain and circulation. This would very quickly be the end of the line if the released microRNA strands were naked when they hit the circulation. But a substantial amount of microRNA is protected, contained within protein complexes or vesicles, keeping the signal alive, at least for a period of time. This mix of passive and controlled release emerged as a major focus and touch-point in the biomarker field, with implications for basic biology and applications in molecular diagnostics.

When You're a MicroRNA Biomarker, How You Travel Matters

Attention to the mechanism by which microRNAs were circulating converged via two different lines of enquiry. There was the question, raised by the circulating RNA studies in the early 2000s, about what allowed microRNAs to be so stable in blood. Biochemical tests had revealed that something was protecting circulating microRNAs from ribonucleases, but what? The other branch of study related to cell-to-cell communication in the immune system. Certain immune cells shuttled material to other cells inside vesicles. The teams working on circulating RNAs took this idea on board as well as some of the methodologies developed by the extracellular vesicle field to answer their questions. Were microRNAs packaged within released vesicles? Could they be taken up by recipient cells? Could they affect protein production once inside? And what proportion of the circulating RNA pool was packaged this way? In pursuing this, researchers from the microRNA field quickly adopted a different approach to the treatment of biofluids. What had been used up until then were solutions and buffers that would extract it all. Any free RNA plus any protein or membrane-enclosed RNA was released for measurement. This missed any carrier mechanism of the circulating microRNA, which could contain additional diagnostic value or mechanistic insights. Searching for microRNA components within vesicles would require some additional steps, to separate and sediment. That advance came in 2007, with research led by a team at Gothenburg University in Sweden. Their study appeared in *Nature Cell Biology* and has been cited by more than 13,000 other papers since.[328] They identified microRNAs inside a type of extracellular vesicle called exosomes.

Exosomes are one of a variety of small membrane-bound vesicles that can be produced by cells. They are part of the wider world of inter-cellular signalling biology, which deals with signals between non-connected cells. This has become a very active field, although the origin, the biogenesis, the release, the mechanism of engaging and ultimately the fate of vesicles remain incompletely understood. All cells appear to be capable of releasing membrane-bound vesicles. And this is not unique to humans or animals – bacteria, archaea, fungi and plants also produce them. Extracellular vesicles are a large and diverse class. They are generated by independent pathways within cells, they vary in size and they contain distinct contents that seem to serve specific purposes. Extracellular vesicles range in size from 50 nanometres to about 1 micrometre. There are two main types. Vesicles that bud-off from the outer plasma membrane of the cell are called microvesicles. Exosomes come from endosomes, a sorting system deep within the cell close to the Golgi apparatus. The endosome system directs materials such as proteins and nucleic acids for release, distribution elsewhere or destruction. Exosomes are formed by inward budding of the endosome membrane and are then temporarily enclosed in a larger structure called a multivesicular body, after which they can be shuttled to the surface for release outside the cell. They are generally smaller than microvesicles, ranging from 50 to 150 nanometres in diameter and about 8 million times less than the volume of a cell. Their function was initially thought to be a form of waste disposal. That view changed following detailed characterisation of the contents of different forms of extracellular vesicle and the effects they can have when they encounter a recipient cell. Current thinking is that they are a sophisticated communication system,[58, 327] a cell-to-cell warning system and a mechanism for priming and coordinating responses within and between tissues in health and disease. The machinery that assembles these structures, decides what is to be packaged inside, what decorates the outside and hence influences their docking to recipient cells, and what triggers their ultimate release, is complex and dependent on the cell(s) and the biological context. For some vesicles, the act of docking to the receiving cell surface appears to be the purpose of the signal, triggering a change in the cell's activation state. But these packages can also be internalised by the recipient cell. The outer chemistry of the extracellular vesicle appears to shape their destiny once inside. Many vesicles appear to be sent straight to lysosomes, a waste disposal system, and likely undergo immediate destruction. But some escape, to release their contents.

Returning to the findings of 2007, after isolating exosomes based on size and surface and inner chemistry, and having cleared away any outer contamination by treating with ribonucleases, the researchers broke the exosomes open and explored the RNA contents.

They found specific types of RNA present. There were a variety of mRNAs and these were functional. That is, when fed into an artificial protein synthesis complex, they generated a protein. And they found microRNAs. More than 100 different microRNAs were identified in exosomes from different cell sources. The levels of some were higher than background levels, indicating that they had been actively concentrated inside; they weren't simply caught up during the packaging step. The conclusion drawn at the time was that exosomes might be used to shuttle microRNAs between cells to adjust the recipient cell's gene expression landscape. This could be a useful way of synchronising cellular activity within a tissue or alerting to the presence of pathogens or abnormal cell states such as cancerous transformation. The study was a major advance, marking the discovery of a new mechanism of cell-to-cell communication and a new horizon for microRNAs. A surge of interest in microRNAs in exosomes followed. But not everyone was convinced.

The AGO Strikes Back

Many researchers embraced the idea of microRNAs being shuttled inside exosomes. There were claims that this was *the* major mechanism of microRNA transport in the circulation. But there were soon to be contrary findings, and the first salvo came from the Seattle group, in 2011.[329] Picking one of the most abundant plasma microRNAs, the team found that 95 per cent of the copies of miR-16 in a plasma sample were not in vesicles but instead separated out with a protein-rich sediment. While they found a few microRNAs that were more enriched in vesicles, many more were in the protein-containing fraction. They proposed that AGOs were the more dominant carriage mechanism. Indeed, when they extracted AGO proteins from plasma samples, and AGO2 in particular, they found them rich with microRNAs. There was now an additional culprit for the stability of circulating microRNAs. And AGOs are particularly well-suited to this task, in terms of protecting any inner contents from the reach of ribonucleases. Their physical shape makes them hardy and the RNA cargo is buried deep in their binding pocket. The balance would tip further towards AGOs with the results of a second paper, published a month later by a team from Heidelberg, Germany.[330] They found that passing blood plasma through a filter to remove the exosome component had a negligible effect on overall plasma levels of miR-16 as well as several other microRNAs. They also found that it was AGO2 to which most of the microRNAs were bound. The conclusions of the two studies were that exosomes were at most a minor contributor to the overall circulating microRNA population. A further cooling of the exosomes-as-microRNA-bearing messengers hypothesis came in 2014.[331] The Seattle team asked a simple question: Assuming there is microRNA in plasma exosomes, and the exosomes reach target cells, is there enough inside to produce an effect on the recipient? The core experiment involved counting the number of exosomes and the number of copies of microRNAs in a biofluid sample. The ratio of microRNAs to exosomes was less than one; that is, exosomes carried, on average, less than a single microRNA each. Barring a mechanism by which exosomes could concentrate in vast numbers on a small number of cells, the findings suggested that the importance of vesicle-delivered microRNAs was overstated and perhaps biologically unimportant. In addition, interrogation of the protein contents of exosomes found little or no AGO proteins inside. Even if they were carrying microRNAs, it was unclear how effective they would be when released into a recipient cell.

Although thinking in the field shifted, much research continued, with studies reporting biological effects of microvesicle-carried microRNAs on target cells in various contexts.

These include examples from the neuroscience field, where microRNA-carrying exosomes have been reported to affect the functions of neurones and glia and processes such as inflammation and tissue repair. It remains an interesting branch of microRNA research. Additionally, there is at least consensus that microRNAs do circulate in extracellular vesicles and this could have diagnostic value regardless of their effects, if any, on recipient cells.

Less-Invasive Sources of Biomarkers

Obtaining plasma and serum to measure circulating microRNA biomarkers requires a blood draw. A needle has to be inserted into your forearm; the procedure is called a phlebotomy. If you've donated blood as an adult or given a sample for another reason, you'll know this is unpleasant enough. For children, it is avoided when possible. There are other patient groups for whom giving blood by this route would rather be avoided, such as the elderly and the frail. If testing for blood-based molecules such as microRNAs were ever to move outside of the hospital setting, including the home, then a minimally or non-invasive route to obtain a microRNA-containing sample will be needed. So, are there ways around? Are there microRNAs in other body fluids that can be accessed less-invasively? This search has been a key undercurrent alongside the other research on microRNA biomarkers. It was another Seattle-based group, teaming up with researchers in Luxembourg and Taiwan, who first reported a broad dive into the full range of body fluids to search for microRNAs.[332] The study included many sources of biofluid that could be non-invasively obtained. Surveying 12 different body fluids, including urine, saliva, tears and breast milk, they reliably detected microRNAs in all of them. The amount and the variety of microRNAs varied among the fluids. Saliva had the most and urine had the least. But urine still contained more than 200 different microRNAs. About 1 in 10 microRNAs were found in all body fluids. Several body fluids, including plasma, contained at least one microRNA unique to that source. Interestingly, when the lists of microRNAs were grouped according to similarity, the most shared microRNAs at the most similar levels were the reproduction-related fluids, which included breast milk, seminal and amniotic fluid. The findings, reported in 2010, opened up the possibility of using less-invasive body fluids for microRNA measurement.

As studies continued, the range of biofluid sources expanded the application of this approach to more diseases and allowed profiling with little direct harm to the patient. If you are interested in biomarkers of kidney function, you might choose urine as your starting material. Oral and mouth-related diseases could perhaps use saliva. One of the most interesting aspects to come out of that study for us was the observation that the microRNA profile in tear fluid was quite similar to that in the brain's cerebrospinal fluid. This raised the exciting prospect that a trace of whatever microRNA changes occur in relation to brain disease might make their way into tear fluid, from where they can be easily and non-invasively sampled. Notably, the retina is part of the CNS and eye researchers have known for some time that the chemical composition of emotion-related tears is different from the content of tears shed for purposes of general eye lubrication or in response to an irritant. Colleagues of mine decided to explore tears as a source of microRNA biomarkers for Alzheimer's disease.[333] The need for biomarkers of Alzheimer's disease is self-evident, not just to help diagnose the condition but so that, if we can catch it early, we have the best chance of interrupting the degenerative process before it becomes too advanced, assuming we can find the drug that can stop it – a search that continues. Early diagnosis is possible, but only through a combination of brain imaging and sampling biomarkers from cerebrospinal fluid, a biofluid that to obtain requires a needle to be inserted into the spine, usually the lower, lumbar region, under local anaesthetic. Searches for a simple-to-access biomarker have focussed on people displaying mild cognitive impairment, a high-risk state for Alzheimer's. But a significant portion of people with mild cognitive impairment do not convert to Alzheimer's disease. Telling the groups apart is an important goal. As part of this effort, the team had already identified a microRNA in the blood that seemed to predict conversion from mild cognitive impairment to Alzheimer's disease (**Figure 8.2**).

Another reason tear fluid was worth studying was because the telltale amyloid protein deposits characteristic of Alzheimer's pathology can be seen in the lenses and the retinas of the eyes of people who develop Alzheimer's. Joining with colleagues from the Severo Ochoa Centre in Madrid, named after the Spanish Nobel prize–winning biochemist, the group set out to measure microRNAs in tear fluid and determine if a profile was unique to people with either mild cognitive impairment or Alzheimer's disease.[333] Tears were gathered by placing a strip of absorbent paper on the lower eyelid for five minutes before dropping it into a tube. There were two main findings. First, the amount of small RNAs in tear fluid was higher in Alzheimer's patients than age-matched healthy controls, with the mild cognitive

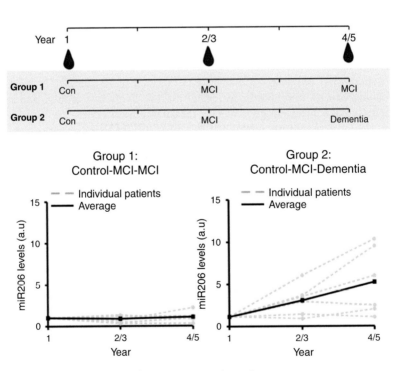

Figure 8.2 A blood-based microRNA predicts conversion to dementia

Plasma miR-206 was analysed in a longitudinal cohort of patients with repeated blood sampling from the same patient over time. Group 1 patients developed mild cognitive impairment (MCI), but this remained stable. Group 2 patients developed MCI, but they progressed to dementia. Levels of miR-206 increased in those who progressed but not those who remained stable, suggesting that it may be a biomarker of conversion.

Source: From Kenny et al., *Biomolecules*, vol. 9, 734 (2019).[334].

impairment group falling midway between. Second, the microRNA profiles were different among the three groups. While the number of specific microRNAs detected was similar, at ~200 or more different microRNAs in the tear fluid from each group, the mild cognitive impairment and Alzheimer's groups had distinct microRNA profiles, with a mix of higher and lower levels of specific microRNAs. The optimal combination of these to separate the groups remains to be determined. Encouragingly, preclinical studies by teams from a set of North American universities have since shown that mice genetically engineered to develop features of Alzheimer's disease produce elevated levels of microRNAs linked to production of the amyloid protein and inflammatory responses within their tear fluid.[335] Together, this may be a promising approach to the identification of biomarkers that would easily scale up, an important factor if we are ever to undertake national-level screening for Alzheimer's and perhaps other conditions in the future.

Researchers have continued to look at ever-smaller and less-invasive sources of microRNA that might have diagnostic use. These include human sweat and exhaled breath condensate. The latter was first reported in 2013 by teams based at research institutes in Delhi, India.[336] The condensate from breath is easy to collect. Simply breathe into a collection tube, then exhaled traces of the fluid lining the airways can be obtained and analysed. The team were able to extract quantities of RNA from healthy volunteers and people with asthma or pulmonary tuberculosis. Within the RNA were several hundred microRNAs. These included known lung-enriched microRNAs and small differences in their levels were found in samples from people with either of the two lung diseases. They also probed the mechanisms responsible for the stability of the exhaled microRNAs. There they found exosomes to be present in the condensate and the main source of the detected microRNAs. So, exosome secretion may reflect disease status, which is encouraging for the use of this non-invasive source of microRNAs as a basis for diagnostic or disease-stage biomarkers. Predictably, use of breath-based microRNAs has also been explored in several lung cancer studies. One study reported changes to a panel of microRNAs that included miR-21 and miR-212 in lung cancer patients.[337] However, they found that incorporating the readings into the clinical profiles of the patients did not add much additional diagnostic yield. Thus, the clinical use of this approach requires further study, particularly as a lung cancer diagnostic. Indeed, the stronger evidence is from a competing approach, using cell-free DNA, which is also detectable in exhaled breath condensate and so far has been found to provide more-accurate disease insights.

How You Travel Matters in Brain Disease

The competing stance of researchers for or against the importance of exosomes versus AGO or other compartments as the conveyors of microRNAs in the circulation had implications for my field. Exosome-carried microRNA could be a biomarker of epilepsy. Comparing the relative amounts of different microRNAs in the vesicle and AGO 'pools' might tell us something new about the disease or provide a basis for a diagnostic test. The first opportunity to tackle this came during the EpimiRNA project. One of the sub-projects was run by my PhD student, an Iraqi doctor named Rana Raoof, who, owing to the unstable situation in her home region at the time, had come to Dublin to study. Her idea was to profile human cerebrospinal fluid for microRNA biomarkers of epilepsy or seizures.[338] Cerebrospinal fluid circulates slowly through the ventricular system of the brain and is in direct contact with brain tissue. This makes it a better source than blood for brain disease biomarkers. Any molecular signal from disease processes may be captured and, since the CNS contains about

150 millilitres of cerebrospinal fluid compared to the 5 litres of blood in a human, it is less diluted. The downside is that cerebrospinal fluid is not routinely collected from epilepsy patients. We had managed to source cerebrospinal fluid samples from about a dozen people with epilepsy and another dozen samples from people who had experienced an episode of status epilepticus. This is a severe seizure lasting more than five minutes. Our expectation was that there would be microRNAs in the cerebrospinal fluid of these two patient groups that were not normally present, or at least that they would be present at higher levels than in healthy controls. We also expected there to be higher amounts of any seizure-released microRNAs in the status epilepticus samples compared to the epilepsy samples owing to the greater seizure burden in the former group.

Working with cerebrospinal fluid is technically challenging. For one thing, RNA levels are vanishingly low. We found that we needed extremely sensitive methods to detect and measure the microRNAs and, since we only had a small amount of cerebrospinal fluid from each patient, we wanted to use as little as possible for profiling. Both issues were solved by a recently developed detection technology called OpenArray; it was specifically designed for small volume samples with low RNA content. We were able to use one-fifth of a millilitre of cerebrospinal fluid, which is more or less a drop of the fluid. The main limitation was that the OpenArray chip could detect only a few hundred human microRNAs, so we would be missing a number of potentially relevant microRNAs. But, overall, it served us well. We obtained a signal for about 50 different microRNAs in the control samples, which were from people who had presented with a headache and had cerebrospinal fluid sampled to check for possible meningitis, but who were later found to be negative. The cerebrospinal fluid samples from the patients, particularly the status epilepticus cases, contained many more microRNAs than the controls. This supported the idea that tissue or cell damage caused by the severe seizure results in a small leak of microRNA into the cerebrospinal fluid. Some were known to be brain-enriched, including miR-9. Another microRNA of note was miR-451a. This is the same microRNA that is blood-enriched and generated via a Dicer-independent pathway. This was only increased in the status epilepticus patients. Its presence in cerebrospinal fluid could, therefore, be owing to the rupture of tiny vessels in the brain. Such vessel damage is something that has been detected in the past in studies of status epilepticus. The elevated presence of miR-451a in cerebrospinal fluid was a potential proxy for vessel damage and the biomarker of having experienced an episode of status epilepticus (see **Figure 8.3A**). Unfortunately, we did not have access to enough clinical information, so could not know if, within the status epilepticus group, levels of the microRNAs were higher in those patients that experienced more-prolonged or more-severe seizures.

There are statistical methods that help assess the sensitivity and the specificity of a biomarker. One of these is a receiver operating characteristic (ROC) analysis and it was a computer scientist, Catherine Mooney, who had joined our team that first applied the tests. Basically, you enter the data on the measured levels of the biomarker (microRNA) and it generates a plot with a curve (imagine the left-half arc of a rainbow). The more area under the curve, the better the sensitivity and the specificity. A perfect biomarker would give an area under the curve of 1.0. A score of 0.5 means that it is no use at distinguishing patients from controls. You start to get excited when you see an ROC with an area under the curve close to 0.9. When we plotted some of the microRNAs we had found in cerebrospinal fluid, either alone or in combinations, by using another statistical technique called binomial logistic regression, we got a result of 0.85. Not bad. This proved, at least in principle, that

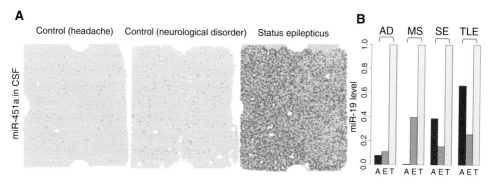

Figure 8.3 MicroRNA biomarkers in human brain fluid

Panel A shows the results of a digital PCR analysis of miR-451a in human cerebrospinal fluid (CSF). The dots in the image panels represent positive signals from amplified miR-451a on a representative chip.

Panel B shows the relative amounts of miR-19b in different fractions (Ago, A; E, exosome; T, total) in CSF from patients with Alzheimer's disease (AD), multiple sclerosis (MS), status epilepticus (SE) and temporal lobe epilepsy (TLE).

Source: Adapted from Raoof et al., *Scientific Reports*, vol. 7, 3328 (2017).[338]

human brain fluid contains a molecular signature of microRNAs that can tell a patient from a control.

Were some or all of these microRNAs in exosomes? Or bound to AGOs? If different cell types contain different capacity to generate extracellular vesicles and contain varying amounts of AGOs, then brain diseases might all look a bit different from each other when we compare the relative amounts of a microRNA between the two pools. We went back to the freezer, taking additional aliquots of cerebrospinal fluid and then split them in half. One sample was processed using a series of centrifugation steps to yield an exosome-enriched vesicle fraction. The other sample we mixed with antibodies against AGO2. We then collected the antibodies, holding onto their AGO2 cargo, by a centrifuge spin. Small RNAs were extracted from both the vesicle 'soup' and the AGO2 pull-down and we measured the levels of three of our best-performing microRNAs from the earlier study. We had also expanded our cerebrospinal fluid collection at this point. One of the hospitals that gave us the cerebrospinal fluid samples from the status epilepticus patients also had a collection of cerebrospinal fluid from other brain diseases. This included samples from people with Alzheimer's disease and multiple sclerosis. Now we had an opportunity to look at whether the amounts of a microRNA in exosomes or AGO2 were not just different between status epilepticus and epilepsy but also different from two other major brain diseases. What we found was interesting. For one of the microRNAs we tested, miR-19b, the cerebrospinal fluid from each brain disease had a different amount of the microRNA in exosomes and AGO2. In the epilepsy and status epilepticus patients there was more microRNA in the AGO2 fraction than in the exosomes. In samples from multiple sclerosis patients, we found the opposite; the microRNA was more abundant in the exosomes and the signal from AGO2 was nearly undetectable. Alzheimer samples also looked different, with only very low amounts in both pools. Most of the microRNA in those samples appeared to be in neither source, circulating in some other form (see **Figure 8.3B**). This suggests that brain diseases produce slightly different mixes of exosome and AGO2-carried microRNA in the cerebrospinal fluid. This is presumably driven by distinct contributions of pathways within and between cells, that is, differences between neurones and glia in terms of how they package and release microRNA, their exosome-producing capacity in the brain and how these cell types are affected by and drive the disease. This disease signature has obvious diagnostic applications. Measuring microRNA and comparing across physical sources could tell these brain diseases apart.

We applied part of the learnings from working with cerebrospinal fluid, namely that the physical way microRNAs circulate has diagnostic value, to a study on blood microRNAs. Raoof's and Mooney's work had identified three microRNAs in plasma that were promising biomarkers of seizures in patients with TLE.[311] Blood samples had been collected on admission of patients to two hospital epilepsy monitoring units. We also collected a further blood sample within 24 hours of a recorded seizure. We found a number of microRNAs whose overall blood levels were different in the post-seizure samples. We then dug into whether measuring these same microRNAs in the exosome-rich vesicle or AGO2 fraction, using the same methods of sample processing as for our cerebrospinal fluid study, enhanced in any way the diagnostic insights. We found that the AGO2 fraction was more useful at confirming a seizure. That is, the microRNA levels within the AGO2 fraction changed in the post-seizure samples. The exosome-rich fraction contained microRNAs, but did not display much difference in microRNA content in the post-seizure sample. The findings backed up what we had seen with the cerebrospinal fluid study, namely that how you measure microRNA biomarkers is as important as which microRNAs you measure. We do not know why the amounts in AGO2 change after a seizure or do not change in the vesicle component, but it could reflect a shedding of cell contents owing to the seizure, which makes its way into the circulation. As with the cerebrospinal fluid tests, these insights should guide the design of any future diagnostic test, for example adding a processing step, to enrich for exosomes or AGO2 (or something else) to get the most accurate result.

Plasma and Serum MicroRNAs as Brain Disease Biomarkers

The search for blood microRNA signatures to diagnose brain disease took hold in the late 2000s and most brain diseases have been extensively studied. The volume of published work is too vast to go into each disease in detail, but it is worth highlighting some examples. A 2013 study in *Genome Biology* reported a panel of 12 microRNAs that included lower levels of some brain-enriched microRNAs that, when measured together in whole blood, could distinguish Alzheimer's disease from healthy controls with sensitivity and specificity above 90 per cent.[339] Blood levels of miR-137 have been found to be elevated in patients with schizophrenia and, in combination with others, might have promise in diagnosis.[340] A study published in *Nature Neuroscience* in late 2021 identified elevated plasma levels of miR-181, one of the most brain-enriched microRNAs and found in motoneurones, as a sensitive and specific predictor of disease progression and the risk of dying, in patients with ALS.[341]

Figure 8.4 provides a conceptual framework for how and why plasma might contain microRNA that could support a diagnosis of epilepsy or recent seizure. The first study to look at the effects of seizures on microRNA profiles in the blood appeared in late 2009.[224] Rats had been given an injection of kainic acid and then blood collected the following day. While the study was rather underpowered, reducing the statistical significance of the findings, they nevertheless found several microRNAs up- or down-regulated in the blood after seizures. The study was also important because it found that the specific combination of up/down microRNAs was not the same in rats that had a stroke or brain bleed. Different

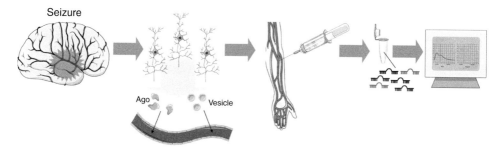

Figure 8.4 Circulating blood-based microRNA biomarkers

This schematic shows the concept behind blood-based microRNA biomarkers of epilepsy. Seizure activity or the inciting insult damages neuronal networks leading to passive and/or active release of microRNA in forms such as AGO-bound or enclosed in exosomes. These enter the circulation because of interruption to the integrity of the blood–brain barrier, and can then be collected in a blood draw. The microRNAs can then be extracted and quantified.

Source: Generated using images from Servier Medical Art. Servier Medical Art by Servier is licensed under a Creative Commons Attribution 3.0 Unported License (https://creativecommons.org/licenses/by/3.0/).

brain diseases have distinct circulating microRNA profiles while a number of blood microRNAs change no matter what the brain injury. In 2015, the first human epilepsy studies were published.[342, 343] Using RNA sequencing, a Chinese team at Qingdao University identified a set of microRNAs that were up-regulated in serum samples from epilepsy patients. Among the elevated microRNAs was miR-146a, one of the first microRNAs linked to epilepsy based on studies of the hippocampus. This was encouraging. The same team also found that a set of microRNAs was elevated in serum from people with drug-resistant seizures compared to well-controlled epilepsy and healthy controls. These were potential biomarkers of recent seizures or a signal from the pathophysiologic changes that drive and sustain treatment resistance. When ROC curves were plotted for individual and combinations of the microRNAs, the sensitivity and the specificity were within a useful range.

In the years since, there have been further advances.[344] Differences in circulating levels of microRNAs have been found that can identify subtypes of epilepsy or known aetiologies and between different seizure types. Researchers have found microRNAs that are different in exosome-enriched fractions of blood in epilepsy patients. Studies have also shown that microRNA profiles adjust upon drug treatment, returning closer to baseline levels when seizure control is achieved. There have also been studies that replicate earlier findings. Some of the same microRNAs have come up time and time again. These include miR-146a, which was reported to be elevated in epilepsy patients in the original 2015 study by the Chinese team, and has since been confirmed to be elevated in at least half a dozen further studies. Elevated levels of miR-129, miR-132 and miR-134, all microRNAs known to be activity-dependent and up-regulated in the brain following seizures, have appeared as up-regulated in blood samples in multiple human studies. Another epilepsy-linked circulating microRNA is miR-106b. This has been reported on separate occasions to be increased in blood samples in both generalised and focal epilepsies. This is the same microRNA that controls the *KCNQ2* transcript that encodes a potassium channel, lower levels of which contribute to hyperexcitability. We are seeing the emergence of a panel of microRNAs that could be specific for epilepsy. But challenges are ahead. One problem is that when samples from controls and patients are compared, there may be a statistical difference, but if you pick out individual data points, you find many patient samples with levels that overlap values in controls. There is significant variability in the baseline levels of these microRNAs and this may be sufficient to obscure a disease signal. Unless there is clear daylight between the two groups, the test will lack accuracy. Another criticism of the results so far is that patient samples are often being compared to healthy controls. This is fine, to a point, but a more difficult test to pass, a higher bar, is whether the microRNA level in epilepsy samples differs from that in patients diagnosed with PNES. Clinically, the two groups can look quite similar and PNES patients may be on some of the same medications. This issue of medication is important, with studies often comparing results in patients who are being treated with ASMs to non-medicated healthy controls. Some of the signal may be drug-related rather than disease-specific. Extracting the disease signal from the noise-generating effects of treatment and co-morbid conditions is essential for progress. So, including samples from PNES patients is a firm test of whether a microRNA panel is really specific or not for epilepsy. We have paid attention to this and included PNES samples in some experiments and have found several plasma microRNAs, including miR-93a and miR-199a, that are different between these patients compared to people diagnosed with epilepsy.[345] But our studies and those from others working on this problem need to be repeated with larger sample groups. One or two studies have reported associations between the level of the circulating microRNA and clinical information such as the patient's seizure burden. When digging into whether microRNA profiles can distinguish specific epilepsy syndromes, the results have been disappointing. That is, while levels of microRNAs such as miR-146a are elevated in epilepsy compared to controls, few studies have identified microRNAs that can distinguish patients with generalised seizures from focal onset, despite the likely differences in the underlying pathophysiology of these syndromes, a mixture of genetics, developmental, environmental, cell and brain region combinations and the differing effect of the seizure on brain networks. Perhaps this is too harsh a judgement. Most of the studies are probably statistically underpowered to identify microRNA levels that distinguish syndrome or treatment–related differences among patients.

Another potential problem is that some of the epilepsy-related microRNAs have also been proposed as biomarkers of other brain diseases. These include miR-132 (mild cognitive impairment), miR-134 (mild cognitive impairment and bipolar disorder), miR-146a (Alzheimer's disease) and miR-106b (Parkinson's disease, Creutzfeldt-Jakob disease). This may not be an issue in most clinical settings, where a microRNA test might be used to confirm whether a seizure has occurred or whether, in a previously diagnosed patient, they are at risk of developing treatment resistance in the future. Moreover, in some of the diseases where the same microRNA has been identified as a potential biomarker, the direction of change is different. For example, levels are lower than controls in the neurodegenerative disease whereas they are higher in epilepsy. So cross-disease findings may not be a barrier to their adoption.

My own team is now working to measure microRNA profiles as soon as possible after a first seizure or epilepsy diagnosis. The goal is to determine whether measuring a panel of microRNAs in blood has any predictive value for the later development of treatment-resistant epilepsy. In another study called SEISMIC, we are looking at whether serum samples taken in an emergency department setting can distinguish epileptic seizures from seizure mimics such as syncope and alcohol withdrawal–related seizures. Knowing which it is would help steer clinical decision-making in a fast-paced hospital setting. One of the most important uses of circulating microRNAs would be if they could predict risk of epilepsy development after a brain injury, as biomarkers of the process of epileptogenesis.[322] Preclinical studies in rodents have identified blood microRNA changes after known triggers of epilepsy such as status epilepticus and traumatic brain injury. If a set of circulating microRNAs reflected this process, it would be a potent enabler of clinical trials for drugs that may prevent epilepsy. Currently, we do not have accurate-enough ways to predict who will and who will not develop epilepsy. These are not simple studies to run because they require cross-neurological care team cooperation to collect samples at the time and at follow-up as well as tracking whether or not epilepsy develops in the intervening months and years. Not impossible, but a challenge. My own optimism that we will find a microRNA-based biomarker of traumatic brain injury–induced epilepsy was recently dampened by preclinical findings. A large multi-centre study in rats led by a team in Finland looked for circulating microRNAs that predict epilepsy after traumatic brain injury.[346] They found that while the plasma microRNA profile two days after injury accurately predicted the extent of the brain tissue damage, it had no predictive value for whether or not the animal would go on to develop epilepsy or the frequency of events in those animals that had spontaneous seizures. Early microRNA profiles in this setting did not seem to capture epileptogenic aspects that could help predict risk.

How can we do better in the future? First, we need to do more large, multi-centre studies to ensure statistically significant findings and reduce the bias and false positives/negatives that come from small, underpowered studies based in a single lab or hospital. The study that identified miR-181 as a biomarker of ALS began with profiling samples from more than 100 patients from several centres. Adoption of proposed standard sampling and analysis pipelines would reduce technical variability. Only a few of the studies have managed to match levels of the circulating microRNAs to clinical variables such as time-from-seizure or seizure burden. This would be important. A slew of other factors need to be controlled for, such as time of day the sample is collected, recent meal, sex, weight, age and race. Studies in other fields suggest that all of these variables can affect the accuracy and the reproducibility of microRNA profiles in blood. Studies need to be planned in advance and include sufficient follow-up time. If you want to find out if measuring blood levels of microRNAs after a first seizure can predict later drug-resistance, you need to coordinate research of scale stretching over several years.

Proving That Circulating MicroRNAs Actually Come from the Brain

One of the questions that has been asked at meetings about microRNAs as biomarkers is to do with the evidence, or lack thereof, that the circulating microRNAs in the blood actually came from the brain. Good point. We could be looking at a signal that is from the periphery, a downstream reaction of the immune or the vascular systems, an effect of the medications, and thus an indirect proxy of what is happening inside the brain. How can we be sure that some or all of the microRNA signal is coming from the brain? We can look at some of the microRNAs found to be elevated in the blood, such as miR-9 and miR-134, and surmise that they must have come from the brain since we know they are made only in the brain. But this is rather unsatisfactory. Any gene, including microRNAs, could switch on in a disease state, appearing in cells that do not normally make them. We began to think of experiments we could perform to resolve this issue. Could we somehow label a microRNA in the brain and then trace it making its way into the circulation? After running through a number of potential strategies, we settled on an idea. Place a chemical tag on a RISC component in brain cells and then track the tagged protein in the blood and analyse its microRNA contents.[347] We knew that Anne Schaefer had previously engineered mice that made AGO2 with an additional amino acid sequence called a FLAG tag. The sequence comprises aspartic acid-tyrosine-lysine-aspartic acid-aspartic acid-aspartic acid-aspartic acid-lysine (shortened as DYKDDDDK) and does not occur in nature. Antibodies can be generated to detect the FLAG sequence so it is possible to separate the tagged form from the natural AGO2. The sequence in the engineered mouse genome was flanked by sites for the Cre recombinase. This meant that we could cross the AGO2-FLAG mice with animals that had Cre under the control of cell type–specific promoters. If the promoters were specific for neurones or glia, the tagged AGO2 would be made inside those cells and nowhere else. Detecting any microRNA attached to FLAG-AGO2 in a blood sample would then prove that circulating microRNAs came from the brain. Anne kindly agreed to send us the mice and we bred them with mice that had been engineered to express Cre, one under the control of a neuronal promoter, the other specific for microglia. Having generated the two trans-genic mice lines, one with AGO2-FLAG in neurones and one with AGO2-FLAG in microglia, we performed some checks (we tried to create an astrocyte version but could not get it to work). Using tissue samples from various organs, we confirmed that AGO2-FLAG was made only in the brain and, within the brain, in either neurones or microglia. Satisfied that we had the tagged AGO2 in the right place, we then used kainic acid to trigger seizures in the mice. Two weeks later, when the mice usually have epilepsy, we took blood samples. After preparing plasma and then mixing this with antibodies to the FLAG tag, we tested the extract for microRNA. We got a signal: a small amount of microRNAs bound to FLAG-AGO2 in the plasma of both types of engineered mice. This was proof that some AGO2 from neurones and microglia makes its way into the circulation after a seizure. It is an important result that links circulating microRNAs to what happens in the brain.

Other Examples of Circulating MicroRNAs as Biomarkers

Let us move away from epilepsy. Used appropriately, radioactivity is a powerful diagnostic tool that saves lives. Nuclear medicine applications range from the tracers used in PET scanning to image amyloid plaques and detect early-onset Alzheimer's disease, to radio-therapy to treat certain cancers. But exposure to high levels of radiation can be fatal in humans. On 11 March 2011, the most powerful earthquake ever recorded in Japan triggered a tsunami that flooded the Fukushima Daiichi Nuclear Power Plant in Ōkuma, Japan. This resulted in the worst nuclear power accident since Chernobyl in 1986. And nuclear power plant disasters are not the only source of devastating radiation exposure. At the time of writing, the Russian Federation, the country with the world's largest stockpile of nuclear weapons, is at war with Ukraine. The threat of the use of nuclear weapons or some kind of nuclear weapons or reactor-related disaster is once again in people's minds.

The immediate threat to life from radioactivity is damage to the bone marrow, which contains regenerating cells termed haematopoietic stem cells. These are the blood cell production sites in the body. If caught in time, people exposed to fatal levels of radioactivity can be saved through a bone marrow transplant. Unfortunately, spotting those in need is not simple. Blood cell markers are not able to predict at an early stage whose bone marrow is irreversibly damaged and resources do not allow widespread bone marrow transplantation. Being able to identify who has or has not received a fatal dose of radiation exposure within the first hours or days would enable triage for bone marrow treatment at a much earlier time. A Polish team, based in Lodz, has been working on this problem with colleagues at the Dana-Farber Cancer Institute at Harvard University. They discovered that circulating microRNAs can identify lethal from non-lethal radiation exposure. The team began with studies in mice, reported in *Science Translational Medicine* in 2015.[348] Exposing mice to different levels of radiation confirmed the clinical experience. That is, for two weeks after total body irradiation, the blood chemistry between mice given a high but non-lethal dose and those that would go on to die remained indistinguishable. They profiled microRNAs in serum samples that were taken from the mice 24 hours after exposure to radiation. A set of microRNAs were found that were at altered levels in the mice given the fatal dose of radioactivity compared to those who would eventually survive. The lethal dose–prediction panel comprised two serum microRNAs that were higher (miR-30a and miR-30c) and three that were lower (miR-187, miR-194 and miR-27a). Two members of the panel, miR-30a and miR-30c, could distinguish the groups up to a week after exposure. So, long before any differences in red and white blood cell counts appear between lethal and non-lethal doses of radiation, serum microRNAs show a difference. Notably, serum microRNA profiles in the mice were also able to distinguish between control mice and animals exposed to the non-lethal dose of radiation, indicating that they are very sensitive indicators of radiation exposure. But do mice react to radiation in the same way as us? To get closer to the answer, the team moved to non-human primates.[349] Similar results were found, albeit the microRNA identities were different. In the non-human primates, the best-performing panel of circulating microRNAs for exposure to fatal versus survivable radiation exposure comprised miR-133b, miR-215, miR-375, miR-30a and miR-126. More recently, the team and their collaborators have been able to part-validate these findings, using serum samples from people who had undergone radiation treatment.[350] The results therefore offer a way to rapidly screen people exposed after a radiation event for health risks. They may also be useful as a guide to radiation dosing in patients.

Point-of-Care

Assuming that one or more microRNAs emerge as suitable biomarkers for a disease or condition, how will a doctor/nurse or, in my own area of interest, epileptologist measure this? If time is not critical, a biofluid sample can be sent off to a centralised testing lab to be processed in a similar way to measuring markers of inflammation, with results being available within a few days. But there are scenarios where point-of-care testing would be preferable, when rapid clinical decisions are needed because time is of the essence and diagnosis could be delivered close to the patient. This might be in an ambulance or the emergency department. In one of the examples used earlier, a microRNA-based test to confirm if a seizure or stroke has occurred would be most useful if it could be administered right there and then, with a result in minutes. Time is key in these situations and a prompt diagnosis would inform treatment decisions and possibly save lives. In resource-poor settings, a point-of-care device would also make sense, avoiding the need to organise and pay for shipping biofluids for off-site testing. There may also be uses in an at-home setting.

For example, if a particular microRNA profile could predict when a seizure is imminent or confirm if a seizure had occurred, and if this could be checked at home, it would empower people living with chronic diseases such as epilepsy that have unpredictable symptoms to make informed decisions such as do I drive today or work from home? At-home tests that confirmed a seizure could replace seizure diaries in clinical trials. The use or context will ultimately inform the design of the device. An at-home device needs to be small, portable and cheap. Likewise in a GP's office. If it is hospital-based, size may be less critical.

Along these lines, there have been exciting advances in technologies and point-of-care devices for circulating microRNAs.[351] The range of options for detection is growing and includes traditional PCR-based methods as well as a version called isothermal amplification, which doesn't require precise temperature controls during amplification and detection of the signal. There are lateral flow-based systems where the microRNA is detected using a chromatographic, similar to home Covid tests. There are nanobead-based methods that conjugate the detection probe to a chemical structure that releases a quantifiable signal upon meeting its microRNA target. This is an area my colleague in Dublin, Robert Forster, has been pursuing in parallel with our efforts to identify the right microRNA biomarkers. His work focusses on electrochemistry and achieving the fastest time-to-answer. An early prototype comprised a three-strand configuration. First, an immobilised capture probe on an electrode surface that is complementary to one-half of the microRNA of interest. MicroRNA strands present in the sample bind to the probe. This leaves a separate section or overhang of the microRNA exposed. The exposed end of the microRNA then binds a second probe complementary to the remaining portion of the microRNA which carries a catalytic particle. This can be made of a material such as platinum, although the optimal chemistry is a subject of ongoing research. The metal particle catalyses the reduction of hydrogen peroxide that is added to the device, generating an electrical current whose magnitude is proportional to the number of microRNA molecules present. This allows rapid quantification of microRNA levels in a sample. The limit of detection is extremely low, in the picomolar (10^{-12} molecules per litre) range, sufficient to detect the microRNA signal in cerebrospinal fluid, one of the lowest-yield biofluids. In the prototype, described in 2015, his team designed a probe to miR-134 and used it to compare levels in a set of patient samples to controls.[352] The detection technology and sensitivity continue to advance. A later version involved a spinning disc device that used centrifugal force to pass the sample, wash buffer and measurement solution over the functionalised electrodes where the microRNA is detected, a process that took about an hour and a half from start to finish.[353] Still a bit slow, but already faster than PCR. Later prototypes have been developed that allow three microRNAs to be measured together, a technique called multiplexing, enabling rapid detection of combinations of biomarkers. This approach and parallel efforts like it promise to have point-of-care devices ready to go by the time the microRNAs to be tested are fully validated. The introduction of biofluid-measured microRNAs and companion point-of-care technology would transform diagnostic care in clinical practice and the home, removing some of the odyssey for healthcare professionals and enabling people living with chronic conditions to exercise more control over their lives.

Reflections

In this chapter we have seen the development of a new scientific focus of microRNA research based around microRNAs' use as circulating biomarkers. The properties of microRNAs as well as how they circulate in biofluids make them highly promising candidates. Altered microRNA profiles define most human diseases spanning cancer to Alzheimer's and, remarkably, clinical and commercial applications of biofluid microRNAs as diagnostic tests appeared within a few short years of those discoveries. Such tests are yet to be adopted beyond specific cancer applications, however, and remain in need of validation and optimisation for sensitivity and specificity. Further mechanistic studies are needed to understand the origins, distribution and effects of circulating microRNA biomarkers. This will be driven both by clinical need and commercial interest; potent partners in developing new technologies.

The discovery of microRNA biomarkers also sparked interest in vesicles as mediators of cell-to-cell communication. The idea that we use microRNAs packed inside vesicles as a method of long-range cell-to-cell communication remains enticing. But it is possible that there is no biological function for this circulating extracellular microRNA in humans. This does not mean that it is not scientifically important or that it doesn't still hold biomarker value or serve a purpose in diagnostics applications. Last, we have seen how computer scientists, materials chemists and nanotechnologists are helping to deliver on the promise of microRNAs as biomarkers, providing the materials and the algorithms needed for rapid and hopefully close-to-patient diagnostic care.

9

Finale and Encore for MicroRNAs

Anytime we do . . . experiments, there are going to be three or four new questions that come up when you think you've answered one.

Carol Greider, Nobel prize in physiology or medicine, 2009

We have covered the origins of microRNA, who discovered them and some of the key experiments performed. We have also seen how a wider scientific community has enthusiastically embraced this new science, driving the early work that unpicked microRNAs' genomic locations, as well as their biogenesis pathway and rules of engagement. This includes uncovering their evolution, tracing them back to the earliest and most simple organisms in Earth's history, and establishing their place in the teeming molecular world inside and outside cells, their fundamental coordinating role adjusting gene expression by fine-tuning protein levels. MicroRNAs supply a missing piece of the puzzle of life, that of how ever-increasing organism complexity is achieved without the need for more 'genes'. They are a solution to the C/G paradox and smoothing the effects of the stochastic nature of transcription to produce a stable molecular landscape. Moving on, we have covered a range of the jobs that microRNAs do, guiding organism development and maintaining healthy tissue function throughout adulthood. We have seen how failures of the microRNA system can wreak havoc on the body, but also how they can be turned into medicines. Last, we have seen the harnessing of microRNAs and technologies for their detection in the tiniest drops of body fluid as a means to test our own health and well-being. Let us finish with a look at some of the latest findings and peek into the future. If I may reuse the orchestra metaphor from the start of the book, it is time for the finale and, I hope you will agree, a short encore if time allows . . ..

First Things First

Before we get to the forward-looking statements, it is worth looking back at some of the missteps of the past so that we do better in the future. The microRNA field exploded in the 2000s, with microRNAs being studied for their general mechanisms, roles in health and disease, and towards applications as therapeutics and diagnostic biomarkers. Technology for their detection and other commercial interests evolved in parallel, becoming a whole sub-industry. Among the many brilliant discoveries, however, there is also some lower-quality research. Lack of rigour and reproducibility will hamper adoption in the health space. Let's fix that as we move forward.[354] First, we need to increase the focus on deducing what is happening in individual cells. Mashing up a piece of tissue and finding higher or lower levels of a microRNA has become an outdated scientific approach as we cannot know if a change in the abundance of a microRNA is being driven by one cell type making much more/less of the microRNA or by multiple cell types making a little bit more/less. And tissue usually contains blood cell components that are mixed in, contaminating the signal or generating spurious conclusions. So, more attention is needed in the microRNA field on discovery approaches that provide cell-level localisation of the microRNA signal and remove sources of microRNA cross-contamination.

There are other sources of error, bias and variability, such as the reagents used to extract the microRNA, the normalisation method used during profiling studies to identify and count microRNAs, and the microRNA-genome alignment tools. More attention to the basal amount of the microRNA relative to its target(s) will avoid wasting effort on biologically meaningless microRNAs or noise in the data. Without careful dosing, the introduction of microRNAs using mimics and over-expression techniques may generate spurious findings because of non-physiologically relevant saturation of real and new targets and pathways, and the triggering of cellular stress responses. We need to apply more sensitive techniques that can assess functioning microRNAs and probe directly the interactions between microRNAs and their targets. Target prediction tools are not yet perfect, particularly when predicting effects or not outside the seed region, and inferring pathway effects of a microRNA should take account of target presence in the sample/model.

During the course of microRNA research, some initially promising findings have ultimately fallen out of favour or been discredited.[354] Either they were over-hyped at the time or later demonstrated to be more likely a technical oddity or an erroneous finding. I expect that such findings will continue from time to time. It is a natural outcome of the scientific system, of always trying to discover the next 'big thing', with our academic funding systems and the super-competitive nature of research. Ten years ago, researchers reported that microRNAs from other species may be functioning inside us, the so-called xenomir hypothesis. The idea was spawned by a 2012 paper and the source of the microRNAs was consumed food, specifically rice.[355] The suggestion was that some microRNAs survive the digestive process to make their way into our bloodstream where they may encounter and target human transcripts to produce biological effects. Other studies suggested environmental sources of microRNAs from other species. While enticing, these ideas have been largely minimalised or refuted in the ensuing years by more rigorous studies that deduced that this was mainly owing to technical issues such as contamination and measurement artefacts. While this has diverted and consumed resources, with researchers trying to replicate findings, it served a purpose of sorts, driving new thinking and refreshing the field. Applying some of the careful approaches considered in this volume will reduce this. We need to keep taking brave leaps, even if sometimes those result in a slip and fall.

Before we leave this section, I want to add one point of reflection. While I am not about to undermine the importance of microRNAs in conferring robustness to the gene programmes that underpin cell functions, we must remember that some pathways can tolerate significant variation in gene expression and still produce the same 'output'. Some classic experiments in the late 1990s showed neural circuits to be surprisingly tolerant of variation in gene expression. That is, despite variation among the levels of different ion channels that underpin the action potential, the firing characteristics of the neural circuit remained stable.[161] This means that multiple configurations of expressed genes were able to produce the same biophysical output. This should be kept in mind and we must be cautious before accepting claims of large phenotypic effects on a brain function coming from a small change to the level of a perhaps low-expressed microRNA.

So, where are things going? What are some of the most exciting recent discoveries? What are some of the next questions to ask? What are the big challenges and opportunities? Here, I intend to look at some of the scientific as well as clinical applications that might emerge in the future. This will naturally be speculative and some of the predictions may fall wide of the mark.

A Final Count

A key objective must be to reach consensus on the number of microRNAs in different organisms, in particular in humans. This sounds straightforward, but it is not. The production of isomirs, RNA modifications, the functionality of passenger strand microRNAs and other matters create a richer microRNA landscape than is strictly encoded in the genome. The microRNA research community has come together several times to reach consensus on nomenclature and the features that define bona fide microRNAs. And yet the number of accepted microRNAs varies depending on who you ask. As covered in Chapter 2, a 2015 study by teams of mainly USA-based researchers at institutes in six different states reported finding more than 3,700 novel microRNAs to add to the list of just over 2,700 in the most up-to-date version (20) of miRbase.[45] The novel microRNAs had been identified by screening 1,323 samples from 13 human cell types. Contrast this with the conclusions of a 2019 study by researchers at the Centre for Human Genetics at Saarland University in Germany.[44] This is a highly reputable group, responsible for various microRNA community tools and tissue atlases. Their starting material was a collection of more than 20,000 human small RNA sequencing samples. They reported the number of true human microRNAs to be 2,300. This is a discrepancy that needs to be resolved.

Everything, Everywhere, All at Once

A general objective must be to detect each microRNA acting on each of its target(s) in specific living cells in real time and measure the effect this produces on proteins. This type of single cell resolution of microRNA function is fundamental to our next level of understanding their actions in health and disease. We can get close to this already, but the full appraisal requires combinations of methods that can simultaneously measure microRNA and mRNA levels, the components of the RISC and microRNA machinery, protein production and intracellular resolution, and monitor that (sub)second to (sub)second. This would make it possible to prove what effect individual microRNAs have on their targets and how this adjusts individual cellular functions within a tissue or network of cells. While this is not yet possible, the pace of technological advances in sensitive RNA and protein detection, tracers for tracking molecular movement and interaction, super-resolution and live-cell microscopy will almost certainly deliver more of this in the coming years.[356] Then we will know what a microRNA is doing in any cell, at any given time. A deep look into the sub-second, sub-cellular world of microRNA.

New Parts of the Pathway

While the biogenesis process for microRNAs is largely understood, new discoveries continue to refine our understanding and show little sign of slowing. These range from studies that deepen our working knowledge of the molecular interactions between proteins and microRNAs, microRNAs and mRNAs, interactions with targets besides mRNAs, through to entirely new discoveries about the process. A 2023 study in *Science Advances* found that a multi-protein complex called *Integrator* controls levels of some microRNAs.[357] Integrator is normally active at sites of transcription in the nucleus, working alongside Pol II. However, the researchers discovered that Integrator components also support a step after Dicer acts but before AGO loading, in which the guide strand to be AGO-loaded and the passenger strand to be degraded are separated. Without Integrator's actions, AGO loading was impaired and microRNAs were destabilised. The study used HeLa cells, so more research will be needed to determine if this is a broadly conserved molecular process and under what conditions it functions. Cell line–based studies must be followed by replication of findings in more physiologically relevant systems. But it moves another step forwards to a complete understanding of the microRNA pathway.

Also in 2023, back-to-back papers in *Nature* from Kim and colleagues at Seoul University in the Republic of Korea reported new insights into how Dicer works.[358, 359] The basic requirements and actions of Dicer are the processing of double-stranded RNA of approximately 22 nucleotides in length, bearing a 2-nucleotide overhang on the 3' end and possessing a terminal loop. The team uncovered an additional feature, specifically a paired G, C or U and a mismatched C or A nucleotide pair, recognised by the RNA binding domain of Dicer. Its presence in the pre-microRNA promotes efficient processing as well as determining the cleavage site. This was not just in human cells; it was found to be the same in the fly version of Dicer, indicating deep evolutionary conservation. In the accompanying paper, the team used advanced electron microscopy to study the shape changes that occur as Dicer is in the act of cutting its substrates. This revealed previously unknown conformational changes of several sub-domains of the enzyme. The details are not important here, but this underscores how new features continue to emerge about the system. And this is just one step in microRNA biogenesis and function. It is likely that attention will continue to be focussed on other aspects with further discoveries yet to be made towards a richer understanding of the mechanisms of microRNA biogenesis.

MicroRNA Therapies

What lies ahead for microRNA-based therapies? In Chapter 7, we covered the development and clinical trial of the first microRNA drug and some of the work in the epilepsy and broader neurology field. There are still no licensed microRNA drugs on the market, although about a dozen microRNA-based therapies are in active clinical development for a variety of conditions. I am optimistic that some will be successful and that others will follow. The mechanistic roles in disease and the pleiotropic actions of microRNAs offer a unique proposition. I have argued the case of TLE, where complex, poly-pathology seems well-suited to the multi-targeting actions of microRNAs. There are also strong microRNA-based drug programmes in other complex health conditions such as heart failure. But microRNA-based therapies also have their critics. How do you predict and control the effects on targets you *don't* want? A counter to this is that unwanted effects of microRNAs on proteins besides the ones you want to modify may fall within a range that cells are able to accommodate or comfortably buffer. We have also seen the idea of target site blockers to hone disruption of microRNA targeting to single interactions. And let us not forget that the effects of traditional small molecule drugs are often far from precise. Valproate, for example, has been used to treat epilepsy for decades. The mechanism of action includes blocking sodium channels and perhaps boosting GABA in the brain. But it also has epigenetic actions which can have broad effects on gene expression.

To fully exploit the potential of microRNA therapies will require both enhancing as well as inhibiting microRNA effects and better systems than we have now for delivery to the right part of the body. This will probably be led by viral vector-based approaches. The same gene therapy backbones that can over-express a microRNA can also be used to deliver sustained knock-down. For example, incorporating antisense sequences and decoy nucleotides into the genome of the virus means that when switched on, they block microRNA activity in the infected cell. Other forms of non-coding RNA could also be coerced to help. There is a large group of non-coding RNAs that form natural circles inside cells. Some contain multiple sequences that recognise microRNAs, meaning that they function as microRNA 'sponges'. Delivery of natural or designed RNA circles could be another way to control excess microRNA activity.

Some rare and single-gene causes of disease are also being targeted with microRNA-based drugs. I am less optimistic about ultimate success here, at least against competition from traditional gene therapy approaches, but time will tell. If a successful microRNA therapy reaches the market, it will probably have an accelerator effect, driving more interest, innovation and investment so that more follow. In addition to getting a microRNA to the right cell, research needs to focus on safety. What are the long-term effects of microRNA modulation in the brain? How does this change as we age? Are their sex differences in how we react to microRNA therapies? If we can crack how to guide microRNA therapies to specific cells, this will create more-precise treatments, allowing lower doses to be used and limiting effects on gene activity in the wrong cells. Gene therapy vectors such as AAVs programmed with cell promoters will help, but there is no equivalent system yet to guide antisense-based microRNA drugs to specific brain cells. Techniques to enhance uptake by cells include attaching chemical and protein 'linkers' and antibodies that are recognised by surface receptors leading to internalisation, or enclosing in a lipid nanoparticle to better penetrate the outer membrane of cells. What other barriers are there? We have seen with the miravirsen story how competing drug modalities can crush promising microRNA-based drugs. There will be strong competition from other RNA medicine–pursuing companies and small molecule approaches. The rise of gene editing tools such as CRISPR offers the ability to correct the problem at source, inserting or deleting nucleotides in the DNA code. If mutations in microRNA genes are found to cause disease in humans, then they might be fixed with technologies such as CRISPR. If these and other hurdles can be overcome, then sometime, perhaps in the not too distant future, we will have a hospital or community-based pharmacy dispensing one or more microRNA-based drugs for a variety of health conditions.

MicroRNA-Based Switches

In Chapter 7, we encountered the idea of using signals within cells as tools to control gene therapies, that is, embedding sequences within a gene therapy that sense ambient levels of something relevant to the disease mechanism. An example is using a gene that switches on only when neurones fire excessively to power-up a potassium channel to suppress activity. MicroRNAs could be one of the ways to switch a gene therapy pay-load on or off. In the setting of epilepsy, you might use a seizure-activated microRNA as the switch. Epileptic activity causes a spike in microRNA levels which then switch on the therapy. After the seizure ends, microRNA levels re-balance and the therapy sets the pause button. This could mitigate against one of the prevailing concerns with gene therapy. That is, the indefinite pumping out of the RNA or protein in the cell, potentially beyond when it is needed or exhausting the host cell's molecular machinery. These types of microRNA-based switch and the molecular circuits they trigger are now being explored for a variety of applications. One of these relates to purification of cells for regenerative medicine. Induced pluripotent stem cells (iPSCs) offer a means to replace lost cells in the body. There are many potential applications: repair of the brain and the heart, restoring pancreatic beta islet cells in type I diabetes patients and many more. Reprogrammed cells can come from the patient who is to be treated, avoiding host/graft incompatibility. There are risks, however. The main one is incomplete differentiation. If a small number of undifferentiated cells remain, they may continue to divide when introduced into the body, becoming cancerous. It is possible to sort and purify the right cells based on surface proteins, but not all cells express unique markers. The methods to do this are also time-consuming and the physical process by which cells are drawn through sorting machines risks leaving biochemical traces that can activate host immune defences. For cell replacement therapy to be viable and reach its potential, other approaches are needed. Researchers at Kyoto University in Japan recently reported using microRNAs to achieve this goal. They took advantage of cell type–specific expression of microRNAs as a selection technique. They attached a sequence for a microRNA specific to the cell type of interest onto an mRNA sequence that coded for a sticky surface protein called CD4.[360] They then introduced this to a batch of cells. Cells that don't make the microRNA, the ones not wanted, make the surface protein. When the cells are passed through a column that binds the surface protein, they are removed. Meanwhile, cells that express the microRNA, the ones to keep, pass through the column and can be collected. The team were able to show that this created a more than 95 per cent pure population of the desired cell type. Using a cardiac cell microRNA as the selection element, the team then showed that a purified population of iPSC-derived heart cells or cardiomyocytes, grafted into the hearts of mice with tissue damage, adhered and formed functioning adult-like muscle tissue. The same team has developed a second microRNA-based switch. A sequence for a microRNA specific to a desired cell type was embedded ahead of the mRNA for a fluorescent reporter. In cells that do not make the microRNA, the reporter is made and the cells 'glow'. When the microRNA is present, marking the wanted cells, production of the reporter is blocked via a microRNA-OFF switch.[361] If the cells are all fed into a cell sorting system, the ones that glow can be kicked out, and the ones that make the microRNA retained. The researchers were also able to flip this around, creating a microRNA-ON switch. We can imagine this helping in the neurology field with, for example, motoneurone grafts, perhaps using a selection sequence for miR-218. While the purity may need to improve further, it is highly scalable and an approach with exciting potential applications in cell and regenerative therapy.

This is one of many examples from the field of synthetic RNA biology that is harnessing microRNAs to perform specific functions in artificial systems. Another recent example relates to improving gene expression efficiency. A recurring problem in the biotechnology field is that, when using a host cell, the gene to be expressed has to compete for access to the same limited molecular machinery as all the endogenous genes. The more of your artificial gene is added, the more you attenuate the cell's own gene expression. The log-jam occurs at both transcriptional and translational steps and creates unpredictable effects on the cells and the yield of the artificial gene product. It is something researchers would like to solve.

A team from the ETH in Zurich recently found a way around, incorporating microRNA sensing elements into artificial gene expression systems to alleviate the problem of resource availability in synthetic biology applications. By engineering circuits that contained a microRNA binding site, they could limit the impact of introduced artificial gene expression in the host cell.[362] Their findings have implications for the choice of cells in gene over-expression studies. Since adapting the sequences may enhance productivity, this could have commercially valuable applications in the biopharmaceutical sector.

MicroRNAs at the Centre of Battles with Invaders

We saw in Chapters 2 and 7 that microRNAs are at the centre of virus–host battles. New discoveries continue to appear with regularity. Last year, for example, a study in *Nature* from researchers in Wurzburg, Germany, reported a new mechanism by which virally encoded microRNAs control their infected hosts.[363] Herpes simplex virus deploys a microRNA from within its genome that latches onto precursor microRNAs in the infected host cells, preventing their maturation. This triggers fragmentation or fission of the host cell's mitochondria, the source of, among things, most of its cellular energy currency, ATP. Mitochondria are also needed for anti-infection responses. The team found that the virus interfered with maturation of a set of microRNAs that normally dampen the molecular machinery that allows break-up of mitochondria. The now unleashed fission process disabled anti-infection pathways and allowed the reactivation of latent virus. The viral microRNA did this by wrapping around the precursor hairpin loop of specific microRNAs, preventing their maturation. This occurred at the level of the microprocessor, the point where Drosha/DGCR8 act, rather than the Dicer step. Virus re-activation may underlie serious health effects, including encephalitis, so the findings have therapeutic applications. The team also found evidence that some endogenous microRNAs in human cells can also work this way, sticking to the hairpin loops in precursors and reducing their maturation. This is microRNAs crossing swords with one another and a new mechanism by which viruses succeed in overcoming host defences.

Viruses hijack the microRNA system in a diversity of ways, delivering their own and interfering with host microRNA mechanisms by sequestering or altering maturation. It is likely that other viral-based microRNA mechanisms will be discovered. Early into the Covid-19 pandemic, teams found that Covid-19 altered the profile of circulating microRNAs in infected people. A recent study began with the reverse approach, deducing specific microRNAs that might explain altered patterns of mRNA expression in the lungs of infected patients. This identified miR-2392.[364] Infecting cells with Covid-19 caused an elevation in miR-2392 levels and levels of miR-2392 were found to be elevated in serum and other biofluids from Covid-19–infected patients. Predicted targets of this microRNA include transcripts that regulate immune and mitochondrial pathways, and treatment of cells with miR-2392 resulted in a gene expression landscape that looked similar to the profile seen when cells were infected by Covid-19. An antimir targeting miR-2392 protected cultured cells against Covid-19 toxicity, indicating possible uses in reducing infection-related side effects. These and other findings suggest that microRNAs represent therapeutic targets for managing Covid-19 and other future infectious outbreaks. Humans are not, of course, the only target of viruses, which infect and devastate organisms. There can be little doubt that microRNA-based battles between host and invader will continue as part of the relentless evolution of the attack and defend armamentarium of life.

Integrating Detection and Deployment of MicroRNAs

New technologies are emerging that allow ever more precise measurement of microRNAs at the lowest imaginable level in cells. The ability to measure the type and the quantity of microRNAs in specific cell types within intact tissue will be a major boost for several fields, including neuroscience. Research has already appeared showing that hundreds of microRNAs can be identified and their levels quantified in single cells. Currently, this is being done by splitting a clump of cells and separating them by channelling them through microfluidic devices, a bit like one-cell-at-a-time water slides. The optimal platform for single cell microRNA analyses, the reproducibility, the limit of detection and various other factors continue to be worked out. It will be transformative if single cell microRNA measurements can be performed on intact tissue sections, particularly in my own field, where brain cell structure, diversity and organisation are highly complex in health and disease. What might we learn about a disease such as epilepsy if we can map the activity of microRNAs within living brain tissue at single cell resolution? Beyond measuring microRNAs in single cells, will it be possible to watch the loading of multiple microRNAs into AGOs in real time within human neurones in relation to changes in activity? Or to track RISCs zeroing in on their targets, picking and choosing which mRNA to target? Can we combine this with tracking the assembly of downstream components that regulate microRNA and mRNA turnover? As such approaches come online, we will have a powerful new toolkit with which to obtain insights into physiological and pathologic processes controlled by microRNAs. Since some disease-relevant microRNAs may be present in cells at very low copy number, the development of new ways to measure microRNAs in cells will help the field of diagnostics. In a recent study from a team at the University of Albany in New York State, a method of microRNA detection was developed with exquisite sensitivity using DNA-based nanoswitches.[365] The basic design comprises a single stranded DNA molecule that is adorned with two microRNA capture strands, designed to bind to the 3' or the 5' end. In the presence of the microRNA to be detected, the two strands are brought together, forming a bridge that creates a circle out of the previously linear structure of the DNA strand. That is, microRNA binding creates a loop of DNA. The number of loops reflects the number of microRNA molecules in a sample. This can then be quantified using DNA-based rather than RNA-based measurements, which are highly sensitive and have extremely low error rates. Since the nanoswitch can be introduced inside living cells, it can accurately measure microRNA abundance. Researchers are going further, however, thinking of the twin applications of microRNA research in health: detection for diagnosis and manipulation for therapeutics. These have generally moved in separate domains of research. But how about combining them and co-developing a microRNA test with a therapeutic? Now, a sub-branch of microRNA research has emerged that is taking this idea into the future. Among the groups competing in this ever more remarkable area, a team from China recently reported in *Science Advances* the creation of molecular tweezers constructed from oligonucleotide struts that formed a three-dimensional pyramid-like structure.[366] Parts of the device contain sequences complementary to microRNAs, enabling it to bind them, while another region contains a light-emitting molecule. Upon binding, the structure changes shape and this increases fluorescence, meaning that binding events that reflect counts of the microRNA can be quantified. The device was small enough to be absorbed by cells, whereupon it became functional, sensing microRNAs which it was programmed to detect. They had in effect created DNA-intelligent machines to monitor for microRNAs in cells. A further modification allowed the deployment of a microRNA-targeting antisense molecule. This and other work reveals the exciting frontiers at which microRNA-based applications may continue to push.

Genetics and Modelling

Most of the major links between microRNAs and disease have come from work on RNA that either directly finds altered amounts of specific microRNAs or infers their gain/loss effects by observing patterns of target mRNA expression. Researchers have also identified genome-level changes to microRNAs, via inherited or new (*de novo*) mutations in DNA sequence. This has been found at both precursor and mature sequence level. But, overall, the major international projects and consortia researching the genetics of diseases such as schizophrenia, autism and epilepsy, for example, remain focused on the protein-coding portion of the genome. Ever-greater numbers of DNA samples are being pooled and meta-analyses performed to create better statistical predictions of how gene variation accounts for disease. We can expect to find evidence that variation in microRNA sequences drives disease risk. But there is inherently more tolerance for DNA code variants for non-coding RNAs such as microRNA than for protein-coding genes. A single base change in a protein coding gene can upset the triplet code and trigger a stop in protein production or insertion of an amino acid that collapses the function of the protein. A nucleotide base change in a microRNA is less likely to have such devastating effects. But perhaps effects have been missed or overlooked? Part of the problem is that predicting the impact, if any, of variants within a mature microRNA remains challenging and more so for variants outside the seed and in precursors of microRNAs. And just because a nucleotide in a microRNA is different does not mean that it will stay that way. As we saw earlier, microRNAs can be edited, so germline changes may not always track all the way through to the final active microRNA. Machine learning and other tools will increasingly improve predictions of the effects of variation in non-coding RNAs, and the structure–function relationship of RNA–protein interactions. So, genetics will have increasingly more to say about the microRNA world. Indeed, a recent genome-wide association study which searched for variants in genes from 40,000 people worldwide with bipolar disorder found a 'hotspot' at the *MIR124* gene locus. This inspired teams from Johns Hopkins University in Baltimore to check for levels of miR-124 in human cell models of schizophrenia and bipolar disorder, which are known to share some genetic risks in common.[367] This revealed that miR-124 was elevated in both models. In contrast, miR-137, which we met previously, was only elevated in the model of schizophrenia. Further screening showed that the elevation in miR-124 in both disorders was unique among tested microRNAs and was also found in patient brain tissue. Combining a measurement of the levels of miR-124 and genetic data explained a significant proportion of risk for the two disorders. Mice engineered to overproduce miR-124 within excitatory neurones in a part of the brain linked to the two disorders, called the medial prefrontal cortex, displayed altered behaviours, including social interactions. How this works remains unclear, but elevated miR-124 was found to change the amplitude of currents in neurones by reducing the amounts of a glutamate-response receptor, a specific change to synaptic communication that could render networks more excitable or disorganised. The findings provide a plausible explanation for some of the shared features of the two disorders and could open up new therapeutic approaches, either targeting the microRNA or rescuing the over-suppression of miR-124 target gene(s).

That study used an innovative approach to model brain disease. The human neurones came from the nasal epithelium of patients. Access to live brain tissue, unlike the situation in the epilepsy field, is rare or impossible for diseases such as schizophrenia. The nasal samples contain neurone-like cells of the olfactory system. Models like this are powerful new resources for discoveries on microRNAs. We have seen throughout the book the advances made using model organisms such as *C. elegans* and mice. They are and will continue to be supplemented or replaced with human models. The technology to make organoids from iPSCs is already game-changing. We can create sophisticated multi-lobe mini-brains. Researchers are even able to interlace brain cells with microscopic blood vessels to create more realistic living systems. Fluorescent markers can then be introduced that glow in response to cell activity, enabling recordings of the activities of hundreds of human neurones at once in real time. Researchers can study how whole networks in the brain change upon changes to microRNA activity. The human models can be seeded by cells from patients that carry a mutation or the mutation can be replicated, using a tool such as CRISPR. But mini-brains do not yet allow us to study behaviours. Model organisms such as mice will continue to play a valuable role here, where we can test their cognition, emotions, curiosity, alertness, sociability and how these vary with age and sex. The future will be a varied blend of these human and other model species, selected to answer the right questions with the best possible tools.

Timing of the Tuning

One of the most interesting biological processes controlled by microRNAs is *circadian rhythm*, that is, our body clock(s). This refers to the 24-hour cycles that regulate alertness and sleep, body temperature, appetite and food intake, and much more. The body's clock system is essential for the correct functioning of multiple systems in our body. We know this because disruption to circadian cycles is associated with obesity, type 2 diabetes and poor mental health. The physiological importance of sleep is increasingly understood. Studies in mice show that the physical spaces between brain cells widen slightly during specific phases of sleep, allowing the drainage of extracellular debris out of the brain. This process, achieved by a specialised vascular system called glymphatics, is impaired by poor sleep.[368] As a result, therapies targeting this system are being looked at as a potential solution to the build-up of extracellular β-Amyloid plaques in Alzheimer's disease. The central synchroniser for our daily cycles is the suprachiasmatic nucleus, found within the hypothalamus in the brain. This coordinates information from specialised ganglion cells in our retina, separate from the rods and cones discussed previously, that are non-image forming and instead feed their signals to this part of the brain. From there, the nucleus triggers the tissue and cell clocks via neural and hormone-based mechanisms. This includes 'sub-clocks' in multiple parts of the body which set circadian processes, including in the cardiovascular and immune systems. The expression of many genes undergoes rhythmic cycling, increasing or decreasing at certain times of the day.

The circadian cycle is set by the oscillating actions of a set of transcription factors. The basic loop involves formation of a complex of two proteins called CLOCK and BMAL1 which then promote expression of two further sets of genes called *PER 1, 2* and *CRY 1, 2*. After these are translated, they translocate to the nucleus and suppress CLOCK/BMAL1 activity. So, the system has built-in negative feedback whereby the PER-CRY complex inhibits transcription mediated by CLOCK and BMAL1. Two further loops support the cycling function and protein degradation also plays a key role. Research several years ago uncovered key roles for microRNAs in regulating levels of the core machinery of the mammalian clock system.[369] For example, the CLOCK-BMAL1 complex promotes transcription of specific microRNAs, including miR-219, and this and other microRNAs display a robust circadian pattern of up- and down-regulation, peaking at different times of the day, in the suprachiasmatic nucleus. Genetic studies in mice show that deletion of core clock components such as the two *Cry* genes stops this microRNA cycling behaviour. MicroRNAs have been found to mediate effects both during light entrainment and in the length of the active phase of the day–night cycle. Thus, there are separate light-responsive microRNAs and clock-regulated microRNAs active in this brain region. Targets of these microRNAs include transcription factors that mediate changes in gene expression essential to the circadian system. MicroRNA-controlled circadian functions are also important outside the brain. Macrophages are a subtype of immune cell that also display circadian cycles, presumably as a way to optimise their activity to the phases in which they are most likely to encounter pathogens. Studies show that a sepsis-like infectious stimulus up-regulates miR-155 which then targets *Bmal1*, resulting in changes to the circadian rhythm and altered macrophage function.[370] Research by my colleagues at RCSI has shown that the physical shape of mitochondria, the engines of cellular energy, changes over a 24-hour period.[371] Mitochondria in immune cells form networks during the rest phase, becoming more disconnected during activity. While the benefits of the connected phase are not yet clear, these and other findings are thought to explain why poor sleep is associated with altered immunity. Indeed, disruption to the clock gene system in specific immune cells renders them less responsive to vaccine exposure. This suggests that tailored timing of vaccinations may enhance protection. These and other findings demonstrate that microRNAs within the suprachiasmatic nucleus and beyond function to fine-tune the gene expression landscape that underlies the central and peripheral control of the circadian-timing process in health and disease. This raises opportunities for therapies based on targeting microRNAs to restore circadian function.

Now, I am bending the rules including this in a 'future' section since the microRNA–circadian link was discovered some years ago. There is extensive ongoing work, however, revealing additional microRNAs underpinning the circadian functions of cells and tissues in a variety of systems. These may also include epilepsy. It has been known for some time that seizures occur in clusters in some patients, including over circadian and multi-dien timescales.[372] This may be influenced by disruption to the clock mechanisms within the brain. Indeed, triggering TLE in rats leads to re-timing of the normal circadian-cycling patterns of gene expression in the hippocampus. This includes transcripts gaining a circadian pattern that normally do not cycle and transcripts that normally cycle losing this ability. Such changes may also underlie why good sleep hygiene has been proven to help reduce seizure occurrence in some people with epilepsy. Is the disturbed circadian gene expression in epilepsy an effect of altered control by microRNAs? Ongoing research is aiming to find out.

Future Diagnostics

How might efforts to develop blood and other biofluid-based biomarkers develop in the next years? For many diseases, there is still much to do in terms of demonstrating reproducibility, refining the set of microRNAs and testing how they perform over time and in different cohorts. By learning how microRNAs circulate and the optimal biofluid that combines least-invasive source with greatest yield of molecular information, then linking all this back to the disease, we are likely to see more microRNA-based diagnostics reaching the clinic. Could microRNA point-of-care tests reach the bedside or the home? Let us jump further into the future. Perhaps, if all the barriers ahead are overcome, we might see a scenario like the following play out one day. A nurse/doctor/specialist, having completed their patient's history taking, clinical examination and perhaps other suitable diagnostic tests, takes a blood or other biofluid sample. The fluid is drawn into a device that separates the cells from the surrounding fluid, passing them over detectors primed for full genome analysis, measurement of mRNAs and specific microRNAs. Perhaps additional chemical modifications, more refined markers of health, are also screened. Within minutes, a reading emerges, revealing telltale patterns that can be integrated with the collected clinical information. Analysing the data in fractions of a second, it generates a risk and disease profile that narrows down the diagnosis. But this is not the end. The results are now forwarded for custom design of a patient-specific RNA medicine, perhaps antimirs or microRNA mimics, which are rapidly synthesised, purified and decanted into an injectable solution. Perhaps this is a difficult case, a profile not seen before, with patterns of gene expression altered that do not line up with any endogenous microRNAs. After studying the profile, an entirely new microRNA is designed to correct the gene profile, perhaps even a cocktail of antimirs that tackle the problem. The patient is treated, sent home and their symptoms resolve. Is this scenario likely? How far into the future? I don't know. Let's wait and see . . ..

Improving the Next Generation?

In Chapter 4, we covered the discovery that microRNAs are present within sperm and, upon fertilisation, appear capable of affecting early gene expression programmes during embryo development. More remarkable still, the composition of sperm microRNAs is sensitive to a variety of environmental exposures, including stress, and the effects of this can be detected in the offspring. If sperm microRNAs can produce intergenerational effects that confer advantages or disadvantages on the 'fitness' of the next generation, this raises the prospect of fertility-related applications. What if we could adjust the sperm microRNA content to enhance or oppose these effects? What if we could cancel out the effects of traumatic experiences on the next generation by adjusting the sperm microRNA content? What if we could enhance beneficial effects conveyed by sperm microRNA, such as resilience to stress or a diabetes-resistant metabolism? This is currently not possible and there may never be a way to achieve the desired effects. Any such technology would also have profound ethical implications. For now, we are left with the thought experiment that we might one day be able to safely tinker with the microRNA contents of sperm or egg cell to influence the behaviours of a future child. But should we, even if we could?

Solutions to Life's Last Challenge?

MicroRNAs appear at the earliest moments of life, as we develop, shaping the gene expression patterns that define who we will become. They are still with us as adults, but are they there at the end and what are they up to? Ageing is something we cannot avoid. As a species, humans are living longer, but can we stay healthy for longer? New research shows that microRNAs have important roles in a process related to cell ageing called senescence. Nicknamed *geromirs*, research has identified changes to levels of certain microRNAs during the ageing process in animals.[373] This includes both higher and lower levels of microRNAs and each body system seems to be associated with specific ageing-related microRNA changes. These microRNA changes represent more than passive biomarkers of ageing, however. Functional studies show that several microRNAs regulate levels of known ageing-related biochemical pathways. There is evidence that the pathway that leads to cellular senescence, the deterioration that accompanies ageing, is druggable. In fact, eliminating senescent cells has been reported to have rejuvenating effects in animals. Since the biochemical pathway of ageing is regulated by specific microRNAs, this raises the exciting prospect that we might, one day, be taking a microRNA-based treatment to prolong life or improve health into our old age.

Other-World MicroRNAs?

MicroRNAs are found in every branch of the tree of multicellular life, even in some unicellular organisms, and in every major ecosystem on Earth. They evolved at the very earliest moments, within the simplest and most ancient forms of eukaryotic life. MicroRNA are present among highly adapted species for extreme conditions, having been recently mapped in the genomes of Antarctic-dwelling icefish.[374] I will finish with a speculation that if extraterrestrial life exists – and I have no doubt that it is out there somewhere – we will find a microRNA-like regulator as part of its alien molecular make-up. As we turn our telescopes and perhaps spacecraft to monitor for signs of life on other planets, it may be that a signature will be found, or a sample one day obtained. Proof of the pervasive nature of these wondrous molecules. Conducting the molecular orchestra in some distant corner of the universe in whatever form of life that takes . . ..

References

1 Lee R. C., Feinbaum R. L., Ambros V. The *C. elegans* heterochronic gene lin-4 encodes small RNAs with antisense complementarity to lin-14. *Cell.* 1993;**75**:843–54.

2 Ambros V. The evolution of our thinking about microRNAs. *Nat Med.* 2008;**14**:1036–40.

3 Wightman B., Ha I., Ruvkun G. Posttranscriptional regulation of the heterochronic gene lin-14 by lin-4 mediates temporal pattern formation in *C. elegans*. *Cell.* 1993;**75**:855–62.

4 Reinhart B. J., Slack F. J., Basson M., Pasquinelli A. E., Bettinger J. C., Rougvie A. E., et al. The 21-nucleotide let-7 RNA regulates developmental timing in *Caenorhabditis elegans*. *Nature.* 2000;**403**:901–6.

5 Pasquinelli A. E., Reinhart B. J., Slack F., Martindale M. Q., Kuroda M. I., Maller B., et al. Conservation of the sequence and temporal expression of let-7 heterochronic regulatory RNA. *Nature.* 2000;**408**:86–9.

6 Ruvkun G. Molecular biology: glimpses of a tiny RNA world. *Science.* 2001;**294**:797–9.

7 Fire A., Xu S., Montgomery M. K., Kostas S. A., Driver S. E., Mello C. C. Potent and specific genetic interference by double-stranded RNA in *Caenorhabditis elegans*. *Nature.* 1998;**391**:806–11.

8 Hamilton A. J., Baulcombe D. C. A species of small antisense RNA in posttranscriptional gene silencing in plants. *Science.* 1999;**286**:950–2.

9 Bartel D. P. MicroRNAs: genomics, biogenesis, mechanism, and function. *Cell.* 2004;**116**:281–97.

10 Brennan G. P., Henshall D. C. MicroRNAs as regulators of brain function and targets for treatment of epilepsy. *Nat Rev Neurol.* 2020;**16**:506–19.

11 Lagos-Quintana M., Rauhut R., Lendeckel W., Tuschl T. Identification of novel genes coding for small expressed RNAs. *Science.* 2001;**294**:853–8.

12 Editorial. Henrietta Lacks: science must right a historical wrong. *Nature.* 2020;**585**:7.

13 Lau N. C., Lim L. P., Weinstein E. G., Bartel D. P. An abundant class of tiny RNAs with probable regulatory roles in *Caenorhabditis elegans*. *Science.* 2001;**294**:858–62.

14 Lee R. C., Ambros V. An extensive class of small RNAs in *Caenorhabditis elegans*. *Science.* 2001;**294**:862–4.

15 Mathews D. H., Sabina J., Zuker M., Turner D. H. Expanded sequence dependence of thermodynamic parameters improves prediction of RNA secondary structure. *J Mol Biol.* 1999;**288**:911–40.

16 Grishok A., Pasquinelli A. E., Conte D., Li N., Parrish S., Ha I., et al. Genes and mechanisms related to RNA interference regulate expression of the small temporal RNAs that control *C. elegans* developmental timing. *Cell.* 2001;**106**:23–34.

17 Ambros V. MicroRNAs: tiny regulators with great potential. *Cell.* 2001;**107**:823–6.

18 Mourelatos Z., Dostie J., Paushkin S., Sharma A., Charroux B., Abel L., et al. miRNPs: a novel class of ribonucleoproteins containing numerous microRNAs. *Genes Dev.* 2002;**16**:720–8.

19 Calin G. A., Dumitru C. D., Shimizu M., Bichi R., Zupo S., Noch E., et al. Frequent deletions and down-regulation of micro-RNA genes miR15 and miR16 at 13q14 in chronic lymphocytic leukemia. *Proc Natl Acad Sci U S A.* 2002;**99**:15524–9.

20 Lagos-Quintana M., Rauhut R., Yalcin A., Meyer J., Lendeckel W., Tuschl T. Identification of tissue-specific microRNAs from mouse. *Curr Biol.* 2002;**12**:735–9.

21 Zeng Y., Wagner E. J., Cullen B. R. Both natural and designed micro RNAs can inhibit the expression of cognate mRNAs when expressed in human cells. *Mol Cell.* 2002;**9**:1327–33.

22 Reinhart B. J., Weinstein E. G., Rhoades M. W., Bartel B., Bartel D. P. MicroRNAs in plants. *Genes Dev.* 2002;**16**:1616–26.

23 Hutvagner G., Zamore P. D. A microRNA in a multiple-turnover RNAi enzyme complex. *Science.* 2002;**297**:2056–60.

24 Lagos-Quintana M., Rauhut R., Meyer J., Borkhardt A., Tuschl T. New microRNAs from mouse and human. *RNA.* 2003;**9**:175–9.

25 Lee Y., Ahn C., Han J., Choi H., Kim J., Yim J., et al. The nuclear RNase III Drosha initiates microRNA processing. *Nature.* 2003;**425**:415–9.

26 Yi R., Qin Y., Macara I. G., Cullen B. R. Exportin-5 mediates the nuclear export of pre-microRNAs and short hairpin RNAs. *Genes Dev.* 2003;**17**:3011–6.

27 Lim L. P., Glasner M. E., Yekta S., Burge C. B., Bartel D. P. Vertebrate microRNA genes. *Science.* 2003;**299**:1540.

28 Kasschau K. D., Xie Z., Allen E., Llave C., Chapman E. J., Krizan K. A., et al. P1/HC-Pro, a viral suppressor of RNA silencing, interferes with Arabidopsis development and miRNA function. *Dev Cell.* 2003;**4**:205–17.

29 Ambros V. MicroRNA pathways in flies and worms: growth, death, fat, stress, and timing. *Cell.* 2003;**113**:673–6.

30 Houbaviy H. B., Murray M. F., Sharp P. A. Embryonic stem cell-specific microRNAs. *Dev Cell.* 2003;**5**:351–8.

31 Krichevsky A. M., King K. S., Donahue C. P., Khrapko K., Kosik K. S. A microRNA array reveals extensive regulation of microRNAs during brain development. *RNA.* 2003;**9**:1274–81.

32 Johnson S. M., Lin S. Y., Slack F. J. The time of appearance of the *C. elegans* let-7 microRNA is transcriptionally controlled utilizing a temporal regulatory element in its promoter. *Dev Biol.* 2003;**259**:364–79.

33 Khvorova A., Reynolds A., Jayasena S. D. Functional siRNAs and miRNAs exhibit strand bias. *Cell.* 2003;**115**:209–16.

34 Lewis B. P., Shih I. H., Jones-Rhoades M. W., Bartel D. P., Burge C. B. Prediction of mammalian microRNA targets. *Cell.* 2003;**115**:787–98.

35 Lim L. P., Lau N. C., Garrett-Engele P., Grimson A., Schelter J. M., Castle J., et al. Microarray analysis shows that some microRNAs downregulate large numbers of target mRNAs. *Nature.* 2005;**433**:769–73.

36 Baek D., Villen J., Shin C., Camargo F. D., Gygi S. P., Bartel D. P. The impact of microRNAs on protein output. *Nature.* 2008;**455**:64–71.

37 Friedman R. C., Farh K. K., Burge C. B., Bartel D. P. Most mammalian mRNAs are conserved targets of microRNAs. *Genome Res.* 2009;**19**:92–105.

38 Gebert L. F. R., MacRae I. J. Regulation of microRNA function in animals. *Nat Rev Mol Cell Biol.* 2019;**20**:21–37.

39 Raj A., van Oudenaarden A. Nature, nurture, or chance: stochastic gene expression and its consequences. *Cell.* 2008;**135**:216–26.

40 Ebert M. S., Sharp P. A. Roles for microRNAs in conferring robustness to biological processes. *Cell.* 2012;**149**:515–24.

41 Li Y., Wang F., Lee J. A., Gao F. B. MicroRNA-9a ensures the precise specification of sensory organ precursors in Drosophila. *Genes Dev.* 2006;**20**:2793–805.

42 Hornstein E., Shomron N. Canalization of development by microRNAs. *Nat Genet.* 2006;**38** Suppl:S20–4.

43 Berezikov E. Evolution of microRNA diversity and regulation in animals. *Nat Rev Genet.* 2011;**12**:846–60.

44 Alles J., Fehlmann T., Fischer U., Backes C., Galata V., Minet M., et al. An estimate of the total number of true human miRNAs. *Nucleic Acids Res.* 2019;**47**:3353–64.

45 Londin E., Loher P., Telonis A. G., Quann K., Clark P., Jing Y., et al. Analysis of 13 cell types reveals evidence for the expression of numerous novel primate- and tissue-specific microRNAs. *Proc Natl Acad Sci U S A.* 2015;**112**:E1106–15.

46 Drouin G., Godin J. R., Page B. The genetics of vitamin C loss in vertebrates. *Curr Genomics.* 2011;**12**:371–8.

47 Moroz L. L., Kocot K. M., Citarella M. R., Dosung S., Norekian T. P.,

Povolotskaya I. S., et al. The ctenophore genome and the evolutionary origins of neural systems. *Nature*. 2014;**510**:109–14.

48 Calcino A. D., Fernandez-Valverde S. L., Taft R. J., Degnan B. M. Diverse RNA interference strategies in early-branching metazoans. *BMC Evol Biol*. 2018;**18**:160–72.

49 Gouzouasis V., Tastsoglou S., Giannakakis A., Hatzigeorgiou A. G. Virus-derived small RNAs and microRNAs in health and disease. *Annu Rev Biomed Data Sci*. 2023;**6**:275–98.

50 Brawand D., Wagner C. E., Li Y. I., Malinsky M., Keller I., Fan S., et al. The genomic substrate for adaptive radiation in African cichlid fish. *Nature*. 2014;**513**:375–81.

51 Mehta T. K., Penso-Dolfin L., Nash W., Roy S., Di-Palma F., Haerty W. Evolution of miRNA-binding sites and regulatory networks in cichlids. *Mol Biol Evol*. 2022;**39**: msac146.

52 Sunkar R., Li Y. F., Jagadeeswaran G. Functions of microRNAs in plant stress responses. *Trends Plant Sci*. 2012;**17**:196–203.

53 He M., Kong X., Jiang Y., Qu H., Zhu H. MicroRNAs: emerging regulators in horticultural crops. *Trends Plant Sci*. 2022;**27**:936–51.

54 Axtell M. J., Bowman J. L. Evolution of plant microRNAs and their targets. *Trends Plant Sci*. 2008;**13**:343–9.

55 Cuperus J. T., Fahlgren N., Carrington J. C. Evolution and functional diversification of MIRNA genes. *Plant Cell*. 2011;**23**:431–42.

56 Taylor R. S., Tarver J. E., Hiscock S. J., Donoghue P. C. Evolutionary history of plant microRNAs. *Trends Plant Sci*. 2014;**19**:175–82.

57 Betti F., Ladera-Carmona M. J., Weits D. A., Ferri G., Iacopino S., Novi G., et al. Exogenous miRNAs induce post-transcriptional gene silencing in plants. *Nat Plants*. 2021;**7**:1379–88.

58 Chen X., Rechavi O. Plant and animal small RNA communications between cells and organisms. *Nat Rev Mol Cell Biol*. 2022;**23**:185–203.

59 Kosik K. S., Nowakowski T. Evolution of new miRNAs and cerebro-cortical development. *Annu Rev Neurosci*. 2018;**41**:119–37.

60 Hu H. Y., He L., Fominykh K., Yan Z., Guo S., Zhang X., et al. Evolution of the human-specific microRNA miR-941. *Nat Commun*. 2012;**3**:1145.

61 Nowakowski T. J., Rani N., Golkaram M., Zhou H. R., Alvarado B., Huch K., et al. Regulation of cell-type-specific transcriptomes by microRNA networks during human brain development. *Nat Neurosci*. 2018;**21**:1784–92.

62 McCreight J. C., Schneider S. E., Wilburn D. B., Swanson W. J. Evolution of microRNA in primates. *PLoS One*. 2017;**12**: e0176596.

63 Bohmert K., Camus I., Bellini C., Bouchez D., Caboche M., Benning C. AGO1 defines a novel locus of Arabidopsis controlling leaf development. *EMBO J*. 1998;**17**:170–80.

64 Tomari Y., Zamore P. D. MicroRNA biogenesis: drosha can't cut it without a partner. *Curr Biol*. 2005;**15**:R61–4.

65 Lee Y., Kim M., Han J., Yeom K. H., Lee S., Baek S. H., et al. MicroRNA genes are transcribed by RNA polymerase II. *EMBO J*. 2004;**23**:4051–60.

66 O'Donnell K. A., Wentzel E. A., Zeller K. I., Dang C. V., Mendell J. T. c-Myc-regulated microRNAs modulate E2F1 expression. *Nature*. 2005;**435**:839–43.

67 He L., He X., Lim L. P., de Stanchina E., Xuan Z., Liang Y., et al. A microRNA component of the p53 tumour suppressor network. *Nature*. 2007;**447**:1130–4.

68 Raver-Shapira N., Marciano E., Meiri E., Spector Y., Rosenfeld N., Moskovits N., et al. Transcriptional activation of miR-34a contributes to p53-mediated apoptosis. *Mol Cell*. 2007;**26**:731–43.

69 Chang T. C., Wentzel E. A., Kent O. A., Ramachandran K., Mullendore M., Lee K. H., et al. Transactivation of miR-34a by p53 broadly influences gene expression and promotes apoptosis. *Mol Cell*. 2007;**26**:745–52.

70 Landgraf P., Rusu M., Sheridan R.,
    Sewer A., Iovino N., Aravin A., et al.
    A mammalian microRNA expression atlas
    based on small RNA library sequencing.
    Cell. 2007;**129**:1401–14.

71 Fiore R., Khudayberdiev S., Christensen M.,
    Siegel G., Flavell S. W., Kim T. K., et al. Mef2-
    mediated transcription of the miR379-410
    cluster regulates activity-dependent
    dendritogenesis by fine-tuning Pumilio2
    protein levels. *EMBO J.* 2009;**28**:697–710.

72 Miller-Delaney S. F., Bryan K., Das S.,
    McKiernan R. C., Bray I. M., Reynolds J. P.,
    et al. Differential DNA methylation profiles
    of coding and non-coding genes define
    hippocampal sclerosis in human temporal
    lobe epilepsy. *Brain.* 2015;**138**:616–31.

73 Borchert G. M., Lanier W., Davidson B. L.
    RNA polymerase III transcribes human
    microRNAs. *Nat Struct Mol Biol.* 2006;**13**:
    1097–101.

74 Filippov V., Solovyev V., Filippova M.,
    Gill S. S. A novel type of RNase III family
    proteins in eukaryotes. *Gene.*
    2000;**245**:213–21.

75 Ruiz-Arroyo V. M., Nam Y. Dynamic
    protein-RNA recognition in primary
    microRNA processing. *Curr Opin Struct
    Biol.* 2022;**76**:102442.

76 Gregory R. I., Yan K. P., Amuthan G.,
    Chendrimada T., Doratotaj B., Cooch N.,
    et al. The microprocessor complex mediates
    the genesis of microRNAs. *Nature.*
    2004;**432**:235–40.

77 Kwon S. C., Nguyen T. A., Choi Y. G.,
    Jo M. H., Hohng S., Kim V. N., et al.
    Structure of human DROSHA. *Cell.*
    2016;**164**:81–90.

78 Partin A. C., Zhang K., Jeong B. C.,
    Herrell E., Li S., Chiu W., et al. Cryo-EM
    structures of human drosha and DGCR8 in
    complex with primary microRNA. *Mol Cell.*
    2020;**78**:411–22 e4.

79 Morlando M., Ballarino M., Gromak N.,
    Pagano F., Bozzoni I., Proudfoot N. J.
    Primary microRNA transcripts are
    processed co-transcriptionally. *Nat Struct
    Mol Biol.* 2008;**15**:902–9.

80 Ha M., Kim V. N. Regulation of microRNA
    biogenesis. *Nat Rev Mol Cell Biol.*
    2014;**15**:509–24.

81 Treiber T., Treiber N., Meister G.
    Regulation of microRNA biogenesis and its
    crosstalk with other cellular pathways. *Nat
    Rev Mol Cell Biol.* 2019;**20**:5–20.

82 Lund E., Guttinger S., Calado A.,
    Dahlberg J. E., Kutay U. Nuclear export of
    microRNA precursors. *Science.* 2004;**303**:95–8.

83 Hammond S. M., Bernstein E., Beach D.,
    Hannon G. J. An RNA-directed nuclease
    mediates post-transcriptional gene
    silencing in Drosophila cells. *Nature.*
    2000;**404**:293–6.

84 Bernstein E., Caudy A. A., Hammond S. M.,
    Hannon G. J. Role for a bidentate
    ribonuclease in the initiation step of RNA
    interference. *Nature.* 2001;**409**:363–6.

85 Hutvagner G., McLachlan J.,
    Pasquinelli A. E., Balint E., Tuschl T.,
    Zamore P. D. A cellular function for the
    RNA-interference enzyme Dicer in the
    maturation of the let-7 small temporal
    RNA. *Science.* 2001;**293**:834–8.

86 Knight S. W., Bass B. L. A role for the RNase
    III enzyme DCR-1 in RNA interference and
    germ line development in Caenorhabditis
    elegans. *Science.* 2001;**293**:2269–71.

87 Shang R., Lee S., Senavirathne G., Lai E. C.
    MicroRNAs in action: biogenesis, function
    and regulation. *Nat Rev Genet.* 2023;**24**:
    816–33.

88 Macrae I. J., Zhou K., Li F., Repic A.,
    Brooks A. N., Cande W. Z., et al. Structural
    basis for double-stranded RNA processing
    by Dicer. *Science.* 2006;**311**:195–8.

89 Chendrimada T. P., Gregory R. I.,
    Kumaraswamy E., Norman J., Cooch N.,
    Nishikura K., et al. TRBP recruits the Dicer
    complex to Ago2 for microRNA processing
    and gene silencing. *Nature.* 2005;**436**:740–4.

90 Liu Z., Wang J., Cheng H., Ke X., Sun L.,
    Zhang Q. C., et al. Cryo-EM structure of
    human Dicer and its complexes with a
    pre-miRNA substrate. *Cell.* 2018;**173**:1191–
    203 e12.

91 Ruby J. G., Jan C. H., Bartel D. P. Intronic microRNA precursors that bypass Drosha processing. *Nature*. 2007;**448**:83–6.

92 Okamura K., Hagen J. W., Duan H., Tyler D. M., Lai E. C. The mirtron pathway generates microRNA-class regulatory RNAs in Drosophila. *Cell*. 2007;**130**:89–100.

93 Berezikov E., Chung W. J., Willis J., Cuppen E., Lai E. C. Mammalian mirtron genes. *Mol Cell*. 2007;**28**:328–36.

94 Cheloufi S., Dos Santos C. O., Chong M. M., Hannon G. J. A Dicer-independent miRNA biogenesis pathway that requires Ago catalysis. *Nature*. 2010;**465**:584–9.

95 Schwarz D. S., Hutvagner G., Du T., Xu Z., Aronin N., Zamore P. D. Asymmetry in the assembly of the RNAi enzyme complex. *Cell*. 2003;**115**:199–208.

96 Sheu-Gruttadauria J., MacRae I. J. Structural foundations of RNA silencing by Argonaute. *J Mol Biol*. 2017;**429**:2619–39.

97 Chandradoss S. D., Schirle N. T., Szczepaniak M., MacRae I. J., Joo C. A dynamic search process underlies microRNA targeting. *Cell*. 2015;**162**:96–107.

98 Bartel D. P. Metazoan microRNAs. *Cell*. 2018;**173**:20–51.

99 Schirle N. T., MacRae I. J. The crystal structure of human Argonaute2. *Science*. 2012;**336**:1037–40.

100 Schirle N. T., Sheu-Gruttadauria J., MacRae I. J. Structural basis for microRNA targeting. *Science*. 2014;**346**:608–13.

101 Leung A. K. L. The whereabouts of microRNA actions: cytoplasm and beyond. *Trends Cell Biol*. 2015;**25**:601–10.

102 Trabucchi M., Mategot R. Subcellular heterogeneity of the microRNA machinery. *Trends Genet*. 2019;**35**:15–28.

103 Meller R., Thompson S. J., Lusardi T. A., Ordonez A. N., Ashley M. D., Jessick V., et al. Ubiquitin proteasome-mediated synaptic reorganization: a novel mechanism underlying rapid ischemic tolerance. *J Neurosci*. 2008;**28**:50–9.

104 Engel T., Martinez-Villarreal J., Henke C., Jimenez-Mateos E. M., Sanz-Rodriguez A., Alves M., et al. Spatiotemporal progression of ubiquitin-proteasome system inhibition after status epilepticus suggests protective adaptation against hippocampal injury. *Mol Neurodegener*. 2017;**12**:21.

105 Ruegger S., Grosshans H. MicroRNA turnover: when, how, and why. *Trends Biochem Sci*. 2012;**37**:436–46.

106 Krol J., Loedige I., Filipowicz W. The widespread regulation of microRNA biogenesis, function and decay. *Nat Rev Genet*. 2010;**11**:597–610.

107 Han J., Mendell J. T. MicroRNA turnover: a tale of tailing, trimming, and targets. *Trends Biochem Sci*. 2023;**48**:26–39.

108 Krol J., Busskamp V., Markiewicz I., Stadler M. B., Ribi S., Richter J., et al. Characterizing light-regulated retinal microRNAs reveals rapid turnover as a common property of neuronal microRNAs. *Cell*. 2010;**141**:618–31.

109 Ramachandran V., Chen X. Degradation of microRNAs by a family of exoribonucleases in Arabidopsis. *Science*. 2008;**321**:1490–2.

110 Han J., LaVigne C. A., Jones B. T., Zhang H., Gillett F., Mendell J. T. A ubiquitin ligase mediates target-directed microRNA decay independently of tailing and trimming. *Science*. 2020;**370**: eabc9546.

111 Bernstein E., Kim S. Y., Carmell M. A., Murchison E. P., Alcorn H., Li M. Z., et al. Dicer is essential for mouse development. *Nat Genet*. 2003;**35**:215–17.

112 Liu J., Carmell M. A., Rivas F. V., Marsden C. G., Thomson J. M., Song J. J., et al. Argonaute2 is the catalytic engine of mammalian RNAi. *Science*. 2004;**305**: 1437–41.

113 Wang Y., Medvid R., Melton C., Jaenisch R., Blelloch R. DGCR8 is essential for microRNA biogenesis and silencing of embryonic stem cell self-renewal. *Nat Genet*. 2007;**39**:380–5.

114 Schaefer A., O'Carroll D., Tan C. L., Hillman D., Sugimori M., Llinas R., et al. Cerebellar neurodegeneration in the absence of microRNAs. *J Exp Med.* 2007;**204**:1553–8.

115 Cuellar T. L., Davis T. H., Nelson P. T., Loeb G. B., Harfe B. D., Ullian E., et al. Dicer loss in striatal neurons produces behavioral and neuroanatomical phenotypes in the absence of neurodegeneration. *Proc Natl Acad Sci U S A.* 2008;**105**:5614–19.

116 Tao J., Wu H., Lin Q., Wei W., Lu X. H., Cantle J. P., et al. Deletion of astroglial Dicer causes non-cell-autonomous neuronal dysfunction and degeneration. *J Neurosci.* 2011;**31**:8306–19.

117 Harfe B. D., McManus M. T., Mansfield J. H., Hornstein E., Tabin C. J. The RNaseIII enzyme Dicer is required for morphogenesis but not patterning of the vertebrate limb. *Proc Natl Acad Sci U S A.* 2005;**102**:10898–903.

118 Hang Q., Zeng L., Wang L., Nie L., Yao F., Teng H., et al. Non-canonical function of DGCR8 in DNA double-strand break repair signaling and tumor radioresistance. *Nat Commun.* 2021;**12**:4033.

119 La Rocca G., King B., Shui B., Li X., Zhang M., Akat K. M., et al. Inducible and reversible inhibition of miRNA-mediated gene repression in vivo. *Elife.* 2021;**10**: e70948.

120 Zhao Y., Ransom J. F., Li A., Vedantham V., von Drehle M., Muth A. N., et al. Dysregulation of cardiogenesis, cardiac conduction, and cell cycle in mice lacking miRNA-1–2. *Cell.* 2007;**129**:303–17.

121 Heidersbach A., Saxby C., Carver-Moore K., Huang Y., Ang Y. S., de Jong P. J., et al. MicroRNA-1 regulates sarcomere formation and suppresses smooth muscle gene expression in the mammalian heart. *Elife.* 2013;**2**:e01323.

122 Jacobs G. H., Williams G. A., Cahill H., Nathans J. Emergence of novel color vision in mice engineered to express a human cone photopigment. *Science.* 2007;**315**:1723–5.

123 Busskamp V., Krol J., Nelidova D., Daum J., Szikra T., Tsuda B., et al. miRNAs 182 and 183 are necessary to maintain adult cone photoreceptor outer segments and visual function. *Neuron.* 2014;**83**:586–600.

124 Lumayag S., Haldin C. E., Corbett N. J., Wahlin K. J., Cowan C., Turturro S., et al. Inactivation of the microRNA-183/96/182 cluster results in syndromic retinal degeneration. *Proc Natl Acad Sci U S A.* 2013;**110**:E507–16.

125 Xiang L., Chen X. J., Wu K. C., Zhang C. J., Zhou G. H., Lv J. N., et al. miR-183/96 plays a pivotal regulatory role in mouse photoreceptor maturation and maintenance. *Proc Natl Acad Sci U S A.* 2017;**114**:6376–81.

126 Schaefer M., Nabih A., Spies D., Hermes V., Bodak M., Wischnewski H., et al. Global and precise identification of functional miRNA targets in mESCs by integrative analysis. *EMBO Rep.* 2022;**23**: e54762.

127 Suh M. R., Lee Y., Kim J. Y., Kim S. K., Moon S. H., Lee J. Y., et al. Human embryonic stem cells express a unique set of microRNAs. *Dev Biol.* 2004;**270**:488–98.

128 Li L., Chen K., Wu Y., Long Q., Zhao D., Ma B., et al. Gadd45a opens up the promoter regions of miR-295 facilitating pluripotency induction. *Cell Death Dis.* 2017;**8**:e3107.

129 Sinkkonen L., Hugenschmidt T., Berninger P., Gaidatzis D., Mohn F., Artus-Revel C. G., et al. MicroRNAs control de novo DNA methylation through regulation of transcriptional repressors in mouse embryonic stem cells. *Nat Struct Mol Biol.* 2008;**15**:259–67.

130 Mansfield J. H., McGlinn E. Evolution, expression, and developmental function of Hox-embedded miRNAs. *Curr Top Dev Biol.* 2012;**99**:31–57.

131 Lutz B., Lu H. C., Eichele G., Miller D., Kaufman T. C. Rescue of Drosophila labial null mutant by the chicken ortholog Hoxb-1 demonstrates that the function of Hox genes is phylogenetically conserved. *Genes Dev.* 1996;**10**:176–84.

132 Yekta S., Shih I. H., Bartel D. P. MicroRNA-directed cleavage of HOXB8 mRNA. *Science.* 2004;**304**:594–6.

133 Yekta S., Tabin C. J., Bartel D. P. MicroRNAs in the Hox network: an apparent link to posterior prevalence. *Nat Rev Genet.* 2008;**9**:789–96.

134 Banisch T. U., Goudarzi M., Raz E. Small RNAs in germ cell development. *Curr Top Dev Biol.* 2012;**99**:79–113.

135 Galagali H., Kim J. K. The multifaceted roles of microRNAs in differentiation. *Curr Opin Cell Biol.* 2020;**67**:118–40.

136 Giraldez A. J., Mishima Y., Rihel J., Grocock R. J., Van Dongen S., Inoue K., et al. Zebrafish MiR-430 promotes deadenylation and clearance of maternal mRNAs. *Science.* 2006;**312**:75–9.

137 Perez M. F., Lehner B. Intergenerational and transgenerational epigenetic inheritance in animals. *Nat Cell Biol.* 2019;**21**:143–51.

138 Dunn G. A., Morgan C. P., Bale T. L. Sex-specificity in transgenerational epigenetic programming. *Horm Behav.* 2011;**59**:290–5.

139 Vagero D., Pinger P. R., Aronsson V., van den Berg G. J. Paternal grandfather's access to food predicts all-cause and cancer mortality in grandsons. *Nat Commun.* 2018;**9**:5124.

140 De Rooij S. R., Bleker L. S., Painter R. C., Ravelli A. C., Roseboom T. J. Lessons learned from 25 years of research into long term consequences of prenatal exposure to the Dutch famine 1944–45: the Dutch famine birth cohort. *Int J Environ Health Res.* 2022;**32**:1432–46.

141 Bale T. L. Epigenetic and transgenerational reprogramming of brain development. *Nat Rev Neurosci.* 2015;**16**:332–44.

142 Gapp K., Jawaid A., Sarkies P., Bohacek J., Pelczar P., Prados J., et al. Implication of sperm RNAs in transgenerational inheritance of the effects of early trauma in mice. *Nat Neurosci.* 2014;**17**:667–9.

143 Ostermeier G. C., Goodrich R. J., Moldenhauer J. S., Diamond M. P., Krawetz S. A. A suite of novel human spermatozoal RNAs. *J Androl.* 2005;**26**:70–4.

144 Liu W. M., Pang R. T., Chiu P. C., Wong B. P., Lao K., Lee K. F., et al. Sperm-borne microRNA-34 c is required for the first cleavage division in mouse. *Proc Natl Acad Sci U S A.* 2012;**109**:490–4.

145 Rodgers A. B., Morgan C. P., Bronson S. L., Revello S., Bale T. L. Paternal stress exposure alters sperm microRNA content and reprograms offspring HPA stress axis regulation. *J Neurosci.* 2013;**33**:9003–12.

146 Rodgers A. B., Morgan C. P., Leu N. A., Bale T. L. Transgenerational epigenetic programming via sperm microRNA recapitulates effects of paternal stress. *Proc Natl Acad Sci U S A.* 2015;**112**:13699–704.

147 Fullston T., Ohlsson Teague E. M., Palmer N. O., DeBlasio M. J., Mitchell M., Corbett M., et al. Paternal obesity initiates metabolic disturbances in two generations of mice with incomplete penetrance to the F2 generation and alters the transcriptional profile of testis and sperm microRNA content. *FASEB J.* 2013;**27**:4226–43.

148 Takahashi K., Yamanaka S. Induction of pluripotent stem cells from mouse embryonic and adult fibroblast cultures by defined factors. *Cell.* 2006;**126**:663–76.

149 Lin S. L., Chang D. C., Chang-Lin S., Lin C. H., Wu D. T., Chen D. T., et al. Mir-302 reprograms human skin cancer cells into a pluripotent ES-cell-like state. *RNA.* 2008;**14**:2115–24.

150 Judson R. L., Babiarz J. E., Venere M., Blelloch R. Embryonic stem cell-specific microRNAs promote induced pluripotency. *Nat Biotechnol.* 2009;**27**:459–61.

151 Yoo A. S., Sun A. X., Li L., Shcheglovitov A., Portmann T., Li Y., et al. MicroRNA-mediated conversion of human fibroblasts to neurons. *Nature.* 2011;**476**:228–31.

152 Jayawardena T. M., Egemnazarov B., Finch E. A., Zhang L., Payne J. A., Pandya K., et al. MicroRNA-mediated in vitro and in vivo direct reprogramming

of cardiac fibroblasts to cardiomyocytes. *Circ Res.* 2012;**110**:1465–73.

153 Nam Y. J., Song K., Luo X., Daniel E., Lambeth K., West K., et al. Reprogramming of human fibroblasts toward a cardiac fate. *Proc Natl Acad Sci.* 2013;**110**:5588–93.

154 Jayawardena T. M., Finch E. A., Zhang L., Zhang H., Hodgkinson C. P., Pratt R. E., et al. MicroRNA induced cardiac reprogramming in vivo: evidence for mature cardiac myocytes and improved cardiac function. *Circ Res.* 2015;**116**:418–24.

155 DeVeale B., Swindlehurst-Chan J., Blelloch R. The roles of microRNAs in mouse development. *Nat Rev Genet.* 2021;**22**:307–23.

156 Zhou Y., Song H., Ming G. L. Genetics of human brain development. *Nat Rev Genet.* 2023.

157 Bystron I., Rakic P., Molnar Z., Blakemore C. The first neurons of the human cerebral cortex. *Nat Neurosci.* 2006;**9**:880–6.

158 Yoo A. S., Staahl B. T., Chen L., Crabtree G. R. MicroRNA-mediated switching of chromatin-remodelling complexes in neural development. *Nature.* 2009;**460**:642–6.

159 Ziats M. N., Rennert O. M. Identification of differentially expressed microRNAs across the developing human brain. *Mol Psychiatry.* 2014;**19**:848–52.

160 Uhlen M., Fagerberg L., Hallstrom B. M., Lindskog C., Oksvold P., Mardinoglu A., et al. Proteomics: tissue-based map of the human proteome. *Science.* 2015;**347**:1260419.

161 Marom S., Marder E. A biophysical perspective on the resilience of neuronal excitability across timescales. *Nat Rev Neurosci.* 2023;**24**:640–52.

162 Baczynska E., Pels K. K., Basu S., Wlodarczyk J., Ruszczycki B. Quantification of dendritic spines remodeling under physiological stimuli and in pathological conditions. *Int J Mol Sci.* 2021;**22**:4053–74.

163 Holt C. E., Martin K. C., Schuman E. M. Local translation in neurons: visualization and function. *Nat Struct Mol Biol.* 2019;**26**:557–66.

164 Perez J. D., Fusco C. M., Schuman E. M. A functional dissection of the mRNA and locally synthesized protein population in neuronal dendrites and axons. *Annu Rev Genet.* 2021;**55**:183–207.

165 Perez J. D., Dieck S. T., Alvarez-Castelao B., Tushev G., Chan I. C., Schuman E. M. Subcellular sequencing of single neurons reveals the dendritic transcriptome of GABAergic interneurons. *Elife.* 2021;**10**:e63092.

166 Lugli G., Larson J., Martone M. E., Jones Y., Smalheiser N. R. Dicer and eIF2c are enriched at postsynaptic densities in adult mouse brain and are modified by neuronal activity in a calpain-dependent manner. *J Neurochem.* 2005;**94**:896–905.

167 Lugli G., Torvik V. I., Larson J., Smalheiser N. R. Expression of microRNAs and their precursors in synaptic fractions of adult mouse forebrain. *J Neurochem.* 2008;**106**:650–61.

168 Thomas M. G., Pascual M. L., Maschi D., Luchelli L., Boccaccio G. L. Synaptic control of local translation: the plot thickens with new characters. *Cell Mol Life Sci.* 2014;**71**:2219–39.

169 Dalla Costa I., Buchanan C. N., Zdradzinski M. D., Sahoo P. K., Smith T. P., Thames E., et al. The functional organization of axonal mRNA transport and translation. *Nat Rev Neurosci.* 2021;**22**:77–91.

170 Bicker S., Khudayberdiev S., Weiss K., Zocher K., Baumeister S., Schratt G. The DEAH-box helicase DHX36 mediates dendritic localization of the neuronal precursor-microRNA-134. *Genes Dev.* 2013;**27**:991–6.

171 Vo N., Klein M. E., Varlamova O., Keller D. M., Yamamoto T., Goodman R. H., et al. A cAMP-response element binding protein-induced microRNA regulates neuronal morphogenesis. *Proc Natl Acad Sci U S A.* 2005;**102**:16426–31.

172 Sambandan S., Akbalik G., Kochen L., Rinne J., Kahlstatt J., Glock C., et al. Activity-dependent spatially localized miRNA maturation in neuronal dendrites. *Science.* 2017;**355**:634–7.

173 Banerjee S., Neveu P., Kosik K. S. A coordinated local translational control point at the synapse involving relief from silencing and MOV10 degradation. *Neuron.* 2009;**64**:871–84.

174 Schratt G. M., Tuebing F., Nigh E. A., Kane C. G., Sabatini M. E., Kiebler M., et al. A brain-specific microRNA regulates dendritic spine development. *Nature.* 2006;**439**:283–9.

175 Park I., Kim H. J., Kim Y., Hwang H. S., Kasai H., Kim J. H., et al. Nanoscale imaging reveals miRNA-mediated control of functional states of dendritic spines. *Proc Natl Acad Sci U S A.* 2019;**116**:9616–21.

176 Stenvang J., Petri A., Lindow M., Obad S., Kauppinen S. Inhibition of microRNA function by antimiR oligonucleotides. *Silence.* 2012;**3**:1.

177 Christensen M., Larsen L. A., Kauppinen S., Schratt G. Recombinant adeno-associated virus-mediated microRNA delivery into the postnatal mouse brain reveals a role for miR-134 in dendritogenesis in vivo. *Front Neural Circuits.* 2010;**3**:16.

178 Siegel G., Obernosterer G., Fiore R., Oehmen M., Bicker S., Christensen M., et al. A functional screen implicates microRNA-138-dependent regulation of the depalmitoylation enzyme APT1 in dendritic spine morphogenesis. *Nat Cell Biol.* 2009;**11**:705–16.

179 Daswani R., Gilardi C., Soutschek M., Nanda P., Weiss K., Bicker S., et al. MicroRNA-138 controls hippocampal interneuron function and short-term memory in mice. *Elife.* 2022;**11**:e74056.

180 Lackinger M., Sungur A. O., Daswani R., Soutschek M., Bicker S., Stemmler L., et al. A placental mammal-specific microRNA cluster acts as a natural brake for sociability in mice. *EMBO Rep.* 2019;**20**:e46429.

181 Soutschek M., Schratt G. Non-coding RNA in the wiring and remodeling of neural circuits. *Neuron.* 2023;**111**:2140–54.

182 Sierra-Paredes G., Oreiro-Garcia T., Nunez-Rodriguez A., Vazquez-Lopez A., Sierra-Marcuno G. Seizures induced by in vivo latrunculin a and jasplakinolide microperfusion in the rat hippocampus. *J Mol Neurosci.* 2006;**28**:151–60.

183 Jimenez-Mateos E. M., Engel T., Merino-Serrais P., McKiernan R. C., Tanaka K., Mouri G., et al. Silencing microRNA-134 produces neuroprotective and prolonged seizure-suppressive effects. *Nat Med.* 2012;**18**:1087–94.

184 Jimenez-Mateos E. M., Engel T., Merino-Serrais P., Fernaud-Espinosa I., Rodriguez-Alvarez N., Reynolds J., et al. Antagomirs targeting microRNA-134 increase hippocampal pyramidal neuron spine volume in vivo and protect against pilocarpine-induced status epilepticus. *Brain Struct Funct.* 2015;**220**:2387–99.

185 Morris G., Brennan G. P., Reschke C. R., Henshall D. C., Schorge S. Spared CA1 pyramidal neuron function and hippocampal performance following antisense knockdown of microRNA-134. *Epilepsia.* 2018;**59**:1518–26.

186 Wayman G. A., Davare M., Ando H., Fortin D., Varlamova O., Cheng H. Y., et al. An activity-regulated microRNA controls dendritic plasticity by down-regulating p250GAP. *Proc Natl Acad Sci U S A.* 2008;**105**:9093–8.

187 Magill S. T., Cambronne X. A., Luikart B. W., Lioy D. T., Leighton B. H., Westbrook G. L., et al. MicroRNA-132 regulates dendritic growth and arborization of newborn neurons in the adult hippocampus. *Proc Natl Acad Sci U S A.* 2010;**107**:20382–7.

188 Hansen K. F., Karelina K., Sakamoto K., Wayman G. A., Impey S., Obrietan K. miRNA-132: a dynamic regulator of cognitive capacity. *Brain Struct Funct.* 2013;**218**:817–31.

189 Chai S., Cambronne X. A., Eichhorn S. W., Goodman R. H. MicroRNA-134 activity in

somatostatin interneurons regulates H-Ras localization by repressing the palmitoylation enzyme, DHHC9. *Proc Natl Acad Sci U S A*. 2013;**110**:17898–903.

190 Gao J., Wang W. Y., Mao Y. W., Graff J., Guan J. S., Pan L., et al. A novel pathway regulates memory and plasticity via SIRT1 and miR-134. *Nature*. 2010;**466**:1105–9.

191 Guedes-Dias P., Holzbaur E. L. F. Axonal transport: driving synaptic function. *Science*. 2019;**366**:eaaw9997.

192 Albertin C. B., Simakov O., Mitros T., Wang Z. Y., Pungor J. R., Edsinger-Gonzales E., et al. The octopus genome and the evolution of cephalopod neural and morphological novelties. *Nature*. 2015;**524**:220–4.

193 Zolotarov G., Fromm B., Legnini I., Ayoub S., Polese G., Maselli V., et al. MicroRNAs are deeply linked to the emergence of the complex octopus brain. *Sci Adv*. 2022;**8**:eadd9938.

194 Yu B., Zhang Q., Lin L., Zhou X., Ma W., Wen S., et al. Molecular and cellular evolution of the amygdala across species analyzed by single-nucleus transcriptome profiling. *Cell Discov*. 2023;**9**:19.

195 Haramati S., Navon I., Issler O., Ezra-Nevo G., Gil S., Zwang R., et al. MicroRNA as repressors of stress-induced anxiety: the case of Amygdalar miR-34. *J Neurosci*. 2011;**31**:14191–203.

196 Volk N., Pape J. C., Engel M., Zannas A. S., Cattane N., Cattaneo A., et al. Amygdalar microRNA-15a is essential for coping with chronic stress. *Cell Rep*. 2016;**17**:1882–91.

197 Issler O., Chen A. Determining the role of microRNAs in psychiatric disorders. *Nat Rev Neurosci*. 2015;**16**:201–12.

198 Cheng Y., Wang Z. M., Tan W., Wang X., Li Y., Bai B., et al. Partial loss of psychiatric risk gene Mir137 in mice causes repetitive behavior and impairs sociability and learning via increased Pde10a. *Nat Neurosci*. 2018;**21**:1689–703.

199 Stark K. L., Xu B., Bagchi A., Lai W. S., Liu H., Hsu R., et al. Altered brain microRNA biogenesis contributes to phenotypic deficits in a 22q11-deletion mouse model. *Nat Genet*. 2008;**40**:751–60.

200 Lopez J. P., Lim R., Cruceanu C., Crapper L., Fasano C., Labonte B., et al. miR-1202 is a primate-specific and brain-enriched microRNA involved in major depression and antidepressant treatment. *Nat Med*. 2014;**20**:764–8.

201 Martins H. C., Gilardi C., Sungur A. O., Winterer J., Pelzl M. A., Bicker S., et al. Bipolar-associated miR-499-5p controls neuroplasticity by downregulating the Cav1.2 subunit CACNB2. *EMBO Rep*. 2022;**23**:e54420.

202 Haramati S., Chapnik E., Sztainberg Y., Eilam R., Zwang R., Gershoni N., et al. miRNA malfunction causes spinal motor neuron disease. *Proc Natl Acad Sci U S A*. 2010;**107**:13111–16.

203 Amin N. D., Bai G., Klug J. R., Bonanomi D., Pankratz M. T., Gifford W. D., et al. Loss of motoneuron-specific microRNA-218 causes systemic neuromuscular failure. *Science*. 2015;**350**:1525–9.

204 Reichenstein I., Eitan C., Diaz-Garcia S., Haim G., Magen I., Siany A., et al. Human genetics and neuropathology suggest a link between miR-218 and amyotrophic lateral sclerosis pathophysiology. *Sci Transl Med*. 2019;**11**:eaav5264.

205 Browne T. R., Holmes G. L. Epilepsy. *N Engl J Med*. 2001;**344**:1145–51.

206 Chang B. S., Lowenstein D. H. Epilepsy. *N Engl J Med*. 2003;**349**:1257–66.

207 Kwan P., Schachter S. C., Brodie M. J. Drug-resistant epilepsy. *N Engl J Med*. 2011;**365**:919–26.

208 Devinsky O., Vezzani A., O'Brien T. J., Jette N., Scheffer I. E., de Curtis M., et al. Epilepsy. *Nat Rev Dis Primers*. 2018;**4**:18024.

209 Sen A., Jette N., Husain M., Sander J. W. Epilepsy in older people. *Lancet*. 2020;**395**:735–48.

210 Chevaleyre V., Piskorowski R. A. Hippocampal area CA2: an overlooked but promising therapeutic target. *Trends Mol Med*. 2016;**22**:645–55.

211 Sommer W. Erkrankung des ammonshorns als aetiologisches moment der epilepsie. *Arch Psychiatr Nervenkr.* 1880;**10**:631–75.

212 Asadi-Pooya A. A., Rostami C. History of surgery for temporal lobe epilepsy. *Epilepsy Behav.* 2017;**70**:57–60.

213 Chun E., Bumanglag A. V., Burke S. N., Sloviter R. S. Targeted hippocampal GABA neuron ablation by stable substance P-saporin causes hippocampal sclerosis and chronic epilepsy in rats. *Epilepsia.* 2019;**60**:e52–7.

214 Blumcke I., Spreafico R., Haaker G., Coras R., Kobow K., Bien C. G., et al. Histopathological findings in brain tissue obtained during epilepsy surgery. *N Engl J Med.* 2017;**377**:1648–56.

215 Blauwblomme T., Jiruska P., Huberfeld G. Mechanisms of ictogenesis. *Int Rev Neurobiol.* 2014;**114**:155–85.

216 Glykys J., Dzhala V., Egawa K., Kahle K. T., Delpire E., Staley K. Chloride dysregulation, seizures, and cerebral edema: a relationship with therapeutic potential. *Trends Neurosci.* 2017;**40**:276–94.

217 Elahian B., Lado N. E., Mankin E., Vangala S., Misra A., Moxon K., et al. Low-voltage fast seizures in humans begin with increased interneuron firing. *Ann Neurol.* 2018;**84**:588–600.

218 Miri M. L., Vinck M., Pant R., Cardin J. A. Altered hippocampal interneuron activity precedes ictal onset. *Elife.* 2018;**7**:e40750.

219 Boison D. The adenosine kinase hypothesis of epileptogenesis. *Prog Neurobiol.* 2008;**84**:249–62.

220 Ziemann A. E., Schnizler M. K., Albert G. W., Severson M. A., Howard M. A., III, Welsh M. J., et al. Seizure termination by acidosis depends on ASIC1a. *Nat Neurosci.* 2008;**11**:816–22.

221 Orr R. S. History of a case of epilepsy, accompanied with fever, inflammation, perforation, and gangrene of the lungs, and also pneumothorax. *Edinb Med Surg J.* 1852;**77**:10–23.

222 Chen Z., Brodie M. J., Liew D., Kwan P. Treatment outcomes in patients with newly diagnosed epilepsy treated with established and new antiepileptic drugs: a 30-year longitudinal cohort study. *JAMA Neurol.* 2018;**75**:279–86.

223 Welch C., Chen Y., Stallings R. L. MicroRNA-34a functions as a potential tumor suppressor by inducing apoptosis in neuroblastoma cells. *Oncogene.* 2007;**26**:5017–22.

224 Liu D. Z., Tian Y., Ander B. P., Xu H., Stamova B. S., Zhan X., et al. Brain and blood microRNA expression profiling of ischemic stroke, intracerebral hemorrhage, and kainate seizures. *J Cereb Blood Flow Metab.* 2010;**30**:92–101.

225 Nudelman A. S., DiRocco D. P., Lambert T. J., Garelick M. G., Le J., Nathanson N. M., et al. Neuronal activity rapidly induces transcription of the CREB-regulated microRNA-132, in vivo. *Hippocampus.* 2010;**20**:492–8.

226 Aronica E., Fluiter K., Iyer A., Zurolo E., Vreijling J., van Vliet E. A., et al. Expression pattern of miR-146a, an inflammation-associated microRNA, in experimental and human temporal lobe epilepsy. *Eur J Neurosci.* 2010;**31**:1100–7.

227 Reschke C. R., Silva L. F. A., Vangoor V. R., Rosso M., David B., Cavanagh B. L., et al. Systemic delivery of antagomirs during blood–brain barrier disruption is disease-modifying in experimental epilepsy. *Mol Ther.* 2021;**29**:2041–52.

228 McKiernan R. C., Jimenez-Mateos E. M., Bray I., Engel T., Brennan G. P., Sano T., et al. Reduced mature microRNA levels in association with Dicer loss in human temporal lobe epilepsy with hippocampal sclerosis. *PLoS One.* 2012;**7**:e35921.

229 Iadarola M. J., Gale K. Substantia nigra: site of anticonvulsant activity mediated by gamma-aminobutyric acid. *Science.* 1982;**218**:1237–40.

230 Tan C. L., Plotkin J. L., Veno M. T., von Schimmelmann M., Feinberg P., Mann S., et al. MicroRNA-128 governs neuronal

excitability and motor behavior in mice. *Science.* 2013;**342**:1254–8.

231 Sosanya N. M., Huang P. P., Cacheaux L. P., Chen C. J., Nguyen K., Perrone-Bizzozero N. I., et al. Degradation of high affinity HuD targets releases Kv1.1 mRNA from miR-129 repression by mTORC1. *J Cell Biol.* 2013;**202**:53–69.

232 Gross C., Yao X., Engel T., Xing L., Danielson S. W., Thomas K. T., et al. MicroRNA-mediated downregulation of the potassium channel Kv4.2 contributes to seizure onset. *Cell Rep.* 2016;**17**:37–45.

233 Kim K. W., Kim K., Kim H. J., Kim B. I., Baek M., Suh B. C. Posttranscriptional modulation of KCNQ2 gene expression by the miR-106b microRNA family. *Proc Natl Acad Sci U S A.* 2021;**118**:e2110200118.

234 Vezzani A., French J., Bartfai T., Baram T. Z. The role of inflammation in epilepsy. *Nat Rev Neurol.* 2011;**7**:31–40.

235 Husari K. S., Dubey D. Autoimmune epilepsy. *Neurotherapeutics.* 2019;**16**:685–702.

236 Kumar P., Lim A., Hazirah S. N., Chua C. J. H., Ngoh A., Poh S. L., et al. Single-cell transcriptomics and surface epitope detection in human brain epileptic lesions identifies pro-inflammatory signaling. *Nat Neurosci.* 2022;**25**:956–66.

237 Roth T. L., Nayak D., Atanasijevic T., Koretsky A. P., Latour L. L., McGavern D. B. Transcranial amelioration of inflammation and cell death after brain injury. *Nature.* 2014;**505**:223–8.

238 Badimon A., Strasburger H. J., Ayata P., Chen X., Nair A., Ikegami A., et al. Negative feedback control of neuronal activity by microglia. *Nature.* 2020;**586**:417–23.

239 Srivastava P. K., van Eyll J., Godard P., Mazzuferi M., Delahaye-Duriez A., Steenwinckel J. V., et al. A systems-level framework for drug discovery identifies Csf1R as an anti-epileptic drug target. *Nat Commun.* 2018;**9**:3561.

240 Iori V., Iyer A. M., Ravizza T., Beltrame L., Paracchini L., Marchini S., et al. Blockade of the IL-1R1/TLR4 pathway mediates disease-modification therapeutic effects in a model of acquired epilepsy. *Neurobiol Dis.* 2017;**99**:12–23.

241 Henshall D. C., Clark R. S., Adelson P. D., Chen M., Watkins S. C., Simon R. P. Alterations in bcl-2 and caspase gene family protein expression in human temporal lobe epilepsy. *Neurology.* 2000;**55**:250–7.

242 Khakh B. S., North R. A. P2X receptors as cell-surface ATP sensors in health and disease. *Nature.* 2006;**442**:527–32.

243 Surprenant A., North R. A. Signaling at purinergic P2X receptors. *Annu Rev Physiol.* 2009;**71**:333–59.

244 Jimenez-Mateos E. M., Arribas-Blazquez M., Sanz-Rodriguez A., Concannon C., Olivos-Ore L. A., Reshcke C. R., et al. MicroRNA targeting of the P2X7 purinoceptor opposes a contralateral epileptogenic focus in the hippocampus. *Scientific Reports.* 2015;**5**:e17486.

245 Engel T., Brennan G. P., Sanz-Rodriguez A., Alves M., Beamer E., Watters O., et al. A calcium-sensitive feed-forward loop regulating the expression of the ATP-gated purinergic P2X7 receptor via specificity protein 1 and microRNA-22. *Biochim Biophys Acta.* 2017;**1864**:255–66.

246 Flores O., Kennedy E. M., Skalsky R. L., Cullen B. R. Differential RISC association of endogenous human microRNAs predicts their inhibitory potential. *Nucleic Acids Res.* 2014;**42**:4629–39.

247 Veno M. T., Reschke C. R., Morris G., Connolly N. M. C., Su J., Yan Y., et al. A systems approach delivers a functional microRNA catalog and expanded targets for seizure suppression in temporal lobe epilepsy. *Proc Natl Acad Sci U S A.* 2020;**117**:15977–88.

248 Monk D., Mackay D. J. G., Eggermann T., Maher E. R., Riccio A. Genomic imprinting disorders: lessons on how genome, epigenome and environment interact. *Nat Rev Genet.* 2019;**20**:235–48.

249 Buiting K., Williams C., Horsthemke B. Angelman syndrome – insights into a rare

neurogenetic disorder. *Nat Rev Neurol.* 2016;**12**:584–93.

250 Valluy J., Bicker S., Aksoy-Aksel A., Lackinger M., Sumer S., Fiore R., et al. A coding-independent function of an alternative Ube3a transcript during neuronal development. *Nat Neurosci.* 2015;**18**:666–73.

251 Campbell A., Morris G., Sanfeliu A., Augusto J., Langa E., Kesavan J. C., et al. AntimiR targeting of microRNA-134 reduces seizures in a mouse model of Angelman syndrome. *Mol Ther Nucleic Acids.* 2022;**28**:514–29.

252 Krook-Magnuson E., Szabo G. G., Armstrong C., Oijala M., Soltesz I. Cerebellar directed optogenetic intervention inhibits spontaneous hippocampal seizures in a mouse model of temporal lobe epilepsy. *eNeuro.* 2014;**1**: ENEURO.0005-14.2014.

253 Avagliano Trezza R., Sonzogni M., Bossuyt S. N. V., Zampeta F. I., Punt A. M., van den Berg M., et al. Loss of nuclear UBE3A causes electrophysiological and behavioral deficits in mice and is associated with Angelman syndrome. *Nat Neurosci.* 2019;**22**:1235–47.

254 Wallace R. H., Scheffer I. E., Barnett S., Richards M., Dibbens L., Desai R. R., et al. Neuronal sodium-channel alpha1-subunit mutations in generalized epilepsy with febrile seizures plus. *Am J Hum Genet.* 2001;**68**:859–65.

255 Escayg A., Heils A., MacDonald B. T., Haug K., Sander T., Meisler M. H. A novel SCN1A mutation associated with generalized epilepsy with febrile seizures plus – and prevalence of variants in patients with epilepsy. *Am J Hum Genet.* 2001;**68**:866–73.

256 Claes L., Del-Favero J., Ceulemans B., Lagae L., Van Broeckhoven C., De Jonghe P. De novo mutations in the sodium-channel gene SCN1A cause severe myoclonic epilepsy of infancy. *Am J Hum Genet.* 2001;**68**:1327–32.

257 Yu F. H., Mantegazza M., Westenbroek R. E., Robbins C. A., Kalume F., Burton K. A., et al. Reduced sodium current in GABAergic interneurons in a mouse model of severe myoclonic epilepsy in infancy. *Nat Neurosci.* 2006;**9**:1142–9.

258 Gerbatin R. R., Augusto J., Morris G., Campbell A., Worm J., Langa E., et al. Investigation of microRNA-134 as a target against seizures and SUDEP in a mouse model of Dravet syndrome. *eNeuro.* 2022;**9**:ENEURO.0112-22.2022.

259 Heiland M., Connolly N. M. C., Mamad O., Nguyen N. T., Kesavan J. C., Langa E., et al. MicroRNA-335-5p suppresses voltage-gated sodium channel expression and may be a target for seizure control. *Proc Natl Acad Sci USA.* 2023;**120**: e2216658120.

260 Rosenthal J. J., Seeburg P. H. A-to-I RNA editing: effects on proteins key to neural excitability. *Neuron.* 2012;**74**:432–9.

261 Eisenberg E., Levanon E. Y. A-to-I RNA editing – immune protector and transcriptome diversifier. *Nat Rev Genet.* 2018;**19**:473–90.

262 Benne R., Van den Burg J., Brakenhoff J. P., Sloof P., Van Boom J. H., Tromp M. C. Major transcript of the frameshifted coxII gene from trypanosome mitochondria contains four nucleotides that are not encoded in the DNA. *Cell.* 1986;**46**:819–26.

263 Nishikura K. A-to-I editing of coding and non-coding RNAs by ADARs. *Nat Rev Mol Cell Biol.* 2016;**17**:83–96.

264 Luciano D. J., Mirsky H., Vendetti N. J., Maas S. RNA editing of a miRNA precursor. *RNA.* 2004;**10**:1174–7.

265 Kawahara Y., Megraw M., Kreider E., Iizasa H., Valente L., Hatzigeorgiou A. G., et al. Frequency and fate of microRNA editing in human brain. *Nucleic Acids Res.* 2008;**36**:5270–80.

266 Ekdahl Y., Farahani H. S., Behm M., Lagergren J., Ohman M. A-to-I editing of microRNAs in the mammalian brain increases during development. *Genome Res.* 2012;**22**:1477–87.

267 Lau, K. E. H., Nguyen N. T., Kesavan J. C., Langa E., Fanning K., Brennan G. P., et al.

Differential microRNA editing may drive target pathway switching in human temporal lobe epilepsy. *Brain Commun.* 2024; **fcad355**:1–17.

268 Stenzel-Poore M. P., Stevens S. L., Xiong Z., Lessov N. S., Harrington C. A., Mori M., et al. Effect of ischaemic preconditioning on genomic response to cerebral ischaemia: similarity to neuroprotective strategies in hibernation and hypoxia-tolerant states. *Lancet.* 2003;**362**:1028–37.

269 Caciagli L., Bernasconi A., Wiebe S., Koepp M. J., Bernasconi N., Bernhardt B. C. A meta-analysis on progressive atrophy in intractable temporal lobe epilepsy: time is brain? *Neurology.* 2017;**89**:506–16.

270 Krutzfeldt J., Rajewsky N., Braich R., Rajeev K. G., Tuschl T., Manoharan M., et al. Silencing of microRNAs in vivo with 'antagomirs'. *Nature.* 2005;**438**:685–9.

271 Hsu S. H., Wang B., Kota J., Yu J., Costinean S., Kutay H., et al. Essential metabolic, anti-inflammatory, and anti-tumorigenic functions of miR-122 in liver. *J Clin Invest.* 2012;**122**:2871–83.

272 Tsai W. C., Hsu S. D., Hsu C. S., Lai T. C., Chen S. J., Shen R., et al. MicroRNA-122 plays a critical role in liver homeostasis and hepatocarcinogenesis. *J Clin Invest.* 2012;**122**:2884–97.

273 Lindow M., Kauppinen S. Discovering the first microRNA-targeted drug. *J Cell Biol.* 2012;**199**:407–12.

274 Spearman C. W., Dusheiko G. M., Hellard M., Sonderup M. Hepatitis C. *Lancet.* 2019;**394**:1451–66.

275 Jopling C. L., Yi M., Lancaster A. M., Lemon S. M., Sarnow P. Modulation of hepatitis C virus RNA abundance by a liver-specific MicroRNA. *Science.* 2005;**309**:1577–81.

276 Henke J. I., Goergen D., Zheng J., Song Y., Schuttler C. G., Fehr C., et al. MicroRNA-122 stimulates translation of hepatitis C virus RNA. *EMBO J.* 2008;**27**:3300–10.

277 Gebert L. F. R., Law M., MacRae I. J. A structured RNA motif locks

Argonaute2:miR-122 onto the 5' end of the HCV genome. *Nat Commun.* 2021;**12**:6836.

278 Gottwein E., Mukherjee N., Sachse C., Frenzel C., Majoros W. H., Chi J. T., et al. A viral microRNA functions as an orthologue of cellular miR-155. *Nature.* 2007;**450**:1096–9.

279 Gorbea C., Mosbruger T., Cazalla D. A viral Sm-class RNA base-pairs with mRNAs and recruits microRNAs to inhibit apoptosis. *Nature.* 2017;**550**:275–9.

280 Ziv O., Gabryelska M. M., Lun A. T. L., Gebert L. F. R., Sheu-Gruttadauria J., Meredith L. W., et al. COMRADES determines in vivo RNA structures and interactions. *Nat Methods.* 2018;**15**:785–8.

281 Crooke S. T., Baker B. F., Crooke R. M., Liang X. H. Antisense technology: an overview and prospectus. *Nat Rev Drug Discov.* 2021;**20**:427–53.

282 Tolstrup N., Nielsen P. S., Kolberg J. G., Frankel A. M., Vissing H., Kauppinen S. OligoDesign: optimal design of LNA (locked nucleic acid) oligonucleotide capture probes for gene expression profiling. *Nucleic Acids Res.* 2003;**31**:3758–62.

283 Lecellier C. H., Dunoyer P., Arar K., Lehmann-Che J., Eyquem S., Himber C., et al. A cellular microRNA mediates antiviral defense in human cells. *Science.* 2005;**308**:557–60.

284 Elmen J., Lindow M., Silahtaroglu A., Bak M., Christensen M., Lind-Thomsen A., et al. Antagonism of microRNA-122 in mice by systemically administered LNA-antimiR leads to up-regulation of a large set of predicted target mRNAs in the liver. *Nucleic Acids Res.* 2008;**36**:1153–62.

285 Elmen J., Lindow M., Schutz S., Lawrence M., Petri A., Obad S., et al. LNA-mediated microRNA silencing in non-human primates. *Nature.* 2008;**452**:896–9.

286 Janssen H. L., Reesink H. W., Lawitz E. J., Zeuzem S., Rodriguez-Torres M., Patel K., et al. Treatment of HCV infection by

targeting microRNA. *N Engl J Med.* 2013;**368**:1685–94.

287 Pedersen I. M., Cheng G., Wieland S., Volinia S., Croce C. M., Chisari F. V., et al. Interferon modulation of cellular microRNAs as an antiviral mechanism. *Nature.* 2007;**449**:919–22.

288 Gebert L. F., Rebhan M. A., Crivelli S. E., Denzler R., Stoffel M., Hall J. Miravirsen (SPC3649) can inhibit the biogenesis of miR-122. *Nucleic Acids Res.* 2014;**42**:609–21.

289 Ucar A., Gupta S. K., Fiedler J., Erikci E., Kardasinski M., Batkai S., et al. The miRNA-212/132 family regulates both cardiac hypertrophy and cardiomyocyte autophagy. *Nat Commun.* 2012;**3**:1078.

290 Rho J. M., White H. S. Brief history of anti-seizure drug development. *Epilepsia Open.* 2018;**3**:114–19.

291 French J. A., Lawson J. A., Yapici Z., Ikeda H., Polster T., Nabbout R., et al. Adjunctive everolimus therapy for treatment-resistant focal-onset seizures associated with tuberous sclerosis (EXIST-3): a phase 3, randomised, double-blind, placebo-controlled study. *Lancet.* 2016;**388**:2153–63.

292 Kotulska K., Kwiatkowski D. J., Curatolo P., Weschke B., Riney K., Jansen F., et al. Prevention of epilepsy in infants with tuberous sclerosis complex in the EPISTOP trial. *Ann Neurol.* 2021;**89**:304–14.

293 Morris G., Reschke C. R., Henshall D. C. Targeting microRNA-134 for seizure control and disease modification in epilepsy. *EBioMedicine.* 2019;**45**:646–54.

294 Ruber T., David B., Luchters G., Nass R. D., Friedman A., Surges R., et al. Evidence for peri-ictal blood–brain barrier dysfunction in patients with epilepsy. *Brain.* 2018;**141**:2952–65.

295 Brennan G. P., Dey D., Chen Y., Patterson K. P., Magnetta E. J., Hall A. M., et al. Dual and opposing roles of microRNA-124 in epilepsy are mediated through inflammatory and NRSF-dependent gene networks. *Cell Rep.* 2016;**14**:2402–12.

296 Wirth T., Parker N., Yla-Herttuala S. History of gene therapy. *Gene.* 2013;**525**:162–9.

297 Ingusci S., Verlengia G., Soukupova M., Zucchini S., Simonato M. Gene therapy tools for brain diseases. *Front Pharmacol.* 2019;**10**:724.

298 Feldman E. L., Goutman S. A., Petri S., Mazzini L., Savelieff M. G., Shaw P. J., et al. Amyotrophic lateral sclerosis. *Lancet.* 2022;**400**:1363–80.

299 Rosen D. R., Siddique T., Patterson D., Figlewicz D. A., Sapp P., Hentati A., et al. Mutations in Cu/Zn superoxide dismutase gene are associated with familial amyotrophic lateral sclerosis. *Nature.* 1993;**362**:59–62.

300 Stoica L., Todeasa S. H., Cabrera G. T., Salameh J. S., ElMallah M. K., Mueller C., et al. Adeno-associated virus-delivered artificial microRNA extends survival and delays paralysis in an amyotrophic lateral sclerosis mouse model. *Ann Neurol.* 2016;**79**:687–700.

301 Borel F., Gernoux G., Sun H., Stock R., Blackwood M., Brown R. H., Jr., et al. Safe and effective superoxide dismutase 1 silencing using artificial microRNA in macaques. *Sci Transl Med.* 2018;**10**: eaau6414.

302 Mueller C., Berry J. D., McKenna-Yasek D. M., Gernoux G., Owegi M. A., Pothier L. M., et al. SOD1 suppression with adeno-associated virus and microRNA in familial ALS. *N Engl J Med.* 2020;**383**:151–8.

303 Walker F. O. Huntington's disease. *Lancet.* 2007;**369**:218–28.

304 Harper S. Q., Staber P. D., He X., Eliason S. L., Martins I. H., Mao Q., et al. RNA interference improves motor and neuropathological abnormalities in a Huntington's disease mouse model. *Proc Natl Acad Sci U S A.* 2005;**102**:5820–5.

305 Valles A., Evers M. M., Stam A., Sogorb-Gonzalez M., Brouwers C., Vendrell-Tornero C., et al. Widespread and sustained target engagement in Huntington's disease minipigs upon intrastriatal microRNA-based gene

therapy. *Sci Transl Med.* 2021;**13**: eabb8920.

306 Bekenstein U., Mishra N., Milikovsky D. Z., Hanin G., Zelig D., Sheintuch L., et al. Dynamic changes in murine forebrain miR-211 expression associate with cholinergic imbalances and epileptiform activity. *Proc Natl Acad Sci U S A.* 2017;**114**:E4996–E5005.

307 Brodie M. J. Sodium channel blockers in the treatment of epilepsy. *CNS Drugs.* 2017;**31**:527–34.

308 Meisler M. H., Hill S. F., Yu W. Sodium channelopathies in neurodevelopmental disorders. *Nat Rev Neurosci.* 2021;**22**:152–66.

309 Rosenberg E. C., Tsien R. W., Whalley B. J., Devinsky O. Cannabinoids and epilepsy. *Neurotherapeutics.* 2015;**12**:747–68.

310 Devinsky O., Cross J. H., Laux L., Marsh E., Miller I., Nabbout R., et al. Trial of cannabidiol for drug-resistant seizures in the Dravet syndrome. *N Engl J Med.* 2017;**376**:2011–20.

311 Raoof R., Bauer S., El Naggar H., Connolly N. M. C., Brennan G. P., Brindley E., et al. Dual-center, dual-platform microRNA profiling identifies potential plasma biomarkers of adult temporal lobe epilepsy. *EBioMedicine.* 2018;**38**:127–41.

312 Benavides-Piccione R., Regalado-Reyes M., Fernaud-Espinosa I., Kastanauskaite A., Tapia-Gonzalez S., Leon-Espinosa G., et al. Differential structure of hippocampal CA1 pyramidal neurons in the human and mouse. *Cereb Cortex.* 2020;**30**:730–52.

313 Richards R. K., Everett G. M. Tridione: a new anticonvulsant drug. *J Lab Clin Med.* 1946;**31**:1330–6.

314 Klitgaard H., Matagne A., Gobert J., Wulfert E. Evidence for a unique profile of levetiracetam in rodent models of seizures and epilepsy. *Eur J Pharmacol.* 1998;**353**:191–206.

315 De Santi C., Fernandez Fernandez E., Gaul R., Vencken S., Glasgow A.,

Oglesby I. K., et al. Precise targeting of miRNA sites restores CFTR activity in CF bronchial epithelial cells. *Mol Ther.* 2020;**28**:1190–9.

316 Shteinberg M., Haq I. J., Polineni D., Davies J. C. Cystic fibrosis. *Lancet.* 2021;**397**:2195–211.

317 Han Z., Chen C., Christiansen A., Ji S., Lin Q., Anumonwo C., et al. Antisense oligonucleotides increase Scn1a expression and reduce seizures and SUDEP incidence in a mouse model of Dravet syndrome. *Sci Transl Med.* 2020;**12**: eabb8920.

318 Qiu Y., O'Neill N., Maffei B., Zourray C., Almacellas-Barbanoj A., Carpenter J. C., et al. On-demand cell-autonomous gene therapy for brain circuit disorders. *Science.* 2022;**378**:523–32.

319 Hogg M. C., Raoof R., El Naggar H., Monsefi N., Delanty N., O'Brien D. F., et al. Elevation in plasma tRNA fragments precede seizures in human epilepsy. *J Clin Invest.* 2019;**129**:2946–51.

320 Matsuura S., Ono H., Kawasaki S., Kuang Y., Fujita Y., Saito H. Synthetic RNA-based logic computation in mammalian cells. *Nat Commun.* 2018;**9**:4847.

321 Pitkanen A., Loscher W., Vezzani A., Becker A. J., Simonato M., Lukasiuk K., et al. Advances in the development of biomarkers for epilepsy. *Lancet Neurol.* 2016;**15**:843–56.

322 Simonato M., Agoston D. V., Brooks-Kayal A., Dulla C., Fureman B., Henshall D. C., et al. Identification of clinically relevant biomarkers of epileptogenesis – a strategic roadmap. *Nat Rev Neurol.* 2021;**17**:231–42.

323 Mandel P., Metais P. Nuclear acids in human blood plasma. *C R Seances Soc Biol Fil.* 1948;**142**:241–3.

324 Gruner H. N., McManus M. T. Examining the evidence for extracellular RNA function in mammals. *Nat Rev Genet.* 2021;**22**:448–58.

325 El-Hefnawy T., Raja S., Kelly L., Bigbee W. L., Kirkwood J. M.,

Luketich J. D., et al. Characterization of amplifiable, circulating RNA in plasma and its potential as a tool for cancer diagnostics. *Clin Chem*. 2004;**50**:564–73.

326 Mitchell P. S., Parkin R. K., Kroh E. M., Fritz B. R., Wyman S. K., Pogosova-Agadjanyan E. L., et al. Circulating microRNAs as stable blood-based markers for cancer detection. *Proc Natl Acad Sci U S A*. 2008;**105**:10513–18.

327 Van Niel G., D'Angelo G., Raposo G. Shedding light on the cell biology of extracellular vesicles. *Nat Rev Mol Cell Biol*. 2018;**19**:213–28.

328 Valadi H., Ekstrom K., Bossios A., Sjostrand M., Lee J. J., Lotvall J. O. Exosome-mediated transfer of mRNAs and microRNAs is a novel mechanism of genetic exchange between cells. *Nat Cell Biol*. 2007;**9**:654–9.

329 Arroyo J. D., Chevillet J. R., Kroh E. M., Ruf I. K., Pritchard C. C., Gibson D. F., et al. Argonaute2 complexes carry a population of circulating microRNAs independent of vesicles in human plasma. *Proc Natl Acad Sci U S A*. 2011;**108**:5003–8.

330 Turchinovich A., Weiz L., Langheinz A., Burwinkel B. Characterization of extracellular circulating microRNA. *Nucleic Acids Res*. 2011;**39**:7223–33.

331 Chevillet J. R., Kang Q., Ruf I. K., Briggs H. A., Vojtech L. N., Hughes S. M., et al. Quantitative and stoichiometric analysis of the microRNA content of exosomes. *Proc Natl Acad Sci U S A*. 2014;**111**:14888–93.

332 Weber J. A., Baxter D. H., Zhang S., Huang D. Y., Huang K. H., Lee M. J., et al. The microRNA spectrum in 12 body fluids. *Clin Chem*. 2010;**56**:1733–41.

333 Kenny A., Jimenez-Mateos E. M., Zea-Sevilla M. A., Rabano A., Gili-Manzanaro P., Prehn J. H. M., et al. Proteins and microRNAs are differentially expressed in tear fluid from patients with Alzheimer's disease. *Sci Rep*. 2019;**9**:15437.

334 Kenny A., McArdle H., Calero M., Rabano A., Madden S. F., Adamson K., et al. Elevated plasma microRNA-206 levels predict cognitive decline and progression to dementia from mild cognitive impairment. *Biomolecules*. 2019;**9**:734.

335 Wijesinghe P., Xi J., Cui J., Campbell M., Pham W., Matsubara J. A. MicroRNAs in tear fluids predict underlying molecular changes associated with Alzheimer's disease. *Life Sci Alliance*. 2023;**6**: e202201757.

336 Sinha A., Yadav A. K., Chakraborty S., Kabra S. K., Lodha R., Kumar M., et al. Exosome-enclosed microRNAs in exhaled breath hold potential for biomarker discovery in patients with pulmonary diseases. *J Allergy Clin Immunol*. 2013;**132**:219–22.

337 Shi M., Han W., Loudig O., Shah C. D., Dobkin J. B., Keller S., et al. Initial development and testing of an exhaled microRNA detection strategy for lung cancer case-control discrimination. *Sci Rep*. 2023;**13**:6620.

338 Raoof R., Jimenez-Mateos E. M., Bauer S., Tackenberg B., Rosenow F., Lang J., et al. Cerebrospinal fluid microRNAs are potential biomarkers of temporal lobe epilepsy and status epilepticus. *Sci Rep*. 2017;**7**:3328.

339 Leidinger P., Backes C., Deutscher S., Schmitt K., Mueller S. C., Frese K., et al. A blood based 12-miRNA signature of Alzheimer disease patients. *Genome Biol*. 2013;**14**:R78.

340 Liu S., Zhang F., Wang X., Shugart Y. Y., Zhao Y., Li X., et al. Diagnostic value of blood-derived microRNAs for schizophrenia: results of a meta-analysis and validation. *Sci Rep*. 2017;**7**:15328.

341 Magen I., Yacovzada N. S., Yanowski E., Coenen-Stass A., Grosskreutz J., Lu C. H., et al. Circulating miR-181 is a prognostic biomarker for amyotrophic lateral sclerosis. *Nat Neurosci*. 2021;**24**:1534–41.

342 Wang J., Tan L., Tan L., Tian Y., Ma J., Tan C. C., et al. Circulating microRNAs are promising novel biomarkers for drug-resistant epilepsy. *Sci Rep*. 2015;**5**:10201.

343 Wang J., Yu J. T., Tan L., Tian Y., Ma J., Tan C. C., et al. Genome-wide circulating

microRNA expression profiling indicates biomarkers for epilepsy. *Sci Rep.* 2015;5:9522.

344 Enright N., Simonato M., Henshall D. C. Discovery and validation of blood microRNAs as molecular biomarkers of epilepsy – ways to close current knowledge gaps. *Epilepsia Open.* 2018;3:427–36.

345 Brennan G. P., Bauer S., Engel T., Jimenez-Mateos E. M., Del Gallo F., Hill T. D. M., et al. Genome-wide microRNA profiling of plasma from three different animal models identifies biomarkers of temporal lobe epilepsy. *Neurobiol Dis.* 2020;144:105048.

346 Heiskanen M., Das Gupta S., Mills J. D., van Vliet E. A., Manninen E., Ciszek R., et al. Discovery and validation of circulating microRNAs as biomarkers for epileptogenesis after experimental traumatic brain injury – the EPITARGET cohort. *Int J Mol Sci.* 2023;24:2823.

347 Brindley E., Heiland M., Mooney C., Diviney M., Mamad O., Hill T. D. M., et al. Brain cell-specific origin of circulating microRNA biomarkers in experimental temporal lobe epilepsy. *Front Mol Neurosci.* 2023;16.

348 Acharya S. S., Fendler W., Watson J., Hamilton A., Pan Y., Gaudiano E., et al. Serum microRNAs are early indicators of survival after radiation-induced hematopoietic injury. *Sci Transl Med.* 2015;7:287ra69.

349 Fendler W., Malachowska B., Meghani K., Konstantinopoulos P. A., Guha C., Singh V. K., et al. Evolutionarily conserved serum microRNAs predict radiation-induced fatality in nonhuman primates. *Sci Transl Med.* 2017;9:eaal2408.

350 Nowicka Z., Tomasik B., Kozono D., Stawiski K., Johnson T., Haas-Kogan D., et al. Serum miRNA-based signature indicates radiation exposure and dose in humans: a multicenter diagnostic biomarker study. *Radiother Oncol.* 2023;185:109731.

351 Dave V. P., Ngo T. A., Pernestig A. K., Tilevik D., Kant K., Nguyen T., et al. MicroRNA amplification and detection technologies: opportunities and challenges

for point of care diagnostics. *Lab Invest.* 2019;99:452–69.

352 Spain E., Jimenez-Mateos E. M., Raoof R., El Naggar H., Delanty N., Forster R. J., et al. Direct, non-amplified detection of microRNA-134 in plasma from epilepsy patients. *RSC Advances.* 2015;5:90071–8.

353 McArdle H., Jimenez-Mateos E. M., Raoof R., Carthy E., Boyle D., ElNaggar H., et al. 'TORNADO' – Theranostic One-Step RNA Detector; microfluidic disc for the direct detection of microRNA-134 in plasma and cerebrospinal fluid. *Sci Rep.* 2017;7:1750.

354 Witwer K. W., Halushka M. K. Toward the promise of microRNAs – enhancing reproducibility and rigor in microRNA research. *RNA Biol.* 2016;13:1103–16.

355 Zhang L., Hou D., Chen X., Li D., Zhu L., Zhang Y., et al. Exogenous plant MIR168a specifically targets mammalian LDLRAP1: evidence of cross-kingdom regulation by microRNA. *Cell Res.* 2012;22:107–26.

356 Vandereyken K., Sifrim A., Thienpont B., Voet T. Methods and applications for single-cell and spatial multi-omics. *Nat Rev Genet.* 2023;24:494–515.

357 Kirstein N., Dokaneheifard S., Cingaram P. R., Valencia M. G., Beckedorff F., Gomes Dos Santos H., et al. The Integrator complex regulates microRNA abundance through RISC loading. *Sci Adv.* 2023;9:eadf0597.

358 Lee Y. Y., Kim H., Kim V. N. Sequence determinant of small RNA production by DICER. *Nature.* 2023;615:323–30.

359 Lee Y. Y., Lee H., Kim H., Kim V. N., Roh S. H. Structure of the human DICER-pre-miRNA complex in a dicing state. *Nature.* 2023;615:331–8.

360 Tsujisaka Y., Hatani T., Okubo C., Ito R., Kimura A., Narita M., et al. Purification of human iPSC-derived cells at large scale using microRNA switch and magnetic-activated cell sorting. *Stem Cell Reports.* 2022;17:1772–85.

361 Miki K., Endo K., Takahashi S., Funakoshi S., Takei I., Katayama S., et al. Efficient detection and purification of cell populations using synthetic microRNA switches. *Cell Stem Cell.* 2015;**16**:699–711.

362 Frei T., Cella F., Tedeschi F., Gutierrez J., Stan G. B., Khammash M., et al. Characterization and mitigation of gene expression burden in mammalian cells. *Nat Commun.* 2020;**11**:4641.

363 Hennig T., Prusty A. B., Kaufer B. B., Whisnant A. W., Lodha M., Enders A., et al. Selective inhibition of miRNA processing by a herpesvirus-encoded miRNA. *Nature.* 2022;**605**:539–44.

364 McDonald J. T., Enguita F. J., Taylor D., Griffin R. J., Priebe W., Emmett M. R., et al. Role of miR-2392 in driving SARS-CoV-2 infection. *Cell Rep.* 2021;**37**:109839.

365 Chandrasekaran A. R., MacIsaac M., Dey P., Levchenko O., Zhou L., Andres M., et al. Cellular microRNA detection with miRacles: microRNA- activated conditional looping of engineered switches. *Sci Adv.* 2019;**5**:eaau9443.

366 Zhou L., Gao M., Fu W., Wang Y., Luo D., Chang K., et al. Three-dimensional DNA tweezers serve as modular DNA intelligent machines for detection and regulation of intracellular microRNA. *Sci Adv.* 2020;**6**: eabb0695.

367 Namkung H., Yukitake H., Fukudome D., Lee B. J., Tian M., Ursini G., et al. The miR-124-AMPAR pathway connects polygenic risks with behavioral changes shared between schizophrenia and bipolar disorder. *Neuron.* 2023;**111**:220–35 e9.

368 Nedergaard M., Goldman S. A. Glymphatic failure as a final common pathway to dementia. *Science.* 2020;**370**:50–6.

369 Cheng H. Y., Papp J. W., Varlamova O., Dziema H., Russell B., Curfman J. P., et al. MicroRNA modulation of circadian-clock period and entrainment. *Neuron.* 2007;**54**:813–29.

370 Curtis A. M., Fagundes C. T., Yang G., Palsson-McDermott E. M., Wochal P., McGettrick A. F., et al. Circadian control of innate immunity in macrophages by miR-155 targeting Bmal1. *Proc Natl Acad Sci U S A.* 2015;**112**:7231–6.

371 Dowling J. K., Afzal R., Gearing L. J., Cervantes-Silva M. P., Annett S., Davis G. M., et al. Mitochondrial arginase-2 is essential for IL-10 metabolic reprogramming of inflammatory macrophages. *Nat Commun.* 2021;**12**:1460.

372 Karoly P. J., Rao V. R., Gregg N. M., Worrell G. A., Bernard C., Cook M. J., et al. Cycles in epilepsy. *Nat Rev Neurol.* 2021;**17**:267–84.

373 Kinser H. E., Pincus Z. MicroRNAs as modulators of longevity and the aging process. *Hum Genet.* 2020;**139**:291–308.

374 Kim B. M., Amores A., Kang S., Ahn D. H., Kim J. H., Kim I. C., et al. Antarctic blackfin icefish genome reveals adaptations to extreme environments. *Nat Ecol Evol.* 2019;**3**:469–78.

Index

Locators in *italics* refer to figures.

Printed in the United States
by Baker & Taylor Publisher Services